Graves' Disease

To Arthur

Graves' Disease

A Practical Guide

by Elaine A. Moore
with Lisa Moore

ILLUSTRATIONS BY MARVIN G. MILLER
FOREWORD BY KELLY R. HALE

McFarland & Company, Inc., Publishers
Jefferson, North Carolina, and London

The information in this book is provided for educational purposes only. It is not intended as a substitute for medical treatment. The procedures and therapies described in this book should be discussed with a medical professional.

While all patient anecdotes are factual, in some instances the names and background of the individual, or both, have been changed to protect their privacy.

Library of Congress Cataloguing-in-Publication Data

Moore, Elaine A., 1948–
    Graves' disease: a practical guide / by Elaine A. Moore, with Lisa
Moore ; illustrations by Marvin G. Miller ; foreword by Kelly R. Hale.
        p.   cm.
    Includes bibliographical references and index.
    ISBN 0-7864-1011-6 (softcover : 50# alkaline paper) ∞
    1. Graves' disease — Popular works.   I. Moore, Lisa.   II. Title.
[DNLM: 1. Graves' Disease — diagnosis.   2. Graves' Disease —
immunology.   3. Graves' Disease — therapy.   WK 265 M821g2001]
RC657.5.G7 M665   2001
616.4'43 — dc21   2001037052

British Library Cataloguing data are available

Manufactured in the United States of America

Cover image © 2001 Artville

*McFarland & Company, Inc., Publishers
    Box 611, Jefferson, North Carolina 28640
    www.mcfarlandpub.com*

Contents

Contents

Acknowledgments

This book could have never existed without the help and support of many people. I particularly want to thank all my friends at http://groups.yahoo.com/group/gravcs_support, http://groups.yahoo.com/group/hyperTHYROIDISM2, and http://groups.yahoo.com/group/graves=ALT=SEARCH, especially Julie, Mary, Randi, Jeannette, Julia and Red.

I'd also like to thank my friend and coworker, Marve Miller, for his generous help in illustrating this project and my daughter Lisa for her help in writing the resource chapter and for her encouragement every step of the way. I'd also like to acknowledge the Mosby Year Book Company, W.B. Saunders Publishing Company, and Lippincott, Williams and Wilkins Publishing Company for their assistance. And special thanks to Kelly Hale at the American Foundation of Thyroid Patients, Nancy Patterson at the National Graves' Disease Foundation and Virginia Ladd at the American Autoimmune and Related Diseases Association. And I can't forget Dr. Noel Rose, Dr. John Kennerdell and Dr. Leslie De Groot for the knowledge they so graciously shared. Also, sincere thanks to Kathy Nelson, Librarian at Eastern Idaho Regional Medical Center.

I'd also like to express my gratitude to my husband Rick, my son Brett and my brothers, Ken, John, Richard and Bob for their support and countless hours of proofreading. And special thanks to my brother Arthur to whom this book is dedicated.

Foreword

Finally, a comprehensive "manual" to navigate Graves' disease. When I was diagnosed with the disease in the early '90s, I was naive, and believed that the medical advice I was being given would "pull me through" and return me to my previous "normal life."

Upon receiving this diagnosis, I requested information, the usual "pamphlet" found in many doctors' offices. The staff looked at me as if I was asking for something quite unique and unheard of. I walked away empty-handed, and all too soon discovered that learning more about Graves' disease would not be so easy.

Quite curious and somewhat distressed, I then began a hyper-mission to research Graves' disease — why me, how to best treat, what to expect, and so on. This thought and effort led to the formation of the American Foundation of Thyroid Patients, a nonprofit organization dedicated to providing education to all patients with thyroid related diseases.

I am impressed and moved that Ms. Moore has shared her knowledge, time, and personal experience of Graves' disease to help others who may find themselves in much the same situation as I once did.

Kelly R. Hale
Founder/President
American Foundation of Thyroid Patients

Introduction

Every science and every inquiry, and similarly every activity and pursuit, is thought to aim at some good.
— Aristotle in *Nichomachean Ethics*

As a child, I rarely procrastinated. Unlike my brothers, I did my chores before going out to play. As an adult, I feared that if I ever fell behind, I'd never catch up. Success and praise or abject failure loomed as the consequences. Never one to regard failure lightly, I hurdled my way through "to do" lists. However, when it came to Graves' disease (GD), my system failed me. Then, I learned that alacrity has its own downside.

In college, years before my GD diagnosis, I learned that GD, a hyperthyroid disorder, results from a defective thyroid gland. At least that's what researchers thought in 1970. Had I known that, since then, GD had been found to have an autoimmune origin, I probably wouldn't have chosen aggressive treatment so hastily. Too late, I discovered that in GD, the thyroid is the victim, not the cause, and that the immune system is at fault.

What I've since also learned is that every incidence of GD is unique, and no one treatment works best for all patients. Unlike diseases that always progressively worsen, symptoms in GD wax and wane with periods of variable severity and remission. Each year, 10 percent to 25 percent of GD patients achieve spontaneous remission. Then again, rarely, symptoms can skyrocket, causing heart problems, and, in rare instances, death.

Besides failing to research GD when it would have most benefited me, I also neglected to consider that certain personality traits I'd developed were actually Graves' symptoms, particularly my impatience and tendency to act impulsively. These very symptoms caused me to regard treatment as a line on a chore list, something to scratch off quickly. Considering the consequences, this is not a method I recommend following.

1

Enticed by reports of beneficial outcomes in other diseases, many Graves' patients are consulting naturopath healers. In chapters 9 and 12, you'll meet patients who've successfully used alternative medicine either alone or to complement conventional therapy. Although all GD patients need to be managed by a conventional or alternative practitioner, patients need to be involved in their own healing plans. Enthusiasm for a particular treatment affects both compliance and outcome.

Comprehensive in scope, this book is intended as a reference to be consulted whenever new issues surface. Several patients who critiqued early drafts worried that certain sections could intimidate some readers. Others insisted the same material was essential. I compromised by including figures to clarify the text, and I attempted to define obscure medical terms with their first use. Where I failed to do so, I apologize and hope I didn't neglect to include any of these words in the glossary. To help decipher the numerous thyroid acronyms we, in writing the resource sections, incorporated a list of acronyms into an encyclopedic medical glossary. This tool follows chapter 13.

One of the major consistencies in thyroidology lies in its inconsistencies. Reviewing the major endocrinology journals and textbooks, I've found many conflicting views, particularly regarding treatment recommendations and diagnostic criteria.

In most instances, I included all views. Where this might have caused ambiguity or added to the confusion, I included the prevailing view. For discrepancies surrounding laboratory tests, I deferred to the pathologists, the doctors who oversee hospital laboratories, and to the research scientists who are instrumental in developing these tests.

Although science has made tremendous strides in elucidating the nature of Graves' disease, there is still much more to be learned. Today's limited information will surely expand as researchers attempt to find not merely a treatment but a cure. In the meantime, I present an overview of current medical findings. And I offer you these suggestions for healing.

1 The Graves' Legacy

A Gravesian Tale

I can rationalize stealing my brother's money by blaming it on my health. Since childhood, light, especially sunlight, has hurt my eyes. And although I loved playing outdoors, I could never keep from squinting even on hazy days. Until my theft, that is. Rifling through photo albums I'm reminded of this. Particularly in several pictures taken with my twin on our third birthday, I appear to be in agony I'm squinting and grimacing so fiercely. It's no wonder that at 7, the age of reason, I stole an older brother's three dollars and ran to Clark's, the corner drugstore, to buy sunglasses I later pretended to find.

Taken by itself this minor transgression isn't important. I eventually repaid my debt. This early glimpse of my peculiar sensitivity to light is important, though, in tracing my Graves' legacy. In the shadows of those childhood photos, I see hints of my current health status. Light sensitivity, after all, is a symptom of autoimmune thyroid disease. And although this book is not about me but about Graves' disease (GD), I open this chapter with several excerpts from my life to illustrate how GD often begins insidiously.

Since childhood, I've been plagued by pollen, plant, food, animal and environmental allergies. After my first shot for poison ivy, I objected, with appropriate hysterics, to any scheduling of doctor appointments including the eye exam my aunts kept insisting I needed. At age 10, I refused to be examined and ran from a dentist's office. The only girl and, with my twin, the youngest, I usually got my way. Until I turned 15.

Then, with wily cunning, my mother gleaned that my monthly menstrual period came, at best, annually. I didn't mind. Mom did. She sent

3

me to the neighborhood doctor, an elderly man who appeared perplexed when I stumbled into his office mumbling that I wasn't to have any shots. After twice appraising my reflexes he said I needed to go downtown for a basal metabolism rate (BMR) test. He also prescribed progesterone pills, which worked so well I quit taking them. And I never told my parents about the BMR, a test that would have likely shown a hypermetabolic state.

A spindly child, I towered over my twin until our teens (children with GD are usually tall). Then, as he grew taller, I packed on 20 pounds seemingly overnight and my stomach always felt disconcertingly hollow. (Weight gain is common in GD teens.) Foiled by food, I learned to smoke and I prayed for the pounds to melt.

In college, I got my wish and didn't mind when my erratic menstrual periods totally vanished. Of greater personal concern, I once broke a tooth while eating a carrot. Shaking his head, my dentist insisted that I had an underlying illness. Never linking my dental health to physical health gone awry, I bought vitamins, fearing that my high sugar diet and lifelong avoidance of both milk and dentists might land me in dentures before I turned 20.

As I studied laboratory medicine, I ran nearly every test available on my own blood except for the one thyroid function test available then, a protein bound iodine. However, discovering my serum potassium was abnormally low, I added mineral supplements to my regimen. By college graduation, my gynecological problems had improved.

I had both of my children in my early 20s. After each pregnancy I suffered from postpartum depression (linked to thyroid autoimmunity) and lost more weight than I'd gained. Besides pounds, I began losing patience. The slightest affront enraged me. By my late 20s I was diagnosed with hypertension. Alarmed, I quit smoking and started aerobics.

By age 40, when I was diagnosed with Graves' disease, my only symptoms were a slightly enlarged thyroid, light sensitivity, slightly elevated resting pulse, restless leg syndrome and occasional irritability. Off all antihypertensive medications, my weight and blood pressure were normal. Allergies were my only significant medical complaint. Alas, a savvy physician's assistant at my allergist's office palpated my neck, noticed that my thyroid was slightly enlarged, and suggested I see an internist.

My laboratory tests showed that I was slightly hyperthyroid. Noting my increased radioiodine uptake test (RAI-U, see chapter 5) of 67 percent, my internist diagnosed GD. I never hesitated when he recommended radioiodine ablation (RAI). And when he mentioned there was a slight possibility I'd become hypothyroid (it's 90 percent), I naively thought this was something a pill could easily fix. A week after I had RAI, when my legs began to itch and swell, I began to regret my haste. Since then, I've never felt as good as I used to.

The Nature and Discovery of Graves' Disease

The past ten years have shown tremendous advances in elucidating the etiology or causes of Graves' disease. According to prevailing theory, in GD the vulnerable thyroid, along with the eye, skin and muscle, is targeted by the immune system, genetic influences, and environmental factors. GD is an autoimmune disease with a multi-genetic component.

In this chapter, I explain how GD follows an unpredictable course, typically characterized by periods of variable severity. GD, as you'll learn, doesn't necessarily progressively worsen, although it may. Nor does it always require aggressive treatment measures. GD does, though, require that patients consult a medical doctor or a practitioner of alternative medicine who can monitor symptoms and prescribe appropriate individualized treatment as needed. Chapter one focuses on symptoms associated with autoimmunity and hyperthyroidism, including myopathy, the muscle disorder associated with GD.

Discovery of Graves' Disease

Graves' disease is named after an Irish physician, Dr. Robert Graves, who in 1835 encountered several women with a cluster of seemingly unrelated symptoms including goiter, palpitations, eye disturbances, weakness on exertion and tachycardia. One woman was said to have had such marked exophthalmos (abnormal protrusion of the eyeball; proptosis) she couldn't close her eyes.

Several years earlier, another Irish physician named Caleb Parry noted similar findings, but his observations weren't published until after his death. His findings include an example of GD being directly related to stress. One patient apparently developed GD after her nanny allowed her to fall down a flight of stairs while in a wheelchair.

A Disease with Many Names

Also in Europe, Baron Carl Adolph von Basedow, who hadn't heard of Dr. Graves' findings, reported similar observations in 1840. Thus, in parts of Europe and Africa and in most German speaking regions, the disease is generally referred to as Basedow's disease, von Basedow's disease, Graves-Basedow disease, or Parry's disease. In the United States, however, Parry's disease occasionally refers to hyperthyroidism associated with toxic multinodular goiter. Graves' disease is also known as exophthalmic goiter and toxic diffuse goiter.

Thyrotoxicosis and Hyperthyroidism

The term thyrotoxicosis (symptoms caused by excess thyroid hormone) was originally chosen because the disease process was thought to involve the thyroid's failure to inactivate a toxic substance it had encountered. In Western countries, 90 percent of the cases of hyperthyroidism (condition of sustained periods of thyrotoxicosis) are caused by GD.

The Epidemiology and Incidence

Graves' disease strikes seven to ten times more women than men. The peak age is between 20 and 40 years although GD may occur at any age. GD is rarely diagnosed in children, although Italian researchers have recently described three unrelated children who developed GD before the age of 3 (see chapter 10),[1] and the number of children with GD appears to be rising. The true prevalence of GD is estimated to be slightly less than 1 percent of the U. S. population. Up to 4 percent of the U. S. population is thought to have subclinical Graves' disease in which the patient has no symptoms but has a suppressed thyroid stimulating hormone (TSH) level.[2]

Although Graves' disease affects fewer men, when it does, the symptoms of Graves' ophthalmopathy are generally more severe.[3] And although thyroid hyperfunction is often more severe in men and muscle disorders are more likely, overall symptoms in men may be less severe.[4] Also, GD usually affects men at a later age (40–65).

The Natural Progression of Graves' Disease

Graves' disease affects the body in many different ways and runs an unpredictable, often erratic course. None of the diagnostic tests, including antibody titers, radioiodine uptake testing or blood hormone levels, can predict the disease course of a particular patient.

Graves' disease, Hashimoto's thyroiditis (HT), Hashitoxicosis, and primary myxedema (atrophic autoimmune thyroiditis), are all autoimmune thyroid diseases (AITD). HT is seen 4 times as often as GD and is responsible for most instances of hypothyroidism. HT is also associated with occasional transient periods of hyperthyroidism that closely resemble GD. In Hashitoxicosis, symptoms of hyperthyroidism may occur concomitantly in patients with HT. All of these conditions may occur at different times in one patient's lifetime. Other variations of these syndromes can also occur including transient thyroid dysfunction occurring independent of pregnancy, as well as in 5 percent to 6 percent of postpartum patients. All of these syndromes are linked by similar thyroid cellular changes, similar immune mechanisms and prevalence in family groups.

The Onset of Hyperthyroidism

The onset of hyperthyroid symptoms in GD is usually gradual, with patients most often complaining of increased nervousness, irritability, fatigue, weight loss and menstrual irregularity. In older patients, cardiovascular and myopathic (muscle involvement) features may predominate while the more typical characteristics may be mild or absent, leading to the term apathetic hyperthyroidism. This term can also refer to the symptoms of withdrawal or depression sometimes seen in this age group. Congestive heart failure may be the initial manifestation in older patients, especially if there is underlying cardiac disease.

The Onset of Graves' Ophthalmopathy and Dermopathy

Graves' ophthalmopathy (GO), an eye disease, pretibial myxedema (PTM), a skin disorder, and acropachy, a soft connective tissue disorder (see chapter 4) may all occur in patients with GD. These independent conditions may begin before or after the thyroid disorder emerges. Although the eye and skin disorders generally occur within 18 months of the thyroid disorder, some patients develop these conditions many years later and most patients not at all. Conversely, the eye disease may show up first and years later hyperthyroidism may develop. On occasion, the eye disease may occur with no evidence of hyperthyroidism (euthyroid Graves' disease).

Spontaneous Remissions

Untreated, hyperthyroidism in GD can spontaneously improve and result in a fairly quick return to normality. Given time, it may also eventually progress to hypothyroidism.[5] GD has been reported to have a spontaneous remission rate of 10 percent to 25 percent per year.[6] Spontaneous hypothyroidism may occur as a natural progression of the disease or a result of the patient developing coincident autoimmune thyroiditis. On the other hand, untreated (as well as treated) hyperthyroidism can, on rare occasions, progress to thyroid storm (described later in this chapter) and cause death.

Untreated, patients may remain chronically hyperthyroid although their course may fluctuate, varying in intensity, and sometimes alternating with long periods of remission. Sometimes thyrotoxicosis persists, varying in severity over time. In others, like me, the course may be cyclic, exhibiting remissions of varying frequency, intensity and duration.

Disability and Mortality

A number of Graves' disease patients, especially those who suffer from severe muscle and cardiac problems, develop symptoms at some point that

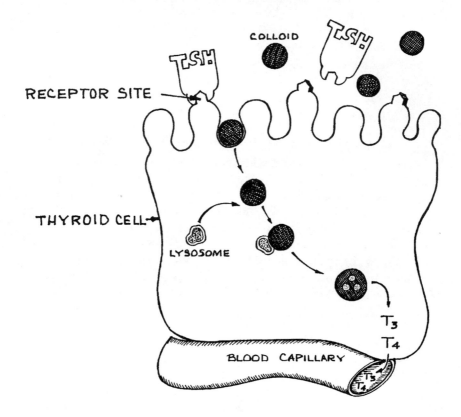

TSH STIMULATING A THYROID
CELL AT A RECEPTOR SITE

COLLOID
TSH
TSH

RECEPTOR SITE

THYROID CELL

LYSOSOME

T₃
T₄

BLOOD CAPILLARY

Thyroid Hormone Release.

prevent them from working. In the United States, thyroid disease is included under the Americans with Disabilities Act of 1990. For general information, answers to specific questions, free materials or information about filing a complaint, call (800) 514-0301 or visit their web site, www. usdj.gov/crt/ada.

The estimated mortality rate from untreated Graves' disease has been reported to be as high as 11 percent.[7] However, death attributable to untreated thyrotoxicosis is rarely seen today and is primarily associated with the elderly. Heart problems, such as myocardial infarction, arrhythmia and heart failure have been responsible for most deaths associated with GD.

Allergic Connections

Of interest, Japanese researchers have recently demonstrated how an elevation of immunoglobulin E (increased in allergies) is also associated with hyperthyroidism in Graves' disease.[8] And in *Japanese Herbal Medicine, The Healing Art of Kampo*, Robert Rister writes that Japanese researchers have linked GD to bouts of severe allergies, specifically to cedar pollen.[9] Perhaps in the future, doctors will sooner consider a diagnosis of GD when they're confronted with patients with severe allergies compounded by weight loss or nervousness or extreme photophobia (light sensitivity).

Manifestations of Graves' Disease

Nervousness, the most common symptom of GD, is often described as a feeling of impending doom or apprehension along with an inability to concentrate. However, not all patients feel nervous. And in some patients, only one terse symptom (out of a potential cornucopia) dominates the clinical picture. Thyroid enlargement (goiter) is the most common manifestation. Goiter occurs in 90 percent of younger patients and 80 percent of older patients. Occasionally, a surreptitiously enlarged thyroid can cause a sense of fullness in the neck or obstructive symptoms. If the thyroid is located behind the tongue, goiter can constrict other organs such a the windpipe.

Symptoms may be attributed to thyrotoxicosis or autoimmunity, or they may be peculiar to GD. The following list describes typical symptoms seen in Graves' patients. Symptoms associated with Graves' eye and skin disease are included in chapter 4.

Symptoms of Graves' Disease
Associated with Hyperthyroidism

Nervousness
Irritability
Depression
Nausea, vomiting
Difficulty sleeping, insomnia
Rapid heartbeat
Shortness of breath (dyspnea)
Edema, especially of ankles
Fine tremor of the hands or fingers
Headaches

Increased sweating
Increased blood pressure
Sensitivity to heat, heat intolerance
Increased temperature
Weight loss despite increased appetite
Goiter
Light or absent menstrual periods
Frequent bowel movements (Note: diarrhea is considered an ominous sign and

may indicate the onset of thyroid storm.)
Increased urination (polyuria)
Fatigue, especially neuromuscular
Restlessness
Hair changes
Muscle weakness, muscle wasting
Emotional disturbances, emotional lability

Increased thirst and appetite	Drug tolerance, increased drug metabolism	Hyperpigmentation of skin
Fertility disorders	Hyperkinesis	Premature graying of the hair
Heart palpitations	Brisk reflexes	Patchy vitiligo (seen in 7 percent of GD patients)
Warm, velvety skin	Hives	
Youthful appearance	Proptosis	
Reduced libido		

Note: The last 2 symptoms listed are associated with autoimmunity. Vitiligo is discussed in chapter 4.

The Pathology of Graves' Disease

Graves' hyperthyroidism results from the direct stimulation of thyroid cells by stimulating TSH receptor antibodies (described further in the next chapter). These antibodies mimic thyroid stimulating hormone (TSH), a pituitary hormone that normally directs the thyroid to produce and release thyroid hormone.

Development of Graves' Ophthalmopathy and Dermopathy

Graves' ophthalmopathy (GO) and dermopathy are both associated with increased production of a congestive mucinous substance known as glycosaminoglycan (GAG). GAG is formed by fibroblasts (immature connective tissue cells that normally differentiate into the cells that form collagen, tendons or fibrous tissue, including orbital or eye tissue).

The primary GAG seen in Graves' disease is hyaluronan. Since hyaluronan accumulation only occurs in the lesions of localized myxedema (see chapter 4) and in the soft orbital tissue of GO, and not in other forms of thyrotoxicosis such as nodular disease, this disturbance is thought to be related to autoimmunity and not thyroid hormone excess.[10]

Other Organ Involvement

Other organs besides the thyroid may occasionally demonstrate lymphocytic infiltration (inflammation), indicating immune system involvement. Patients with GD may have an enlarged thymus gland or spleen (splenomegaly) and enlarged lymph nodes.

Severe thyrotoxicosis may also cause degeneration of skeletal muscle fibers, fatty infiltration or diffuse fibrosis of the liver, decalcification of the skeletal bone, and loss of body tissue, causing symptoms similar to that seen in wasting.

Metabolic Changes

Metabolism refers to both catabolism, in which substances are broken down into smaller parts, and anabolism, in which the body combines small substances such as minerals to build a larger compound such as bone tissue. In catabolism, energy is released, whereas anabolism requires energy. Metabolism in GD is accelerated with patient frequently appearing restless, anxious or just plain "wired." Excess catabolism and energy production contribute to the nervous anxiety and insomnia associated with GD. Most patients lose weight despite an increased appetite and food intake. However, approximately 10 percent of patients with GD gain weight. Weight gain in GD is most often seen in teens.

In general, the cells in the thyrotoxic state burn so much fuel that normal sources can't keep up with the body's demands. Eventually, the body begins to use its own muscle and fat for energy via a process called gluconeogenesis or "new glucose" formation.

Gluconeogenesis and Protein Metabolism

The glucose produced by gluconeogenesis (process by which compounds are broken down to form glucose) is metabolized quickly to produce a chemical known as adenosine triphosphate (ATP), the body's main source of energy. When glucose stores are depleted, the body begins breaking down protein, ravaging it from muscles, including heart muscle. In metabolizing protein, nitrogen is released. This nitrogen is transferred to the liver where it is converted into the compounds creatine and urea. Elevated blood urea nitrogen (BUN) and creatine can cause nausea or headache. Over time, chronically high blood levels of these compounds may lead to uremia or kidney damage.

Blood Lipids and Biliary Secretion

Thyroid hormone also breaks down fat into fatty acids and glycerol, which is used to produce more ATP. Patients with GD usually consume all fatty acid reserves and have free fatty acid deficiencies. Free fatty acids are one of the main sources of energy used by thyroid cells, especially during prolonged periods of increased respiration. Thyroid hormones also enhance the body's lipolytic (ability to break down fat) action on other fat soluble hormones such as catecholamines. This may contribute to weight loss. Thyroid hormone stimulates the metabolism of cholesterol to bile acids. Consequently, a low serum cholesterol level is characteristic of thyrotoxicosis.

Bile acids are necessary for proper fat digestion, including secretion of gastric juices. Reduced bile acid output may contribute to the frequent defecation and steatorrhea (condition of increased fat content in stools) often seen in GD.[11]

Insulin Resistance and Drug Metabolism

Thyrotoxicosis is an insulin-resistant state similar to Type 2 diabetes. To meet its increased glucose demands, the body uses whatever sources it can find. Glucose utilization by thyroid cells is also enhanced in active GD and contributes to the diminished reserves.[12] With its own demands, the thyrotoxic body becomes insensitive to the normal regulatory effects of insulin, resulting in a state of insulin intolerance. Compensatory increases in insulin secretion (in response to the rise in blood glucose) are a result of the body's effort to maintain a normal blood glucose level.

The metabolism and excretion of many drugs are accelerated in the thyrotoxic state. Consequently, a number of medications require an increase in dosage to work effectively in patients with thyrotoxicosis.[13] Faster metabolism of alcohol makes its effects noticeable sooner, and many GD patients report experiencing alcohol intolerance.

Nutrient Deficiencies

Bodily reactions that we take for granted (like breathing) require many different nutrients. In GD, the body's cells consume increased oxygen, depleting nutrient supplies. The increased bowel motility seen in GD and the associated gluten sensitivity (see chapter 6) both contribute to malabsorption of nutrients. Specific nutrient deficiencies cause new symptoms and aggravate others. The minimal daily requirement (MDR) applies to the requirements of normal metabolism. Graves' disease essentially has its own MDR.

Symptoms Caused by Vitamin Deficiencies

VITAMIN A

Deficiencies of vitamin A may cause diminished adaptation to darkness in some patients (night blindness). Both thyroxine (thyroid hormone) and vitamin A share the transport protein transthyretin, or TTR (protein that transports hormones within the body). Excess thyroid hormone binds to most of the TTR, preventing vitamin A's absorption and its conversion from carotene. Vitamin A and vitamin B2 (riboflavin) are essential for proper thyroid function.[14]

VITAMIN D AND CALCIUM

Disturbances in vitamin D and calcium metabolism are also seen in GD. Normally, once peak bone mass (primarily under genetic control) is achieved, the bone mass remains stable for years although resorption and formation are constantly occurring. In resorption, osteoclast cells cause bone to break down. In bone formation, osteoblasts form bone. Thyroid hormones directly stimulate bone resorption, resulting in hypercalcemia (elevated serum calcium) as calcium is released from bone. This condition is reversed when thyroid balance is restored. Severe hypercalcemia may cause vomiting, anorexia, polyuria and occasionally impairment of renal function.[15]

PARATHYROID HORMONE AND VITAMIN D

Calcium regulates the release of parathyroid hormone (PTH) from the parathyroid glands. Hypercalcemia causes decreased PTH secretion or transient hypoparathyroidism. Vitamin D supplementation counteracts the rapid calcium excretion, restoring normal calcium levels. Vitamin C and K levels (needed for bone matrix synthesis) must also be adequate.[16]

The resultant low PTH levels interfere with the body's conversion of vitamin D (which is dependent on adequate PTH). Diminished intestinal absorption of vitamin D results in increased urinary calcium loss. A slight increase in thyroid hormone levels can initiate this process, which can ultimately result in osteoporosis.

VITAMINS C, E AND B

Deficiencies of both vitamins C and E cause thyroid cell hyperplasia (increase in cell number due to excessive cell proliferation), raising thyroid hormone levels. Changes in lipid metabolism and malabsorption of fat soluble vitamins cause vitamin E deficiencies. According to Dr. Stephen Langer, a combination of vitamin E and C deficiencies may cause hyperthyroidism. He proposes that, in a number of instances where patients had their thyroid glands removed or destroyed, vitamin supplementation may have resulted in a cure.[17]

Thyroid hormones regulate the conversion of dietary riboflavin (vitamin B2) into its two active flavin coenzymes. Enzyme activity is increased by thyroid hormones. Consequently, vitamin B2 reserves are diminished in thyrotoxicosis. Vitamin B2 also regulates reproductive organs, and deficiencies can cause reproductive problems.

Vitamin B12 and vitamin B3 (niacin) cannot be properly absorbed unless the thyroid is functioning properly. B12 deficiency can cause mental illness, neuralgia and other neurological disorders. Niacin is needed for the proper metabolism of carbohydrates, proteins and fat. Serum concentrations of vitamin B12 and folic acid are often low in thyrotoxicosis. However, the cause may also be related to a concurrent autoimmune condition. The prevalence of the autoimmune disorder pernicious anemia (PA) is increased and the metabolism of folic acid is accelerated in Graves' disease.[18]

Thiamine (vitamin B1) deficiency, recognized as a cause of high output cardiac failure, occurs in thyrotoxicosis since vast quantities of B1 are used and excreted. Dr. Arem, in *The Thyroid Solution*, recommends that patients with an overactive thyroid increase their consumption of both vitamin B1 and vitamin B6 (pyridoxine).[19] The marked vitamin B6 deficiencies seen in thyrotoxicosis may contribute to muscle weakness.

Symptoms Caused by Mineral Deficiencies

BONE LOSS

GD generally causes increased excretion of calcium and phosphorus and demineralization of bone. These changes may result in conditions of weak, soft or brittle bone such as osteitis fibrosa, osteomalacia or osteoporosis. As GD is treated, bone changes generally resolve, especially in premenopausal women.

In young individuals, normal bone formation usually compensates for bone loss. In fact, in children, hyperthyroidism is associated with increased skeletal growth, and hypothyroidism is associated with reduced growth.[20] Thyroid hormones are critical for cartilage growth and differentiation and they enhance the response to growth hormone. The risk of developing secondary osteoporosis is greatest in postmenopausal women who may also have primary osteoporosis. Hyperthyroidism also causes collagen fiber breakdown. Collagen is the primary component of the matrix or inner layers of bone tissue.

IODINE, MAGNESIUM, COPPER, MANGANESE, ZINC

Minerals utilized in the production and metabolism of thyroid hormone include manganese, iron, phosphorus, calcium, magnesium, sulfur, zinc, copper and selenium. Iodine is one of the primary components of thyroid hormone. However, excess iodine can trigger or exacerbate GD symptoms and strong iodine solution can reduce symptoms (see chapters 3 and 7). Proper absorption of iodine requires adequate magnesium.

High levels of zinc are associated with hyperthyroidism. Of particular importance is the balance between zinc and copper, which is normally 8:1. This balance is essential for proper functioning of the hypothalamic-pituitary-thyroid axis that regulates thyroid levels in the blood, and for production and metabolism of thyroid hormone.[21] As zinc levels rise, copper levels are low relative to zinc, upsetting the critical balance. Elevated zinc levels are associated with hyperthyroidism, whereas high copper levels are seen in hypothyroidism.

CALCITONIN AND CALCIUM REGULATION

Calcitonin, a thyroid hormone produced by C cells in the thyroid (see chapter 3), promotes anabolism by regulating calcium's role in forming bone tissue. In hypercalcemia, which occurs in approximately 27 percent of hyperthyroid individuals,[22] the thyroid gland secretes excess calcitonin. Calcitonin increases the activity of the bone producing cells known as osteoblasts and reduces activity of the osteoclasts, which break down bone. Calcitonin reduces serum calcium levels by promoting calcium absorption and bone development. The function of calcitonin is directly opposite that of PTH.

Essential Fatty Acids

Essential fatty acids (EFAs) are not produced in the body. They must be derived from diet. Hyperthyroidism causes EFA deficiencies. Both the thyroid gland and the brain require sufficient EFA's to function properly. In *Solved: The Riddle of Illness*, Dr. Stephen E. Langer reports that laboratory rats deprived of EFA become hyperactive with excessive thyroid hormone production.[23] EFA deficiencies may cause cardiovascular and circulatory abnormalities, acne, eczema, failure of wounds to heal, mental deterioration, fatty liver and atrophy of exocrine glands. Essential fatty acids, including omega-3, omega-6, and omega-9 fatty acids, are found in varying types and quantities in evening primrose oil, marine fish oil, borage oil and flaxseed oil. Omega-3 is especially deficient in GD.

Nervous System Effects

Emotional Lability and Mental Symptoms

A frequent complaint of GD patients (or their friends and relatives) is emotional lability. Symptoms include hysterical outbursts, mood disorders and crying for no apparent reason. Periods of depression may alternate with periods of elation.

The mental symptoms of hyperthyroidism may precede the physical symptoms, and they may be more pronounced, confusing diagnosis. Hyperthyroidism is associated with elation, which can reach manic proportions and cause hallucinations. The transition from slightly manic (hypomanic) to manic behavior may be gradual or abrupt. Its onset may concur close to the initial diagnosis of GD or be delayed until long afterward.[24] In rare cases of hyperthyroidism, severe psychic disturbances may occur. Bipolar and mood swing disorders, and schizoid or paranoid reactions, may also emerge.

Tremor, Hyperkinesis and Nervousness

Often, there is a fine rhythmic tremor of the hand or tongue, or tightly closed eyelids. Patients with convulsive disorders tend to have seizures more often. Hyperkinesis refers to increased and sometimes involuntary erratic muscle movement. Patients with hyperkinesis can't sit still. This is exemplified in table drumming, tapping feet and jerky, exaggerated, aim-less movements. Hyperkinesis is generally more severe in children. Hyperkinetic or frenetic (frenzied) behavior, thought and speech patterns are also common symptoms.

Many of the symptoms in GD are similar to those of sympathetic ner-vous system activation. However, sympathetic nervous system activity is not increased in thyrotoxicosis. Rather, it seems that thyroid hormones exert effects similar to but separate from those of the body's major cate-cholamines, epinephrine and norepinephrine. Because beta adrenergic antagonists relieve or alleviate symptoms of adrenergic stimulation such as eyelid retraction, tremor, excessive sweating and tachycardia, it's thought that thyrotoxicosis in GD is associated with increased beta adrenergic activity.

The widespread distribution of thyroid hormone receptors in the brain makes it likely that alterations in cerebral metabolism are induced by thyroid hormone excess, despite the fact that oxygen consumption in the brain is not altered.[25] (See chapter 3.)

The Reproductive System in GD

The occurrence of amenorrhea (absence of menstrual periods) result-ing from GD was one of the major symptoms originally reported by Dr. Robert Graves. Since then, other related effects have been noted, includ-ing anovulation (absence of ovulation), oligomenorrhea (decreased or scant menses), and menorrhagia (profuse menstrual flow), which is more often seen in hypothyroidism. Prepubertal girls with thyrotoxicosis may expe-rience a slightly delayed menarche.

Reproductive problems of miscarriage, implantation failure and in vitro fertilization failure are associated with autoimmune thyroid disease (AITD) and are more often seen in hypothyroidism. At Finch University of Health Sciences in Chicago, researchers have found that thyroid autoantibodies present in AITD cause certain changes in the reproductive system. The presence of thyroglobulin autoantibodies (see chapter 6) ulti-mately results in the production of tumor necrosis factor (TNF), which has the potential to damage the embryo and the placental cells that attach the fetus to the uterus.[26] (Also see chapter 10.)

In GD, the body's conversion of androgens to estrogens may be increased due to changes in protein binding. Consequently, circulating estradiol levels are occasionally increased in thyrotoxic men. As a result, men with GD may have symptoms of increased estrogen biologic activity. Gynecomastia (excessive development of breasts in males), spider angi-omas and a decrease in libido are frequent complaints.[27]

Muscular and Digestive System in GD

Patients with GD frequently exhibit muscle weakness and fatigue. Thyrotoxic myopathy, the muscle involvement that resembles wasting, is generally limited to proximal muscle (proximal thigh as compared to distal calf), and its severity appears out of proportion to overall loss of weight. Weakness is most prominent in the pelvic and shoulder girdles and the proximal muscles of the limbs. The shoulder and hand muscles undergo the most obvious atrophy, although the facial muscles may also be affected. Patients with GD often experience difficulty climbing stairs because of weak leg muscles.

Some reduction in the power of muscle contraction is thought to occur in nearly all patients with GD.[28] One of the earliest physiologic measurements of muscle function, the deep tendon reflex test, is increased in GD. In recent years, skeletal muscle has been found to be a site of thyroid hormone metabolism.

Digestive Disturbances

Digestion in GD is usually accelerated. Bowel movements tend to be increased (hyperdefecation), although rarely causing diarrhea. Rapid digestion causes malabsorption (nutrients aren't absorbed from food) and steatorrhea (excess undigested fat in stools). Weight loss is caused by increased caloric requirements and malabsorption. Malabsorption with its subsequent nutrient deficiencies also triggers food cravings.

Liver disease is often seen in thyrotoxicosis, but it's uncertain if thyroid hormone is responsible or if the cause is associated autoimmune liver disease (see chapter 6). Gluten sensitivity, which is also known as celiac disease, is seen in patients with GD more frequently than in the normal population (see chapter 6).

The Cardiovascular System in Graves' Disease

Thyroid hormone exerts its strongest effects on the heart. Increased circulatory demands cause changes in the heart's rate and rhythm. Palpitations, those vigorous, rapid pounding heart beats experienced by many GD patients, are caused by the increased force of cardiac contraction. Cardiovascular findings include a wide pulse pressure, sinus tachycardia, exercise intolerance and atrial arrhythmias (especially atrial fibrillations). Another common symptom is dyspnea or shortness of breath.

An overactive thyroid can cause irregular heartbeat. One of the first cardiovascular changes due to GD is decreased systemic vascular resistance, which causes increased blood flow to the skin, muscles, kidney and

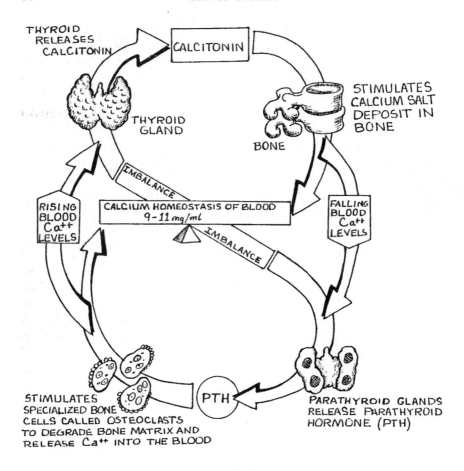

THYROID
RELEASES
CALCITONIN

CALCITONIN

STIMULATES
CALCIUM SALT
DEPOSIT IN
BONE

THYROID
GLAND

BONE

IMBALANCE

RISING
BLOOD
Ca++
LEVELS

CALCIUM HOMEOSTASIS OF BLOOD
9–11 mg/ml

FALLING
BLOOD
Ca++
LEVELS

IMBALANCE

STIMULATES
SPECIALIZED BONE
CELLS CALLED OSTEOCLASTS
TO DEGRADE BONE MATRIX AND
RELEASE Ca++ INTO THE BLOOD

PTH

PARATHYROID GLANDS
RELEASE PARATHYROID
HORMONE (PTH)

Calcium Regulation

heart, increasing cardiac output. As a result the skin may feel flushed and the palms may appear red, warm and moist. Thyroid hormone is a vasodilator and acts directly on vascular smooth muscle, relaxing it while causing an increase in systolic blood pressure, heart rate and cardiac contractility.

Electrocardiographic tracings often demonstrate sinus tachycardia (rapid heart beat). Another 10 percent to 15 percent of GD patients are reported to have atrial fibrillation, although this condition is seen more often in elderly patients in whom it is more difficult to reverse. Atrial muscle refers to the two upper heart chambers (known as atrium, plural atria; the lower chambers are called ventricles, their contractions are ventricular contractions).

In atrial fibrillation, the atria beat wildly and rapidly hundreds of times each minute. Many of these impulses activate the ventricles to contract rapidly too. Consequently, the heart weakens, causing shortness of breath and dizziness. The blood begins to pool in the legs as the overtaxed atria fail to empty completely. The remaining atrial blood becomes stagnant and prone to clots. If a clot breaks free it can block an artery, cutting off the blood supply to major organs. In the brain this causes stroke, which is again more likely to be seen in elderly patients. Complications of atrial fibrillation may lead to heart failure.

Patients with Graves' disease may also have a higher prevalence of mitral valve prolapse, a slight heart valve deformity that causes a heart murmur. For most people, this causes no symptoms, but for some patients it can cause chest pain and a rapid heartbeat. Mitral valve prolapse associated with GD may be due to genetic factors, as this finding has also been demonstrated in patients with chronic autoimmune thyroiditis.[29]

Thyroid Storm (Thyrotoxic Crisis)

Five weeks after receiving radioiodine treatment for Graves' disease, Sharon, a legal secretary living on the East Coast, bolted awake from sleep unable to stop coughing. Trembling, she took her pulse and stopped counting when she reached 150. Between coughs she dialed 911 and was advised to report to the nearest emergency room (ER).

Sharon never once suspected that her symptoms were related to her radioiodine ablation. A smoker, Sharon thought smoking was to blame. Her claim to fame, she says, was overhearing the ER nurse comment, "I've never seen a heart rate that high."

Admitted to the cardiac ward where she remained for several days, Sharon learned that she had an infection that caused her thyroid "to kick up a little." On constant heart monitors, she received intravenous heparin and breathing treatments as well as a daily barrage of laboratory tests. When she was discharged from the hospital with 12 medications and three pages of instructions, her thyroid levels were still off the charts.

Immediately following her radioiodine treatment five weeks earlier, Sharon was armed with beta blockers, prednisone and the heart medication digoxin, and she was told to return in three months to have her thyroid levels checked. The possibility of complications was never mentioned. She was never verbally warned that she might develop any problems, despite having a history of atrial fibrillation related to Graves' disease.

Although, she developed mild thyroid eye disease after her radioiodine ablation and experienced thyroid storm, Sharon emphasized that she has no regrets. She wrote, "I am pro–RAI for certain people, myself included. With all the things that happened, I truly believe it was my only viable option. In fact, I believe I would have died without RAI."

Sharon admits that because of insurance regulations, she switched doctors so many times in the years before her diagnosis that it would have been impossible for any one doctor to realize all of her symptoms. She'd had GD symptoms for ten years, including irregular periods, irritability, heat intolerance, depression and heart problems. Her heart rate was usually higher than 110. At work she couldn't sit still and became furious if someone pointed this out. Extreme hunger caused her to gain 15 pounds. In retrospect, she says that she was partly responsible for her GD becoming so severe. She says she should have listened to her body more closely and pushed harder for a referral to an endocrinologist after her diagnosis since her symptoms were severe.

What Is Thyroid Storm?

Thyroid storm is a relatively rare, life-threatening crisis characterized by exaggerated signs of hyperthyroidism. Approximately 1 percent to 2 percent of patients with hyperthyroidism progress to thyroid storm. Since laboratory tests can't diagnose thyroid storm (which is related to the effects, not the levels, of thyroid hormone), diagnosis is based on symptoms. There is evidence that an increased number of binding sites for circulating catecholamines (such as epinephrine) in thyrotoxicosis induces the symptoms associated with thyroid storm.[30] It has also been suggested that infections (the most common trigger) may reduce serum binding of the thyroid hormone thyroxine (T4), allowing more free T4 to be available to the body's cells.

Warning Signs

Although thyroid storm occurs suddenly, there are usually warning signs, such as fever with a temperature greater than 37.8 C (100 F), tachycardia usually out of proportion to fever, elevated heart rate, central nervous system dysfunction including psychosis, nausea, vomiting, diarrhea, and, in severe cases, jaundice. However, in elderly patients with apathetic hyperthyroidism, symptoms of psychosis aren't as pronounced, and fever, if present, isn't as high. Weakness, emotional apathy and confusion may predominate.

Many patients with thyroid storm report a recent dramatic weight loss of more than 40 pounds. Other typical symptoms include palpitations, chest pain, emotional lability with a wide variation of emotions and mood swings, dyspnea, diaphoresis (sweating, often profuse), dehydration, thyromegaly, exophthalmos, widened pulse pressure, congestive heart failure, tremor, weakness, shock, atrial fibrillation refractory to digitalis, myopathy, periodic paralysis, edema, psychosis, anxiety and disorientation.[31]

Diagnosis is based on symptoms. Although laboratory tests usually indicate thyrotoxicosis, blood levels don't show specific changes. Laboratory support usually also consists of electrolyte levels, renal and liver function tests and a plasma cortisol level.

Causes of Thyroid Storm

A number of precipitating factors have been reported, including:

- Pulmonary infection (most common causes are pharyngitis or pneumonia)
- Diabetic ketoacidosis, hyperosmolar coma and insulin induced hypoglycemia
- Surgical treatment of hyperthyroidism; other surgical procedures
- Abrupt withdrawal of antithyroid medication
- Radioactive iodine ablation
- Excessive palpation of the thyroid gland in hyperthyroid patients
- Emotional stress
- Thyroid hormone overdose
- Cardiovascular events
- Toxemia of pregnancy, and labor
- Pulmonary thromboembolism

Treatment

Therapy is directed at supportive care and thyroid hormone reduction. Beta adrenergic blocking agents (propranolol, metoprolol, etc.) are the mainstay of therapy. Antipyretics (to reduce fever) are indicated, but aspirin should be avoided since it may increase thyroid hormone levels. Anti-thyroid medications are used to inhibit new thyroid hormone synthesis. Iodide agents, such as Lugol's solution, effectively block thyroid hormone release. They should be administered one hour after the loading dose of antithyroid medications so that the iodide itself isn't available for new hormone synthesis.

How to Get Emergency Help

Due to the variable nature of GD, troubling symptoms occasionally emerge suddenly with the most alarming changes invariably occurring "after hours." Often, not knowing if their symptoms are thyroid related, patients seek advice on one of the many internet bulletin boards. Last year, when Susan, a young woman living on the East Coast, was having trouble distinguishing color and experiencing blurred vision on a Saturday night, another patient suggested that the problem was caused by too much prednisone.

Aware of the implications, I suggested Susan call her ophthalmologist immediately. I explained that if he wasn't available or "on call," one of his associates would be covering his practice. I told her that he might direct her to the emergency room and meet her there. However, her physician outdid himself and agreed to meet her at his office although it was already 10 P.M., saving her an emergency room charge. His exam showed optic nerve compression and her prednisone dose was increased to reduce the swelling.

I mention this as a reminder that not all opinions expressed on Internet bulletin boards are reliable. The thyroid boards are intended to offer support and share experiences, not dispense medical advice. I also describe this incident to remind patients that their doctor or one of his or her associates is always on call. It's best to call your doctor when emergencies come up. In most instances, he can evaluate your symptoms over the phone and prescribe medicine or send you to a local hospital for an outpatient lab test.

Other Complications and Disorders Associated with GD

Hypokalemic Periodic Paralysis (HPP) and Thyrotoxic Periodic Paralysis

Hypokalemic periodic paralysis (HPP), a condition of severely depressed serum potassium, may occur together with thyrotoxicosis, and its severity is accentuated by the thyroid disorder. HPP is particularly common in Asian people, although this prevalence appears to be decreasing. This is thought to be a result of dietary changes, particularly less reliance on carbohydrates. It is seen infrequently in whites and rarely in Hispanic and black patients.[32]

Thyrotoxic periodic paralysis is characterized by attacks of muscular weakness or flaccid paralysis that last for several hours up to a few days. Most thyrotoxic patients with this disorder have GD. The episodes of muscle weakness are invariably associated with a decrease in serum potassium concentration (hypokalemia), although the potassium level may not be subnormal. Both HPP and thyrotoxic periodic paralysis are also associated with increased ingestion of carbohydrates. Episodes may be precipitated by ethanol, strenuous exercise in hot weather and by the administration of insulin or acetazolamide.

Edema

Patients with thyrotoxicosis may develop edema (fluid retention). If heart problems are also present, edema may exacerbate cardiac symptoms.

Typically, fluid retention in GD occurs as a pitting edema involving the hands, ankles, legs and sacrum. Patients may also develop severe periorbital edema that requires blepharoplasty, an eye surgery designed to reduce the skin lag around the eye. Edema in GD results from renal salt and water retention caused by the reduction in effective arterial volume. This fluid retention may also contribute to an increase in blood volume and venous pressure.[33]

Parathymic Syndromes

Tumors of the thymus gland are associated with autoimmune diseases including myasthenia gravis, Graves' disease, Type 2 autoimmune polyglandular syndrome (see chapter 6) and Addison's disease.[34]

Parathyroid Hormone Disorders

Transient and permanent disorders of both hypoparathyroidism and hyperparathyroidism may occur spontaneously in patients with Graves' disease. These disorders may also occur as a consequence of treatment for hyperthyroidism.

Exophthalamos, Pretibial Myxedema and Osteoarthropathy (EMO) Syndrome

In 1967, a syndrome of exophthalmos, pretibial myxedema and osteoarthropathy or acropachy (EMO syndrome) occurring together in patients with GD was reported. Most patients with EMO have high titers of thyroid stimulating antibodies. One recent study also reports an association with a heart condition called papillary fibroelastoma.[35]

2 *The Autoimmune Nature of Graves' Disease*

Chapter two focuses on the immune system's role in the development of Graves' disease. Specifically, it explains how various immune system components coordinate their efforts to produce the autoantibodies responsible for the hyperthyroidism of GD.

Graves' disease is considered a disorder of hyperimmunity since immune system cells overreact and produce autoantibodies. However, a depressed number of T suppressor cells (immune system cells that normally prevent autoantibody production) is considered the cause of GD.

Autoimmune Disease in Women

The American Autoimmune Related Disease Association (AARDA), in an internet publication, *Autoimmunity: A Major Women's Health Issue*, reports that the diagnosis of autoimmune disorders is particularly difficult in women, the gender most likely to be affected (women account for 75 percent to 90 percent of autoimmune diseases).[1] Often, AARDA reports, women's concerns are not taken seriously. Gail Devers, in testifying at a 1999 congressional hearing, described how her diagnosis took more than two years.

A survey by AARDA has shown that over 65 percent of patients with autoimmune diseases have been labeled hypochondriacs or chronic complainers sometime during the earliest stages of their illness.[2]

The Role of Emotions, Personality and Stress

In 1935, Dr. Walter Cannon, a Harvard physiologist, reported that the various bodily systems work together to achieve self-maintaining health, a condition he termed homeostasis.[3] A few years later, Dr. Franz Alexander, a Chicago psychiatrist, made the bold statement that many diseases were caused, not by external, mechanical, chemical factors or microorganisms, but by the continuous functional stress found in everyday life.[4]

Exploring this concept, psychosomaticists (doctors specializing in the effects of the mind on disease) in the 1950s found seven distinct conditions that were caused or triggered by psychosomatic ailments, including GD and rheumatoid arthritis. Hans Selye, working at McGill University in Montreal, found the underlying cause of these disorders to be stress. The rats used in Selye's experiments were found, at autopsy, unchanged on the outside. Inside their bodies, however, their glands were atrophied (wasted away).[5]

Many doctors and scientists, including Norman Cousins, who successfully treated his own autoimmune arthritis with stress reduction, have demonstrated how stress and emotions affect the immune system. Psychoneuroimmunology (PNI) is a scientific discipline that originated at Harvard University in the 1980s. PNI explains the interrelationship between the mind, the brain, and the immune system.

The Immune System

Immune system components include:

1. The lymphatics including lymph nodes and lymph fluid
2. Organs such as the bone marrow, spleen, thymus, tonsils, skin and gut; organs serve as production sites and warehouses for the various types of lymphocytes
3. Immune system cells, primarily lymphocytes and macrophages
4. Powerful chemicals and protein components such as complement and cytokines that are released during an immune response

The immune system protects the body from foreign (non-self) antigens by producing antibodies and causing inflammation. The immune system also destroys mutagenic (tumor producing) and autoreactive cells, cells that are destined to become autoantibodies and attack one's own body.

Concept of Self

An important concept in immunity is the concept of self. The "self" that identifies our body's tissues and cells as "our own" refers to the unique molecular configurations that characterize an individual's bodily cells. These unique cell surface markers are a result of our genetic legacy. Any other genetic markers are considered "non-self" or foreign when recognized by immune system cells. Our survival depends on the immune system's ability to recognize foreign antigens and distinguish them from molecules that are "self."

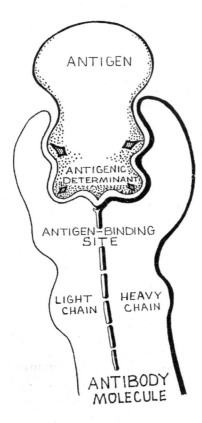

Antigen and Antibody Binding

Antigens

Antigens are substances capable of triggering an immune response. An antigen can be a virus, a bacterium, a grain of pollen or dander, a fungus or one of their protein particles. Human tissue cells from another individual can trigger an immune response serious enough to cause rejection of an organ transplant. Even food can have antigenic properties if the protein molecules aren't first digested and broken down into their primary, non-antigenic amino acid building blocks. Antigenic determinants or epitopes are the specific parts of an antigen molecule that determine or cause a specific immune response.

Antibodies

Antibodies are protective proteins produced in response to an antigen stimulus. Antibodies have the ability to bind to and inactivate the specific antigens that caused their production. For example, children with chicken pox form antibodies to varicella (chicken pox) as their body attempts to fight the infection. On subsequent exposures, antibodies provide these children immunity from contracting chicken pox again. The body's supply of antibody molecules outnumbers immune system cells by about 100 million to one.[6]

Antibody molecules are unique in that their surface has concave regions or indentations that function as combining sites for the very antigens that caused their production. All antigens have protruding regions on their surfaces that are uniquely shaped to fit antibody combining sites precisely, just as a key fits a lock. Antibodies are derived from immuno-globulin (Ig), a specific type of protein with antibody activity. Therefore, the words antibody and immunoglobulin are often used interchangeably. The word immune is derived from Latin and means "exempt" or "free from." If we have immunity we're resistant or immune to these foreign antigens since our antibodies can destroy them.

ANTIBODIES AND PROTEIN MOLECULES

An antibody's unique specificity (telling it what substance to react with) is a result of its particular protein composition. The body's 23 different amino acids are the building blocks of protein. Protein mole-cules are complex compounds containing the elements carbon, hydrogen, nitrogen, oxygen and various elements. Proteins are polymers or chains composed of polypeptides (long-chain amino acids joined by peptide link-ages or bonds). When two amino acids combine to form a chain, a pep-tide is formed. Ten or more peptides form polypeptides. When protein breaks down, polypeptides are released.

IMMUNOGLOBULIN STRUCTURE AND PRODUCTION

The basic immunoglobulin unit consists of two light (L) and two heavy (H) polypeptide chains linked by disulfide bonds. In addition, immunoglobulins have an accessory J polypeptide chain, variable carbo-hydrate groups, constant and variable region domains, and usually three different genetic markers. Consequently, by virtue of varying a few basic ingredients, the body is capable of producing 10^6 to 10^9 different antibody molecules.

There are five immunoglobulin isotopes or subclasses, IgA, IgG, IgM, IgE and IgD, and among these classes there are subdivisions. Eighty per-cent of the body's antibodies, including the thyroid antibodies seen in Graves' disease, are derived from immunoglobulins of the IgG class. Immunoglobulins are constantly being produced and broken down in the body. The various immunoglobulin classes have their own half-lives (time when the original amount is reduced by 50 percent). The half life of IgG immunoglobulins in serum is 23 days.[7] IgG is the only immunoglobulin able to pass through the placenta.

Autoantibodies

With so many antigens to recognize and so many antibodies capable of being synthesized, it's not surprising that immune cells sometimes err. Due to a defect in immunologic tolerance (normally, we don't react with self molecules), the immune system produces autoantibodies directed against one's own body. Autoantibodies may be directed against cellular

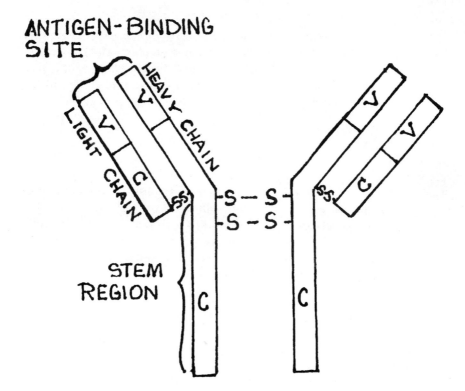

ANTIGEN-BINDING SITE

ANTIBODY MOLECULE

V = VARIABLE AMINO ACIDS

C = CONSTANT REGION

Antigen Binding Site

components scattered throughout the body (seen in systemic autoimmune diseases) or they may be organ specific.

    Even when autoantibodies are organ specific, they're produced against specific cell components rather than entire organs. For instance, thyroglobulin autoantibodies (often seen in GD) are directed against thyroglobulin, a substance found inside the follicle sacs that make up the thyroid gland. All of the various antibodies which react with thyroid components (thyroglobulin, TPO, etc.) are commonly referred to as thyroid antibodies.

Autoimmunity and Antibody Production

Although autoantibodies are present in 20 percent of the population, the National Institute of Health reports that approximately 3 percent of the inhabitants of North America and Europe develop autoimmune disorders.[8] Individuals in Third World countries rarely develop autoimmune diseases. One who develops autoantibodies experiences an autoimmune response or is said to have autoimmunity. The specific autoantibody produced is influenced by genes and environmental influences.

Circulating Immune Complexes

Besides their usual role of attacking cellular components, autoantibodies can form immune complexes (CICs). Rather than binding to cell receptors, autoantibodies may link with their antigenic component or immune system chemicals such as complement and travel through the body. Often, the presence of CICs is associated with disease severity.

Development of Autoimmune Disease

Autoimmune diseases develop when autoantibodies present in the body begin to cause certain symptoms related to the autoimmune disease they're associated with. If the immune system underreacts or fails to recognize a foreign antigen (such as bacteria) within the body, infection results.

Then again, if the immune system underreacts to an abnormal antigen that is part of the body, the result is cancer, in which abnormal body cells are allowed to freely proliferate. If the immune system overreacts in response to an external antigen such as pollen, allergy results. If it overreacts in response to self, or to triggers that cloud its perception of self, autoimmune disease results.

Natural Autoimmunity

As Dr. Noel Rose, a professor of molecular microbiology, immunology and Pathology at Johns Hopkins University, explains we all have some degree of natural autoimmunity. It's only in a minority of cases that autoimmunity causes disease. Treating autoimmune disease by destroying the organ targeted by autoantibodies, he cautions, doesn't stop the disease process.

He emphasizes, "In my opinion, the only way we're going to develop really effective treatments will be to treat the cause of the disease, not the symptoms. The symptoms are late; the symptoms are at the end of the train of events."[9]

Etiology of Autoimmune Thyroid Disease

The primary disorder in immunoregulation that leads to autoimmune thyroid disease hasn't yet been identified. Current theory includes a deficiency of T suppressor cells along with increased antibody production. Multiple genes are involved. Thus, autoimmunity tends to cluster in families, although family members may all develop different autoimmune diseases. In one family a mother may develop GD, her son juvenile diabetes, her sister pernicious anemia, and her father Hashimoto's thyroiditis (disorder of hypothyroidism).

Individuals with GD or other autoimmune thyroid diseases are said to have glandular autoimmune disease. Thus, they're more likely to develop other autoimmune diseases affecting the pancreas, thyroid gland, adrenal glands and the gastric parietal cells because these organs all developed from the same tissue, the endoderm.[10]

Immune System Regulation

CHRONOBIOLOGY AND AGE

The powers of the immune system ebb and flow according to internal and external clocks known as circadian rhythm. Typically, the immune system peaks at 7 A.M. Throughout the day, the immune system slows down, dropping to its lowest point in the afternoon and early evening.[11] In addition to this normal diurnal variation, the immune system chronobiology can be profoundly affected by environmental factors and stress.

The immune system also changes with age. Newborns aren't born with developed immune systems. Only at about age two can the immune system be considered fully functioning. After about age 60, immune powers, especially that of suppressor T cells, begin to decline. While neither immunoglobulin levels nor B cells decline, a qualitative shift in the immune response makes them less effective.

DIETARY AND DRUG INFLUENCES

Diet influences immune function. Nutrients such as selenium, manganese, magnesium, copper, calcium, zinc and vitamin C are needed for the production of certain immune cell components. Sugar and saturated fat have been found to affect immune system scavenger type cells known as macrophages by altering their cellular membrane, thereby reducing their sensitivity and effectiveness and depressing immunity.

Certain drugs, including herbs, also have an immune system effect. Hormones also have an influence. Estrogen is a potential trigger of Graves' disease. Increased estrogen levels are thought to account for the more aggressive immune systems seen in women.

RACE AND SEX

Race and sex also make a difference. In one study of a healthy biracial population, African Americans have been found to have slightly more of one type of IgA, IgM and IgG than whites.[12] A triracial study in Druban, Natal, has shown that Bantu male adults have significantly higher levels of IgM than comparable whites in their communities.[13]

GENETIC AND ENVIRONMENTAL AUTOIMMUNE INFLUENCES

There are three generally accepted ways to prove the genetic basis of autoimmune disease. First is family clustering. About 15 percent of patients with GD have a relative with GD, and about 50 percent of relatives of patients with GD have circulating thyroid autoantibodies.[14] The second is a genetic component, and the third is that autoimmune diseases can be found in animals in instances where the necessary breedings can be demonstrated.

Genetic control of the immune system is governed by several different genes, including genes of the major histocompatability complex (MHC) described in chapter 7. Just as some individuals are genetically predisposed to developing allergies, not a specific allergen, individuals with certain MHC genes may develop any of a number of different autoimmune diseases associated with these genes.

Environmental factors and stress also have a profound immune effect. Stress, in particular, suppresses the immune system, and a reduced number of suppressor T cells is related to autoimmune disease development. Dr. Joan Borysenko, a cancer cell biologist and psychologist, says that the stress of taking final exams can wipe interferon levels down to zero.[15] Interferon, described later in this chapter, causes the release of certain cytotoxic cells that would also ordinarily stop the autoreactive process.

Although the National Institute of Health advises that doctors warn patients of their autoimmune disease triggers we're rarely warned. Certain environmental agents referred to as xenobiotic agents are capable of causing immune system effects in humans. Xenobiotics include mercury, iodine, vinyl chloride, organic solvents, silicon, canavanine, ultraviolet radiation, silica and cigarette smoke, which has been found to produce cadmium and formaldehyde. There is growing evidence that women exposed to diethylstilbesterol (DES) have a greater likelihood of developing autoimmune diseases such as Hashimoto's thyroiditis and Graves' disease.[16]

DRUG RELATED LUPUS

The heart medication procainamide and other medicines may cause an autoreactive process resulting in the presence of antinuclear antibodies (ANA) and antibodies to single stranded DNA (ssDNA Ab),[17] causing a disorder called drug related lupus (DRL). DRL is responsible for a syndrome similar to that of idiopathic systemic lupus erythematosus, although symptoms of DRL usually resolve after the drug is stopped. Many other drugs including antithyroid drugs and beta blockers are associated with DRL.

Immune System Strategies

The immune system employs two broad strategic defense mechanisms known as cell-mediated and humoral immunity. Defense strategies involve a cascade of steps coordinated by various interrelated immune system cells and chemicals. These strategies can be compared to the way a traffic system works at midnight, turning green for approaching traffic, thereby affecting movement in the opposite path.

Cell-mediated Immunity

In cell-mediated immunity, innate immune system cells, primarily T cell lymphocytes, coordinate their efforts to recognize and attack foreign antigens. Cell-mediated reactions also release potent chemicals known as cytokines that help fight off viruses and tumor cells. Innate defenses are non-specific. They may be as simple as epithelial cells in the skin acting as barriers, preventing entry of all foreign antigens.

Humoral or Acquired (Adaptive) Immunity

In humoral immunity, special molecules, such as B lymphocyte cells, produce antibodies directed against foreign antigens. Acquired immunity is a late stage development caused by adaptation and is only found in vertebrates. Humoral immunity can recognize specific antigens, remember antigens previously encountered, and move quickly, particularly against infection. This rapid response is produced by the body's humours or vital fluids that carry antibodies where they're needed.

Cells of the Immune System

Originating as primitive bone marrow stem cells, immune system cells develop and differentiate into specialized cells. All the cells in an individual's body have identical genetic factors. In virtually all cell lines except for lymphocytes, every member of a given population has the same constitution and functions as every other member.

Lymphocytes

The key cells of the immune system, lymphocytes develop in two primary locations in the body, the bone marrow and the thymus. These sites

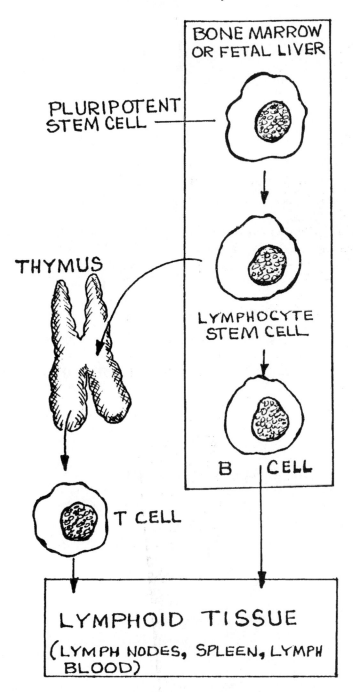

Lymphoid Tissue

are called primary lymphoid tissue. Lymphocytes are also discretely distributed in secondary lymphoid tissue such as the skin, where they bar entry by foreign substances. Hardly stagnant, lymphocytes circulate throughout the body 50 times daily and remain continuously in the circulation for only 30 minutes at a stretch, time spent searching for foreign antigens.

Lymphocytes contain subsets known as T and B cells. T cells, which are immune system scouts, can be further divided into CD4 suppressor and CD8 helper cells. B cells are directly involved in autoantibody production. The cellular interaction between T and B cells is required for complete expression of the immune response.

Lymphocyte cells differ from one another. Each T cell has a surface protein receptor that causes it to recognize specific antigens and react against them. One T cell might watch for viruses while his neighbor scouts for pollen. T cells don't produce antibodies. Their power lies in their capacity to release cytokines (described later in this section).

The Lymphatic System

In the immune response, lymphocytes aggregate where they're needed. The system in which lymphocyte-rich lymph fluid moves through the body is known as the lymphatic system. The lymphatic system is responsible for routing lymph from lymphatic capillaries through lymph nodes that serve as ambush points for foreign antigens. The lymph nodes respond to antigenic stimuli by releasing additional lymphocytes into the bloodstream.

T Cell Lymphocytes

T lymphocyte cells originate in the bone marrow and migrate to the thymus where they mature. T cells (along with macrophages) are responsible for scouting out foreign antigens. T cells respond (by proliferation) to HLA genes (genes that regulate the immune system, described in chapter 7). Consequently, T cells form antigen presenting complexes with the expressed HLA gene determinants. After recognizing specific foreign antigens, T cells are responsible for presenting them to B cells via this complex.

T Helper and Suppressor Subsets

As they mature in the thymus, T cells express functional markers by which they become either helper or suppressor cells. T cells with CD4 markers become helper cells, and CD8 T cells become suppressor cells. Although they both scout for foreign antigens, helper cells aid in antibody production, and suppressor cells normally stop inappropriate activity such as autoantibody production. Both types of T cells release chemicals called cytokines in response to foreign antigens. Cytokines, in turn, alert other cells to attack or retreat.

T Helper Subsets

Depending on the cytokines available, T helper lymphocytes can develop into Th1 or Th2 cells. Normal individuals have a good balance between the two. Th1 cells promote cellular immunity and anti-cancer and anti-viral responses. Th1 cytokines such as IL-2 and IFN-gamma predominate in organ specific autoimmune diseases, such as Graves' Disease.

Th2 cells promote humoral immunity and are more often associated with normal immune responses such as mild allergic reactions and asthma. Th2 cytokines such as the interleukins IL-4, IL-5 and IL-10 are associated with systemic autoimmune disorders.

B Cell Lymphocytes

B cells can produce antibodies because they have available immuno-globulin (Ig) on their cell membranes. There is diversity regarding the type of antibodies that B cells can synthesize and release. There are many different types of B lymphocytes, and those that bear immunoglobulins form merely 10 percent to 15 percent of the circulating blood lymphocytes.

Before B cells produce antibodies, they must determine the specific antibody they need to produce. B cell differentiation can be divided into two stages. The initial stage involves the antigen-independent generation of diversity or proliferation, commonly called clonal expansion. Here, responding to a stimulus, B cells divide and form many clones or families of identical cells.

The second stage is regulated by antigen triggering, T cell interactions, and macrophages, a type of scavenger white blood cell. This stage occurs predominantly in the secondary lymphoid organs (like the thyroid). Here, the immature B cells are activated by antigens to become reactive B cells with new functions, such as secreting cytokines or displaying markedly different behavior toward other cells. Activated B cells may also differentiate into plasma cells (capable of secreting antibodies) and memory cells.

Specialized Immune System Components

Cytokines (Lymphokines)

Cytokines are water soluble, biologically active hormone-like proteins derived from lymphocytes in the bone marrow. Acting as messengers, cytokines cause the proliferation of new cells during an immune response. The subject of much current research, cytokines are roughly divided into several categories, including the interleukins, interferons, B cell growth and differentiation factors, tumor necrosis factor (TNF) and several other factors.

Also known as lymphokines and effector molecules, cytokines regulate the severity of the immune response. Cytokines also stimulate immature leukocyte growth and differentiation. These functions can also be described as pro-inflammatory or anti-inflammatory responses. These apparently easygoing effector molecules may affect or be affected by other lymphocytes, other leukocytes (white blood cells) and other tissue cells.

Although the roles of interleukin-2 and interferon-gamma are not clearly understood, some researchers report that these cytokines may be present at higher levels in GD than in other disturbances of hyperthyroidism. In one study where levels of these cytokines were normal in GD patients and low in patients with non-autoimmune hyperthyroidism, there was no difference between treated and untreated GD patients.[18] Of interest, the immune altering drugs such as interferon and interleukin have been found to trigger the development of Graves' disease.[19]

Natural Killer and Killer Lymphocytes

NK or natural killer cells can be distinguished from other types of cytotoxic cells (cells with destructive properties) because they mediate cytotoxic reactions without prior antigenic sensitization (recognition is sufficient). NK cells are capable of destroying tumors and virally transformed cells. Certain NK cells (CD 56+ variety, CD 19+5+ variety) are activated during autoantibody synthesis. The finding of increased NK cell activity against the placenta in some GD patients has led to fertility treatment advances.[20]

Another type of cytotoxic lymphocyte known as K or killer lymphocytes mediates cell destruction in the presence of certain antibodies (antibody dependence). Both NK and K cells also have the ability to spontaneously kill other cells, especially those expressing HLA antigens such as orbital and thyroid fibroblasts.

NK Cells in Graves' Disease

Normally, NK cells help destroy autoreactive cells before autoantibodies are formed. In one study, when patients with GD were analyzed according to their thyroid status, NK activity was significantly depressed in hyperthyroid patients before treatment and in hyperthyroid and euthyroid patients receiving antithyroid drugs, when compared to normal subjects. GD patients who became hypothyroid after radioiodine or thyroidectomy had normal NK activity. NK activity in GD patients was not affected by levels of serum thyroxine, the presence of ophthalmopathy, or thyroid antibody titers.[21] Thus, regardless of disease severity, patients with active GD have lower levels of NK cells.

Cytotoxic T Lymphocytes in Autoimmune Thyroid Disease

Cytotoxic T cells promote the development of autoimmune thyroid disease. However, there are differences in GD and Hashimoto's thyroiditis (HT). In HT, there appears to be increased activation of cytotoxic T cells. Consequently, there is more thyroid cell mediated destruction in HT than GD.

Phagocytes

Phagocytes, members of a group of non-lymphocyte white blood cells, also play an important role in immune system function. The most important phagocytes are neutrophils, macrophages and monocytes. Migrating from blood into the tissues in response to an infection, phagocytes ingest and digest foreign particles. In tissues, monocytes develop into phagocytic cells called macrophages.

Complement

In an immune response, lymphocytes rush to the site and release many chemicals, including complement. The complement system includes numerous proteins that are involved in inflammatory processes and phagocytosis (process where one cell engulfs another). But whereas antibodies lock on to specific receptors on the surface of invading cells, complement proteins attack any particle considered foreign. Some diseases, such as hereditary angioedema (hives), are cause by the body's inability to turn off complement once it has been activated.[22]

The Lymphatic/HLA Interaction

When T cells recognize foreign antigens, they respond to their body's immune system HLA antigens by proliferating. Specific HLA genes are associated with a certain cluster of autoimmune disorders including Graves' disease (see chapter 7). The target antigen and an HLA gene form a complex on specifically designated antigen presenting cells. Presented with this antigen presenting complex, and influenced by the body's immunoglobulin genes, stimulated B cells recognize what type of antibody to make.

The Immune Response

The immune response has two stages. First, the nonspecific effectors, including cytokines, macrophages, natural killer cells, polymorphonuclear leukocytes and complement, attack potential pathogens. These soluble mediators may play a major role in the initiation and development of autoimmunity. The second stage involves T cell activation and antibody production.

T Cell Activation and the Role of Cytokines

The first step in T cell activation occurs when B lymphocytes are stimulated by an antigen and the cell line multiplies. Macrophage cells are then activated to produce a soluble product called lymphocyte activating factor (LAF) or interleukin-1 (IL-1), a type of cytokine needed for T cell growth. The elevated levels of IL-6 and IL-8 cytokines seen in hyperthyroid patients are evidence of the ongoing autoimmune process in Graves' disease.

IL-1, produced in the first step, is required for the second step in T cell activation. IL-1 induces a subpopulation of T cells with specific receptors for another soluble factor called T cell growth factor (TCGF) or interleukin-2 (IL-2). Helper T cells are then activated by a complex of antigen plus IL-1 to produce receptors (binding sites) for IL-2.

The binding of IL-2 molecules to the specific receptor sites on T cells induces cell proliferation. Once T cells acquire the receptors for IL-2, they no longer require the presence of antigen for continued proliferation. Thus, once the process has begun and T cell activation is complete (autoreactive T cells are formed), an antigenic response is no longer required for autoantibody production.

Loss of Tolerance in Autoimmunity

Normally, the immune system has self-tolerance, meaning it tolerates its own cells and doesn't react with them. Autoimmunity is related to a loss of self-tolerance. Three basic mechanisms normally prevent autoreactive lymphocytes from developing.

These are (1) clonal deletion or physical elimination, (2) clonal anergy that reduces cell responsiveness, and (3) suppression or destruction of autoreactive lymphocytes by other cytotoxic lymphocytes such as NK cells. Cytotoxic cells normally are able to prevent autoimmunity by secreting certain cytokines that have negative regulatory effects. This results from cross linking of surface receptors, or by the creation of anti-autoantibodies (anti-idiotypes).

Lymphocytic Infiltration in Graves' Disease

B cells culled from the thyroid gland in GD patients have been shown to secrete thyroid autoantibodies in vitro (outside of the body). This implies that lymphocytes in GD may be pre-activated. The thyroid in GD, when observed in surgical specimens, is characterized by an irregular lymphocytic infiltration and an increased number of thyroid cells suggesting that the thyroid itself is the major site of TSH receptor antibody synthesis.

Current Theories Regarding Autoimmunity

According to current theory, the reduced number of suppressor T cells may represent a reduced number of developed cells. Immature T cells that bind antigen in the absence of second signal may be desensitized rather than deleted (the phenomenon of anergy). Deletion and anergy may account for the reduced immune suppression. In addition, people with HLA-DR3 antigens (seen in GD) have been shown to have reduced suppressor T cell activity, making them susceptible to developing autoimmune conditions.

Abnormalities in Apoptosis

B cells and T cells that interact with antigens in the absence of the appropriate second signal are usually deleted by apoptosis (programmed cell death or suicide, a normal cellular event), but they may survive in a desensitized state of anergy. The number of cells suspended into a state of anergy or removed by apoptosis may also account for reduced number of T suppressor cells. A certain amount of apoptosis is critical to health. When this process malfunctions, too little programmed cell death may contribute to cancer and autoimmune diseases, while too much causes neurodegenerative diseases.[23]

The Role of Soluble Fas Ligand in Decreased Apoptosis

One current research thread focuses on the role of soluble Fas ligand (molecule capable of binding to another molecule in the immune reaction), a member of the CD95 receptor/ligand system. The Fas ligand (FasL) protein causes apoptosis in susceptible cells by reacting with its receptor, Fas. Both Fas and FasL have roles in immune system regulation, deletion of self-reactive lymphocytes and T cell mediated cytotoxicity. However, the increased levels of soluble Fas (sFas), rather than FasL seen in GD, causes suppression of the body's normal Fas mediated apoptosis. Instead of Fas ligand destroying autoreactive cells, soluble Fas prevents FasL from doing its job.

Recent studies demonstrate a significant increase in soluble Fas (sFas) in patients with untreated Graves' disease. sFas, which may be induced by inflammatory cytokines, is a splicing form of Fas that suppresses apoptosis by competitive binding with Fas ligand.

In one study, after six to eight weeks of treatment with ATDs, serum sFas levels declined in GD patients who were euthyroid for more than three years when compared to untreated GD patients. High levels of sFas, which is also found in thyroid tissue, cultured thyrocytes and intrathyroidal lymphocytes, is associated with high levels of TSH receptor antibody titers. Since Fas-mediated apoptosis may be responsible for the deletion of B cells activated by peripheral self-antigens, increased sFas would block this process. The B cells that escape deletion may be the cause of TSH receptor antibody synthesis in GD.[24]

Other factors influencing apoptosis include loss of self-tolerance, hormonal influences and environmental and viral triggers. Viruses may lead to organ damage and trigger the release of antigens that could evoke an autoreactive process, causing chronic inflammation even after the viral infection has subsided (also see chapter 7).

3 Engine and Fuel: The Thyroid and Its Hormones

This chapter describes thyroid anatomy and physiology and discusses the thyroid's role as an endocrine gland participating in both the body's network system and the pituitary-hypothalamic-thyroid axis. This chapter also includes sections on the role of iodine and goitrogens and a description of the primary thyroid disorders.

Historical Overview

For many years, no one realized that the thyroid existed or that iodine was essential for health. Had you lived in 13th century Europe, especially near the Alps, chances are you would have had a goiter (although in this iodine depleted region it's unlikely that GD would have been the cause). Although it's now known that both thyroid hormone excess and deficiency can cause goiter, back then, no one had even heard of the thyroid.

Prior to the 19th century, physicians attributed all diseases to afflictions of one of the four vital bodily fluids or humors (the heart's blood, the brain's phlegm, the liver's yellow bile, and the spleen's black bile). Goiters were considered a result of excess phlegm, and treatments involved conglomerations aimed at phlegm reduction.

Thyroid function wasn't clearly understood until 1895. Then, researchers at the Mayo Clinic isolated the active iodine substance in the thyroid gland and named it thyroxine.[1] Since, researchers have learned that the thyroid is an endocrine gland and that its hormones are critical to life.

41

The Body's Network System

Emotional disturbances are often the most prominent symptoms of GD. Julia A, a friend from Spain, commented that at the height of her GD, she felt like a dynamo. This she didn't mind. However, she was irritable, behaving, she says, as if she always had a toothache. Frazzled nerves and irritability can be caused by both hormonal influences on the brain and feelings of exhaustion.

To understand how thyroid hormone affects the brain, we need to understand the body's network system. The body has three major communication systems that work like a highway interstate system linking one state to another. The endocrine, immune and nervous systems communicate with one another extracellularly (away from their cellular origin), sending messages throughout the body from one organ to another.

1. The Nervous System

    The nervous system transmits electrochemical signals back and forth between the brain and the tissues of various organs, or between tissue of one organ to tissue of another via reflex circuits. For instance, when you burn your finger, signals are sent to your brain, and when you receive the message, you experience pain. The nervous system relays its messages instantly through impulses traveling across neurons.

2. The Endocrine System

    The endocrine system releases hormones into the circulation and activates functional changes peripherally (away from the hormone's origin). For example, thyroid hormone made in the thyroid gland can circulate and activate receptors in the brain, affecting mood. Hormones must travel through the blood and lymphatic system to reach their target cells, making their responses slower than neural reactions.

3. The Immune System

    The immune system distinguishes self from non-self (foreign substances like bacteria and viruses) and protects the body against these foreign threats. In response to bodily threats, most people scream or flee, whereas immune system cells respond by producing antibodies in an effort to protect us. When the nervous system perceives stress, it communicates this to the immune system, causing changes in immune system cells.

The Endocrine System

The glands of the endocrine system produce and release potent chemical messengers known as hormones in response to internal and external stimuli. Internal stimuli include chemicals known as neurotransmitters. External stimuli include weather, temperature, altitude and stress. Hormones activate or suppress specific cell functions.

Most hormones, including thyroid hormones, are amino acid derivatives or peptides, the building blocks of protein. Besides this group, there is another class of hormones composed of steroid derivatives of cholesterol. Here, there are two subsets, those with an intact steroid nucleus such as adrenal and gonadal steroids, and those in which the steroid's B ring has been cleaved, such as the hormone we call vitamin D.

Each hormone controls a variety of different functions. For example, upon hearing an explosion, your adrenal glands respond, releasing adrenaline. The hormone adrenaline increases heart rate and blood pressure, ensuring that the body's muscles get extra oxygen. Adrenaline also enables the blood to clot easier, preventing excess bleeding in the event of injury. The science that studies the endocrine glands and their hormones is known as endocrinology. Physicians who specialize in this field are known as endocrinologists.

The glands of the endocrine system include the thyroid, adrenals, parathyroid, pituitary, ovaries and testes, thymus pineal and islet of Langerhans in the pancreas.

Anatomy of the Thyroid Gland

Normally weighing less then an ounce, the thyroid is the largest endocrine gland. Like the other endocrine glands, the thyroid is a ductless gland, meaning it can release hormones directly into the blood circulation. The thyroid, which has the same consistency as muscle tissue, is located directly below the larynx or Adam's apple in the neck. Supported by cartilage, it is attached to the trachea and suspended from the larynx. Upon swallowing, the thyroid follows the larynx's movement, moving upward. The first gland to emerge in fetal development, the thyroid normally weighs about 20 grams or two thirds of an ounce and is generally larger in women than in men.

Capsule and Lobes

A thin reddish brown fibrous capsule covers the entire gland. Flexible, this capsule sends out septa, finger-like projections that invaginate the gland and form pseudolobules. Anteriorly (in front), the capsule is smooth, glistening and free. Posteriorly (rear), the capsule is continuous with the trachea's connective tissue, sharing its consistency. The thyroid is composed of two butterfly shaped lobes that lie astride the trachea just above the breast bone. The lobes are connected by a 2 to 6 mm thick band of tissue

ENDOCRINE GLANDS

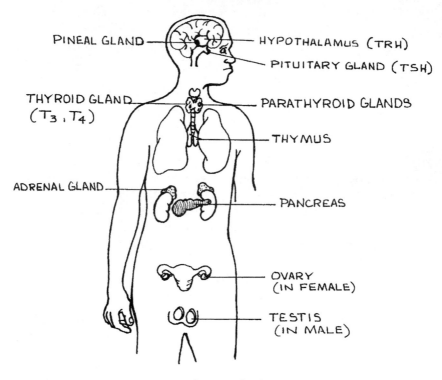

PINEAL GLAND

HYPOTHALAMUS (TRH)

PITUITARY GLAND (TSH)

THYROID GLAND
(T₃, T₄)

PARATHYROID GLANDS

THYMUS

ADRENAL GLAND

PANCREAS

OVARY
(IN FEMALE)

TESTIS
(IN MALE)

Endocrine Glands

called the isthmus. The lobes are approximately 4 cm long, 2 cm wide, and 20 to 40 mm thick. A smaller centrally located pyramidal lobe may also be present.

Thyroid Development

During fetal development, the thyroid gland originates from the base of the tongue (see chapter 10). Embryologically, the thyroid begins to form when endoderm cells of the pharynx (alimentary canal organ between the cavity of the mouth and the esophagus) begin migrating upward into the neck. The migratory tract of the developing thyroid gland is called the thyroglossal duct. Normally, this duct atrophies but it may remain as a fibrous band known as the pyramidal lobe. A remnant of thyroid fetal development, the pyramidal lobe is still attached to the embryonic thyroglossal duct. Although it is said to be present in 80 percent of the population,[2] the pyramidal lobe is normally not palpable or felt during a thyroid exam. It is most often enlarged and palpable in GD.

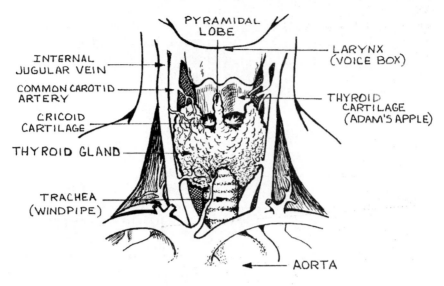

The Thyroid

Thyroid Gland Structure

The structure of the thyroid is unique for an endocrine gland. Microscopically, the thyroid consists of follicles or sacs of varying size. Each thyroid lobe is divided into lobules that are composed of 20 to 40 spherical follicles, each with an average diameter of 30 μm. In the adult male there are 3 X 10^6 follicles. A stroma (supporting framework) of connective tissue containing the capillaries, lymphatics, nerve fibers, larger blood vessels and occasional clusters of lymphocytes keeps the follicles intact.

The thyroid is supplied with blood from four thyroid arteries that provide a blood flow per gram of thyroid tissue greater than that of any other organ in the body. A system of thyroid lymphatic vessels courses between the follicles, ultimately draining into the deep cervical and pretracheal lymph glands, which are occasionally enlarged in Graves' disease.

The interfollicular spaces (spaces between thyroid follicles) and their contents have elasticity of volume to accommodate the continuously changing size of the follicles typically seen in GD. Following a temporary stage of hyperactivity, the connective tissue may increase and enclose isolated follicles, producing nodules or pseudoadenomas.[3]

Goiters

An enlarged thyroid gland may be visible as a goiter. A home test for detecting an enlarged thyroid is to observe one's neck in the mirror while drinking a glass of water. While swallowing, an enlarged thyroid can some-

THYROIDS OF THE ANIMAL WORLD

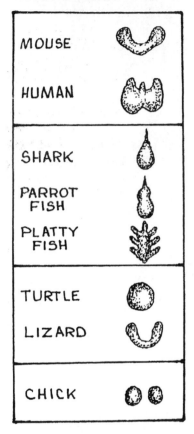

MOUSE

HUMAN

SHARK

PARROT FISH

PLATTY FISH

TURTLE

LIZARD

CHICK

Animal Thyroids

times be observed as it visibly rises. An enlarged thyroid may on occasion swell and press against the trachea or larynx, causing the feeling of having something stuck in one's throat.

Goiters may occur in both hypo-thyroidism, as the thyroid expands in its efforts to trap more iodine, and in hyperthyroidism as the size and number of cells increase in response to excessive stimulation. Goiter in Graves' disease is usually termed diffuse and toxic, although one or more of the following functional adjectives may apply:

Aberrant — associated with ectopic thyroid tissue, occurring away from the usual neck location

Basedow's — colloid filled goiter that becomes hyperfunctional after iodine administration

Cystic — containing cysts formed by mucoid or colloid degeneration

Diffuse — even distribution of iodine uptake, homogeneous

Endemic — occurring in areas of iodine deficiency

Exophthalmic — in association with eyeball protrusion or exophthalmos

Intrathoracic — when part of the gland is situated in the thoracic cavity (chest area)

Lymphadenoid — infiltrated with lymphocytes; seen in Hashimoto's disease

Multinodular — containing circumscribed nodules within its substance

Substernal — when part of the enlarged gland is situated beneath the sternum

Retrosternal — when part of the enlarged gland is behind the sternum

Toxic — seen in Graves' diseases; associated with Graves' hyperthyroidism

Toxic multinodular — hyperthyroidism arising in a multinodular goiter, usually long-standing; also known as Plummer's disease

Vascular — primarily caused by a dilation of thyroid blood vessels.

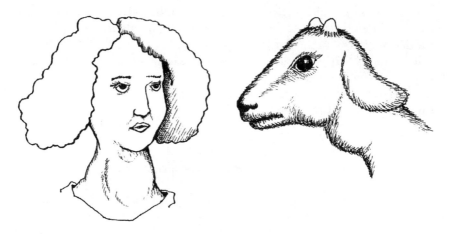

Left: *Hyperthyroid Goiter: A condition commonly seen in Graves' Disease caused by hyperplasia and hypertrophy of thyroid follicular cells.* Right: *Hypothyroid Goiter: A condition seen in young animals with iodine deficiency; goiter occurs as the thyroid cells enlarge in their effort to trap more iodine.*

Microscopic View of the Thyroid Gland

Viewed microscopically, a cross section of thyroid tissue reveals an abundance of hollow spherical follicles or sacs of varying sizes. Each follicle is lined by a layer of active cuboidal epithelial cells, and each follicle contains a central storage lumen filled with colloid secreted by the epithelial cells. Colloid is a gelatinous protein substance to which thyroid hormone is bound and carried throughout the body. Each follicle is enclosed by a basement membrane.

The main

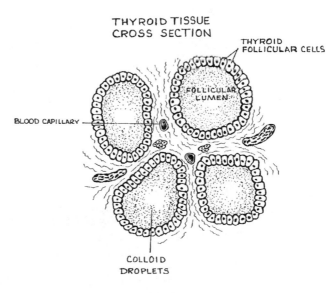

Thyroid Follicular Cell

constituent of colloid is thyroglobulin, a complex glycoprotein that acts as a warehouse for thyroid hormone. Thyroglobulin also serves as a matrix for thyroid hormone synthesis. This extracellular (outside of the follicular cell) storage of thyroglobulin in the follicle lumen is essential for maintaining constant blood levels of thyroid hormone. Along with thyroglobulin, thyroid colloid constitutes a store of smaller amounts of iodine and thyroid hormone precursors.

THYROID FOLLICULAR (FOLLICLE) CELLS

Thyroid follicular cells are functionally the most important thyroid cells. All of the thyroid's metabolic functions, including its growth and pro-

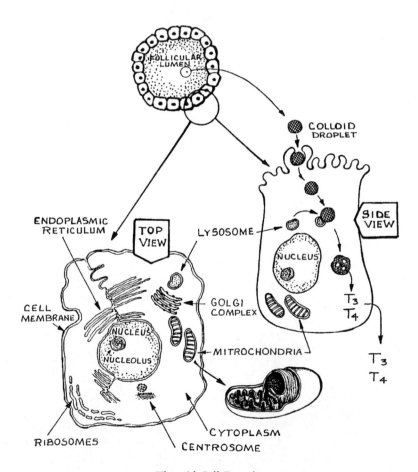

Thyroid Cell Function

duction of colloid and thyroid hormone, are controlled by the pituitary hormone known as thyroid stimulating hormone (TSH, thyrotropin) described later in this chapter. Thyroid follicle cells in the basement membrane trap iodine from the blood. Iodine is then secreted from the follicular cell into the follicular lumen where it is available for thyroid hormone synthesis.

Thyroidal follicular cells are cuboidal to columnar although their shape changes in relation to the TSH secretion. Within the follicular cell cytoplasm (area between the cell membrane and nucleus), there are long profiles of rough endoplasmic reticulum and a large Golgi apparatus for synthesis and packaging of substantial amounts of protein. Numerous lysosomal bodies present in the cell cytoplasm secrete thyroid hormones.

PARAFOLLICULAR OR C CELLS

The parafollicular or C cells (interfollicular cells, light cells) are a separate group of thyroid cells that secrete the hormone calcitonin. C cells are situated either within the follicular wall beneath the basement membrane or between follicular cells. C cells are located in the upper poles of the thyroid lobes, and they are sparse, constituting less than 0.1 percent of the thyroid cells. C cells secrete calcitonin in response to hypercalcemia (high blood calcium levels). The secretion of calcitonin lowers blood calcium levels.

OXYPHIL CELLS

Oxyphil cells (oncocytes, Askanazy cells, Hürthle cells) are enlarged follicular cells characterized by granular cytoplasm filled with swollen mitochondria and large nuclei. They're commonly seen in long-standing GD, autoimmune thyroiditis, thyroids damaged by radiation, Hashitoxicosis, neoplasms and some adenomatous nodules.

The Thyroid in Graves' Disease

In active Graves' disease, the appearance of the thyroid gland changes. The thyroid follicles increase in size to keep up with the increased demand for hormone production. This results in extensive hypertrophy (increase in size) of the follicular cells and hyperplasia (abnormal increase in number of cells).

Consequently, in its hyper state, the thyroid is composed of crowded clusters of columnar follicular cells that form papillary "tufts." These tufts push into the lumen's colloid space (in a process called pinocytosis), leaving small holes or vacuoles and watery to absent colloid. These papillary projections may mimic those seen in papillary carcinoma, a form of thyroid cancer.[4] Despite these bizarre cellular changes, there is little evidence that the thyroid hyperplasia of untreated GD increases the incidence of thyroid cancer.[5]

In Graves' disease, the thyroid is diffusely enlarged to a moderate degree although it may enlarge up to several times its normal size. The capsular covering is smooth and vascular, and its texture may be soft or rubbery. The enlargement is usually symmetrical, but the right lateral lobe may be larger than the left. The thyroid gland is often infiltrated by lymphocytes, and both T and B cells have been identified with T cells predominating.

THYROID NODULES

A recent study described the increased incidence of thyroid nodules in Graves' disease patients. Of 468 patients with GD, 60 were found to have a coexistent thyroid nodule. Of these 60 patients, six patients, none of whom had multiple nodules, were found to have thyroid cancer. Fifty percent of the nodules present in patients subsequently treated with radioiodine or antithyroid drugs disappeared or decreased in size during follow-up.[6] The overall results of this study confirm previous studies demonstrating that thyroid cancer may be more common among patients with Graves' disease than in the general population and the disease course in GD patients with thyroid cancer may be more aggressive.[7]

However, in long term mortality studies of treated patients (cooperative study follow-up described in chapter 8), an increased rate of thyroid cancer mortality is associated only with patients treated with radioiodine. The thyroid cancer mortality rate is not increased in Graves' disease patients treated with surgery or antithyroid drugs.

Parathyroid Glands

The four (occasionally more) parathyroid glands are usually situated on the posterior surface of the thyroid gland immediately adjacent to the recurrent laryngeal nerves. Parathyroid glands are usually found on the thyroid lobe tips, within 1 cm of the inferior thyroid artery. Independent of the thyroid, the parathyroid glands regulate levels of calcium and phosphorus and secrete parathyroid hormone (PTH).

The Role of Iodine

Although iodine is of particular importance in GD, its role appears to be duplicitous. In *The Nature Doctor*, Dr. H.C.A. Vogel, writing in 1951 Switzerland, credits the introduction of iodized salt in Switzerland with the development of GD in genetically predisposed individuals. He writes, "Experience shows that if such people take the slightest amount of iodine they experience palpitations."[8]

Paradoxically, iodine in high concentrations (much higher than diet

THYROID AND PARATHYROID GLANDS

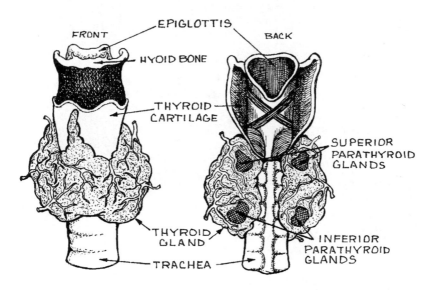

Parathyroid Glands (adapted from Structure & Function of the Body, *9th Edition, by Gary A. Thibodeau, published by Mosby Year Book in 1992).*

might provide) is known to inhibit the release of thyroid hormone. In fact, iodine (in strong solution) has its place in the treatment of hyperthyroidism associated with Graves' disease. Excess iodine also causes some GD patients to have an unnatural desire for prolonged sleep. This tendency is thought to be caused by calcium deficiency more than iodine excess.[9]

Iodine Transport and Organification

Iodine is the rate-limiting substance in thyroid hormone production because it represents 67 percent of the molecules in thyroxine. The process by which the thyroid takes up iodine from the blood is known as iodine transport, in which iodine enters the thyroid follicular cell by a plasma membrane "iodide pump." Free iodide ions are converted to organic iodine in a process known as organification. Inorganic iodide ions must be oxidized (by oxygen or hydrogen peroxide) to a higher oxidation state (iodine) before they can bind with the amino acid tyrosine to form thyroid hormone.

The amount of iodide that is concentrated is regulated by the hormone thyrotropin (TSH) produced in the pituitary and by an internal system known as autoregulation (described later in this chapter). Iodine concentration also occurs outside of the thyroid, in the gastric mucosa,

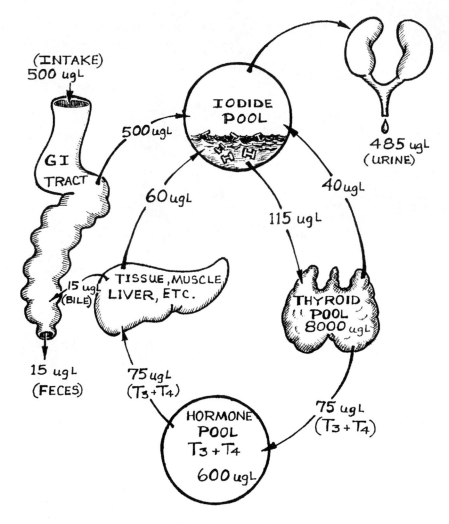

Daily Iodine Metabolism

mammary glands, salivary glands, choriod plexus (infoldings of blood vessels of the pia mater in the brain that secrete cerebrospinal fluid), placenta and skin.•

Impediments to Iodine Absorption and Concentration

Occasionally, patients with a certain metabolic defect lack the ability to concentrate iodide into iodine and are consequently unable to synthesize thyroid hormone. Also, certain anions, such as perchlorate, thiocyanate, fluoride, lithium and pertechnetate, act as competitive inhibitors of iodide transport by the thyroid. Perchlorate, a known anti-thyroid compound found in the American fertilizer supply, is also a component of rocket fuel. The addition of perchlorate to water and fertilizers containing nitrate, another known mild anti-thyroid compound, is associated with hypothyroidism.[10]

Dietary Sources of Iodine

Iodine is abundant in lobsters, shrimp, oysters, iodized salt, milk and in lesser amounts in certain fruit. Plants and animals grown near the ocean have the highest iodine concentrations. The amount of iodine required for adequate thyroxine synthesis varies from one individual to another. The recommended daily allowance (RDA) for iodine is 150 mcg.

Thyroid hormone accounts for 90 percent of the body's iodine content. The rest of the body's iodine is distributed among several organs (the sites of extrathyroidal iodine organification mentioned earlier). Because it is concentrated in mammary glands, iodine is present in breast milk. Cows' milk being contaminated with excess iodine is known to cause hyperthyroidism. Evidence suggests that iodine has a role in the development of autoimmune thyroid disorders. This is demonstrated by the mild cases of GD seen in iodine deficient areas such as Greece. Also, iodine deficiency is associated with a higher remission rate in GD patients who are treated with antithyroid drugs.[11]

Iodine Excess

Excess dietary iodine can increase or decrease hormone synthesis depending on a person's iodine status, thyroid status and individual sensitivity. Excess iodine can cause goiter as well as rashes, asthma and acne. Considering that iodine is present in not only food, but in many vitamin and mineral supplements, kelp extracts and certain drugs used for respiratory and heart problems, it's not difficult to unintentionally ingest excess iodine.

The typical adult iodine intake in the United States is 240 to 740 mcg/day. Iodized salt contains 76 mcg/gram. Kelp contains about 150 mcg/tablet. The quantity of iodine required to suppress radioiodine uptake to <2 percent is more than 15 mg/day or 15,000 mcg/day. This is 100 times greater than the minimal daily requirement and 20 times more than a diet with a heavy salt concentration. Amounts greater than 150 mcg/day may trigger symptoms of hyperthyroidism in sensitive individuals.

Although iodine in excess of 150 mcg stimulates the thyroid, saturated iodine solution of potassium iodide (SSKI) with 47 mg or 47,000 mcg/drop or Lugol's solution with 7.8 mg/ drop[12] has an opposite effect that inhibits the production and release of thyroid hormone. This effect is enhanced in hyperthyroidism (also see chapter 9).

Goitrogens

Iodine deficiencies can also result from eating large quantities of goitrogens, foods containing chemical compounds that block iodine absorption. Goitrogens include: cabbage and other members of the Brassica family, turnips, mustard greens, pears, kale, spinach, peaches, almonds and the cyanoglucosides, which include cassava, maize, bamboo shoots, sweet potatoes and lima beans (also see chapter 9).

Effects of Soy on Iodine Absorption

Soybean extracts also cause iodine deficiency by decreasing the amount of iodine that is absorbed from the intestine. In the 1950s, soy protein was found to cause goiter and iodine deficiency in infants fed soy formula. The problem was corrected by adding supplemental iodine to the soy formula.[13] Recent research, however, finds that a problem with soy still exists. Soy isoflavones inhibit thyroid peroxidase, an enzyme essential for the body's synthesis and metabolism of thyroid hormone. Unfermented products such as tofu, soymilk, texturized soy protein, and soy protein isolate are reported to pose the most risk.[14]

Anti-thyroid Substances

Anti-thyroid substances are substances that prevent the thyroid gland from utilizing iodide brought in by the blood (e.g., pertechnetate and perchlorate). When the consequences of this were realized, antithyroid drugs (ATDs) were developed for therapeutic use. ATDs include thiocyanates, thiourea derivatives and aniline derivatives.

Pituitary-Hypothalamic-Thyroid Axis and Thyroid Hormone Regulation

Thyroid function also depends on the proper function of the pituitary gland and the hypothalamus and their ability to produce and release certain hormones. The hypothalamus in the brain ensures that sufficient thyroid hormone is available for the body's needs. When it senses a decrease in metabolism, it activates the pituitary-hypothalamic-thyroid axis, a negative feedback mechanism, in its attempt to maintain normal thyroid hormone levels.

Regulatory Hormones

The biosynthesis and release of thyroid hormones from thyroglobulin stores are controlled by thyrotropin (thyroid stimulating hormone [TSH]), a hormone synthesized in the anterior pituitary gland and the

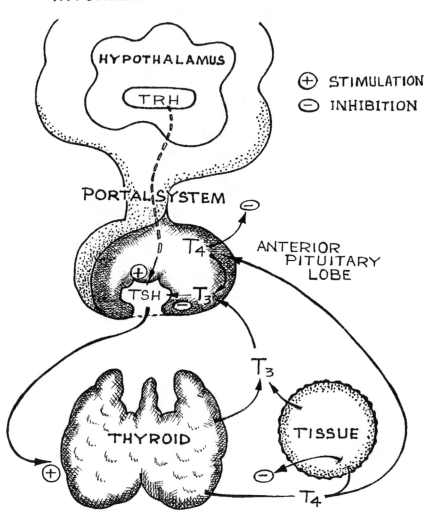

THYROID HORMONE PRODUCTION IN THE
HYPOTHALAMIC-HYPOPHYSEAL-THYROID AXIS

The Pituitary Hypothalmic Thyroid Axis

placenta, and thyrotropin releasing hormone (TRH) synthesized in the hypothalamus. Several accessory circuits involving other neurotransmitters (norepinephrine, ATP, somatostatin), prostglandins and iodine work in tandem with these hormones to regulate thyroid hormone synthesis and release.

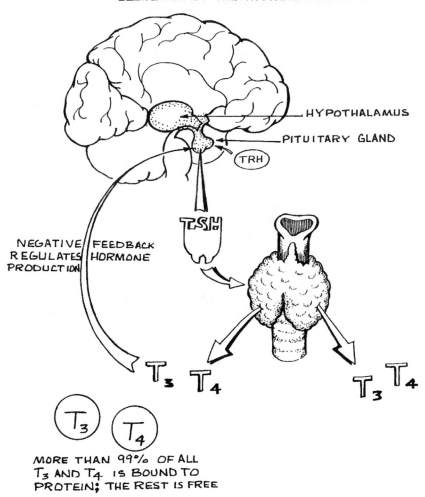

IN THE BRAIN THE HYPOTHALAMUS AND
THE PITUITARY GLAND CONTROL THE
SECRETION OF THE THYROID HORMONES.

HYPOTHALAMUS

PITUITARY GLAND

TRH

TSH

NEGATIVE FEEDBACK
REGULATES HORMONE
PRODUCTION

T_3 T_4

T_3 T_4

T_3 T_4

MORE THAN 99% OF ALL
T_3 AND T_4 IS BOUND TO
PROTEIN; THE REST IS FREE

Thyroid Hormone Regulatory System

The Hypothalamus and Thyrotropin Releasing Hormone

The hypothalamus is a distinct region located in the forebrain or dien-cephalon, located above the pituitary gland. Often referred to as the "old" or original brain, it is the seat of primitive instincts needed for survival of a species, regulating appetite, thirst, sleep, procreation and self-defense. The hypothalamus regulates and coordinates many endocrine functions, especially through its control of the pituitary gland.

When the hypothalamus detects low thyroid levels in the blood, or in response to increased bodily demands such as exposure to cold, it releases thyrotropin releasing hormone (TRH). TRH, along with several different neurotransmitters such as somastatin, orders the pituitary to release thyroid stimulating hormone (TSH). TRH has also been found in the central nervous system, in regions of the cerebral cortex, neurohypophysis, pineal gland, nerve endings and spinal cord, suggesting that TRH may also act as a neurotransmitter outside of the hypothalamus. TRH has also been identified in pancreatic cells and in certain parts of the gastrointestinal tract,[15] suggesting that TSH release is also influenced by nutrient requirements.

The Pituitary and Thyroid Stimulating Hormone (TSH, Thyrotropin)

Located deep inside the head, the pituitary gland or hypophysis lies behind the nasal cavities and directly below the hypothalamus. The pituitary

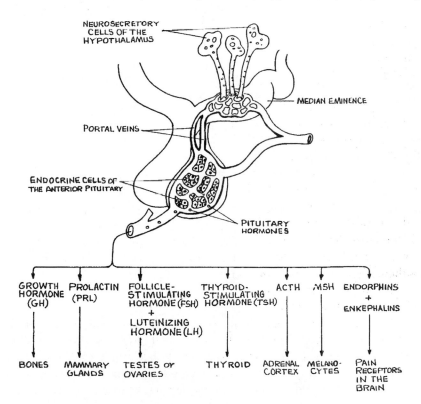

Anterior Pituitary Hormones

is also directly linked to the hypothalamic region of the brain via the central nervous system.

The pituitary governs the activity of the thyroid, the supradrenal gland and the sex glands. The pituitary may be divided into an anterior or front lobe known as the adenohypohysis, an intermediate lobe, and a posterior or neural lobe. Often referred to as the master gland, the pituitary is merely the size of a pea, yet its anterior and posterior lobes each produce hormones that control a diverse array of bodily functions.

Most of the hormones produced in the adenohypophysis are trophic hormones, which means that they stimulate other hormones or glands. For instance, TSH released by the pituitary gland stimulates the thyroid gland to produce and release thyroid hormone. TSH is a glycoprotein hormone that has two subunits. The alpha subunit is similar to the reproductive hormones, including human chorionic gonadotropin (hCG). The beta subunit is different in that it has action specific for the thyroid gland.

Normally, TSH is released continuously in response to the body's needs and peaks between 11 P.M. and 4 A.M. to 6 A.M. The lowest levels of TSH are seen in the late afternoon or early evening. The amount of TSH released by the pituitary is affected by various factors, including the amount of thyroid hormone present in the circulation, influences of hypothalamic TRH, somatostatin and dopamine, diet, the body's energy needs, medications, initial altitude adjustment and body temperature.

Physiology of the Thyroid Gland

The function of the thyroid gland is to collect and concentrate iodide from the blood, convert it to thyroid hormone, store some of this hormone as thyroglobulin, and secrete the rest into the blood for distribution as needed. The thyroid produces thyroxine (T4) and also makes small amounts of the more potent triiodothyronine (T3). However, T3 is primarily made by deiodination (cleaving of an iodine molecule) of thyroxine after its release from the gland. In addition to T3, roughly equal amounts of the biologically inactive hormone reverse T3 or rT3 are also produced in the deiodination process. Conversion of T4 to T3 or rT3 occurs primarily in the liver.

A variety of nutritional and metabolic factors influence activity of iodothyronine monodeiodinase enzymes, which are necessary for the peripheral production of T3. This is clearly seen in the syndrome of non-thyroidal illness, typically when patients are hospitalized for an unrelated systemic illness. In this situation, cytokines or nutritional deficiencies or both inhibit T3 conversion from T4.

The fundamental biochemical effect of thyroid hormone is to increase

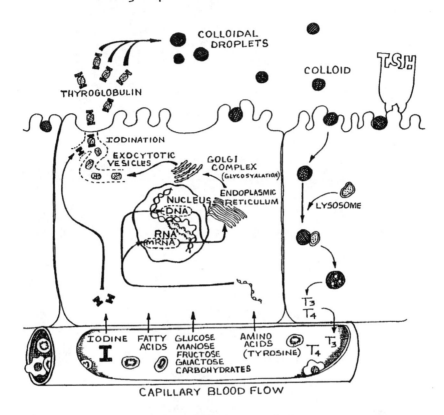

PRODUCTION OF THYROGLOBULIN
AND T₃, T₄ IN THE THYROID CELL

Thyroid Hormone Synthesis

the speed of the normal metabolic processes in all cells of the body except the thyroid gland itself and possibly the anterior pituitary. Normally, the thyroid gland produces adequate hormone for the body's needs and responds to factors such as exercise, stress, medications and diet.

The Mystery of Thyroid Hormones

Confucius once said, "We fear the most that which we little understand." This is often the case when patients are initially diagnosed with an unfamiliar disease. Suddenly they are hurled into a new world with its own language. The thyroid mystery is further aggravated by nomenclature. Each thyroid hormone is known by several different names.

1. Thyroxine (T4, L-thyroxine, levothyroxine or thyroxin)
   Thyroxine is the most abundant thyroid hormone, being 10

Thyroid Hormone Synthesis

to 20 times more abundant than T3. Having four iodine atoms, it is also known as tetraiodothyronine or T4. T4 is generally used in referring to the laboratory test, and levothyroxine (Levoid, Levothroid, Levoxine, Synthroid) refers to the replacement thyroid hormone.

     T4 is eliminated from the body slowly and has a half-life of six to seven days (half-life represents the time it takes for the concentration to be reduced by 50 percent). In hyperthyroidism the half-life is shortened to three to four days, and in hypothyroidism, the half-life may be as long as nine or ten days. These changes are due to altered rates of metabolism. With increased protein binding as in pregnancy, the half-life is increased. One third to one half of the T4 that is secreted is converted to T3.[16]

2. Triiodothyronine (triiodothyronine sodium, liothyronine)

Triiodothyroine, having three iodine atoms, is also known as T3. Discovered nearly 50 years after thyroxine, it's the active thyroid hormone with calorigenic activity five to ten times that of T4.[17] A small amount of T3 is made by the thyroid, and the rest is produced by T4 in a peripheral (away from the thyroid) process called deiodination.

As a medication, T3 can be found as the sodium salt liothyronine alone (in Cytomel and Triostat) or in combination with thyroxine in several preparations including glandular preparations. T3 is less avidly bound to protein and has a half life of one to two days.[18]

The substances 3, 5, 3′–Triiodothyronine and 3, 3′, 5′–Triiodothyronine represent two distinct isomers of T3 found in the body (these are subtypes of T3 unrelated to rT3). Each isomer exerts its hormonal influence on different body organs, and each T3 isomer is converted from T4 with the assistance of a different type of 5′–deiodinase enzyme.[19]

3. Reverse T3 (rT3)

Reverse T3 (rT3) represents an alternative pathway for the deiodination of T4. Normally, T4 loses one iodine atom and is converted to roughly equal amounts of T3 and rT3. But in certain conditions, rT3 predominates. rT3 differs from T3 in that iodine is cleaved from the inner ring of T4, rather than the outer ring. RT3 is metabolized faster than T3 although it is calorigenically inactive. rT3 is increased in the fetus and newborn and in certain non-thyroid disorders including cirrhosis, neoplastic disease, starvation and burns. It is also increased in hyperthyroidism and decreased in hypothyroidism.

The increased conversion to rT3 is thought to be a protective mechanism. When the body is in a low metabolic state, the need for T3 is decreased. Then, an excess of T3 could have detrimental cardiac effects, whereas rT3 is not used as a source of energy.

4. Diiodotyrosine (DIT)

Diiodotyrosine is a hormone produced during thyroid hormone synthesis. Having two iodine atoms, it is also known as T2 and is thought to be responsible for stimulating the production of 5′–deiodinase (monodeiodinase),[20] an enzyme composed of several subtypes necessary for the synthesis of T4 to T3 in peripheral tissue. T2 is stored in the thyroglobulin of the thyroid follicles and is used to make T3 and T4 as needed.

4. Monoiodotyrosine (MIT)

Monoiodotyrosine, another precursor hormone produced

during thyroid hormone synthesis, contains one iodine atom. MIT is stored in the thyroglobulin of thyroid follicles to be used as needed in the synthesis of T3 where it couples with DIT.

5. Other Iodotyronines and Iodotyrosines

Single iodine atoms are capable of combining with tyrosine in other parts of the body such as the stomach, producing iodotyronine and iodotyrosines. Iodotyronines such as the acids TETRAC and TRIAC have biologic activity, 11 percent and 21 percent respectively, of the calorigenic activity of T4. T⁰ is considered biologically inactive.[21]

6. Calcitonin

Calcitonin is a hormone produced in the parafollicular cells (C cells) of the thyroid. Calcitonin regulates the amount of calcium within cells and is important in preserving bone mass. Besides the thyroid, calcitonin is produced in extrathyroidal C cells in multiple organs throughout the body such as the brain, urinary bladder, thymus and lungs.

The Metabolic Effects of Thyroid Hormones

Thyroid hormones enhance oxygen consumption of most body tissues and increase the body's metabolic rate, known as the Basal Metabolic Rate (BMR). The BMR is determined by measuring the body's oxygen consumption. Before blood tests for thyroid function were developed, the BMR was the primary diagnostic thyroid test. Thyroid hormones increase the metabolism of carbohydrates, lipids and protein, and are essential for the development and proper function of the central nervous system. The thyroid hormone T3 also interacts with neurotransmitters in the brain to affect mood and emotion.

Starvation and fasting cause decreased levels of total T3 within 24 to 48 hours. Free unbound T3 is also reduced due to reduced peripheral conversion. This state is reversed by carbohydrates but not by pure protein or fat. This explains the lowered T3 levels seen in carbohydrate restricted diets.[22] In these conditions, the body appears to fall into its protective state of producing rT3, rather than T3.

Conditions affected by thyroid hormone include metabolic rate, body temperature, muscle tone and vigor, growth hormone secretions, cholesterol levels and mood.

Physiological Effects of Thyroid Hormone

The specific physiologic effects of excess thyroid hormone can't be stated simply because increased activity of certain cells may influence other bodily systems, including other endocrine organs, which further complicates matters. For example, thyroid hormone affects growth hormone produced in the pituitary gland. Consequently, children with thyrotoxicosis grow more rapidly than normal children. However, accelerated growth is reversed with antithyroid treatment, and treated children exhibit a normal height.[23]

Cell Receptors and Thyroid Hormone Activity

The primary effects of hormones are physiological changes caused by hormonal interaction with the body's cells. The term receptor denotes the specific component of the cell with which hormones interact. Receptors can be extroverts, hanging out on the cell's surface, or recluses, hiding in the cell's nucleus.

Cell receptors perform two functions. They recognize and bind specific substances such as hormones. Then they translate this information into a cellular signal or transcription message that affects cell function.

Receptors can't leave cells and incite changes. So they act subtly, sending secret messages (like, turn up the heat) to target cells. Since receptors can't talk, they communicate by causing changes in the protein, which activate genes of target cells, turning them on or off. These transcription messages are recognized by the cells as commands. This results in the functional changes associated with the hormone. Thyroid hormone also causes direct or non-transcriptional changes.

Cell Receptor Agonists and Antagonists

Most hormone receptors are proteins capable of recognizing and responding to specific molecules. For example, thyroid hormone seeks out open thyroid hormone receptors as it circulates through the body. Thyroid receptors shouldn't let anything but thyroid hormone bind. However, sometimes receptors are fooled. In Graves' disease, the receptors are tricked by TSH receptor antibodies. Substances able to bind to receptors and mimic the effects of the intended hormone are termed agonists.

Other compounds are able to bind to receptors but they don't mimic the intended hormone's action. Instead, they interfere with the binding of the intended substance. Such compounds, which have no intrinsic regulatory activity but produce effects by inhibiting action, are termed antagonists. TSH receptor antibodies in Graves' disease may act as agonists or antagonists depending on their specific type (stimulating, binding or blocking).

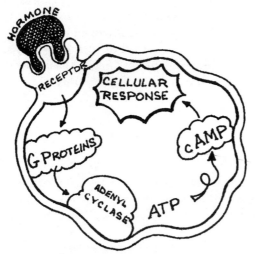

cAMP MEDIATED RESPONSE
OF THYROID HORMONE

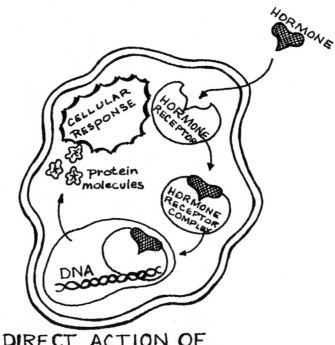

DIRECT ACTION OF
THYROID HORMONE

Thyroid Hormone Action

Endocrine Disruptors

Although hormones were once considered to fit receptors much like a lock fits a key, in recent years researchers have found that receptors aren't that discriminating. Some chemicals known to mimic hormones have structures with little or no resemblance to the intended hormone. The role of hormonal disruptors is discussed later in this chapter.

Action of Thyroid Hormones

How thyroid hormones exert their influence isn't totally clear. Thyroid hormones are known to interact with receptors on the cell nucleus and on the cell membrane. T3 has been shown to cause changes in gene transcription, possibly by activating binding sites that had been repressed, or by causing the release of certain enzymes. T4 also binds to these receptors, but it does so with a much lower affinity than T3. It's commonly suspected that T4 acts as a prohormone with changes in gene transcription solely due to the effect of T3.

Thyroid receptors are also found in the cellular cytoplasm (area of the cell between the nucleus and the cell membrane) and on mitochondria. Mitochondria, cellular substances that have recently been found to be loaded with DNA, are also rich in fats, proteins and enzymes. Most of the body's total oxygen consumption occurs in the cell's mitochondria. Here, about 40 percent of the energy derived from the metabolism of food is trapped and stored in the form of adenosine triphosphate (ATP) for use in a wide variety of energy-requiring cellular functions.

OXYGEN CONSUMPTION

Approximately 30 percent to 40 percent of the increase in the body's consumption of oxygen caused by thyroid hormone is due to stimulation of heart muscle. The liver, kidneys and skeletal muscle are also stimulated by thyroid hormone to use more oxygen. Several organs, including the brain, gonads and spleen, are unresponsive to these calorigenic effects of thyroid hormone. Their oxygen utilization is not affected by thyroid hormone.

THYROID HORMONE'S DIRECT ACTION ON CELLS

Thyroid hormones are fat soluble, which allows them to directly enter into cells and react with specific thyroid hormone receptors. The complex formed by receptor and hormone can migrate to the cell nucleus where it locks onto a specific sequence of DNA, causing direct genetic changes.

THE ROLE OF SECONDARY MESSENGERS

Thyroid hormone can also cause indirect effects with the assistance of a secondary messenger. Secondary messengers are often used to expedite the effects of thyroid hormone. Both the adenylyl cylase and the phospholipase C signaling pathways appear to mediate effects of TSH on thyroid function in human beings.

CYCLIC AMP

Thyroid hormone may also act as a "first messenger" by delivering its message to a specific thyroid receptor found on the outer surface membrane of a cell. This "hormone receptor complex" activates a protein in the cell membrane known as "G" protein. G protein activates a membrane-bound enzyme (chemical catalyst responsible for most chemical reactions in the body) known as adenyl cyclase. Adenyl cyclase, in turn, catalyzes the conversion of the energy molecule adenosine triphosphate (ATP) into a "second messenger" known as cyclic AMP (cAMP). In what is called a "cAMP mediated action," thyroid hormone works indirectly via this second messenger.

PHOSPHOLIPASE C (PIP2)

At higher concentrations than those required to stimulate cyclic cAMP formation, TSH causes activation of a secondary messenger known as phospholipase C. This results in hydrolysis of polyphosphatidyl inositols, increased cytoplasmic Ca^{2+} and activation of protein kinase C allowing thyroid hormone to cause indirect physiological changes.

Hormone Receptors

Hormones (from Greek, set in motion or urge forth) act as messengers by binding to specific hormone receptor sites on cells throughout the body. Besides causing change through gene transcription, thyroid hormone, primarily T3, interacts with receptors on mitochondria and plasma membranes producing non-transcriptional changes.

When the thyroid's receptor system is working properly, thyroid hormone works by binding open thyroid receptors of specific cells. For instance, circulating thyroid hormone in the blood activates thyroid receptors in the heart, ordering it to beat faster.

Receptor sites can be opened or closed depending upon the cells' needs. However, when chronically deprived of its hormone, receptor sites can malfunction and shut down even after the hormone is restored to normal levels. In the case of hypothyroidism, or when TSH receptor binding antibodies are present, treatment may be ineffective due to closed or blocked receptor sites despite normal thyroid hormone levels.

Besides thyroid antibodies, a number of drugs are thought to interfere with the binding of thyroid hormone to receptors. The anticonvulsant phenytoin (Dilantin) has been shown to interfere with binding of T3 to thyroid receptors in the pituitary. Non-steroidal anti-inflammatory drugs (NSAID's) and excess free fatty acids prevent T3 from binding to nuclear receptors.[24]

In addition to specific hormone receptors, the body contains a number of orphan receptors, cell receptors whose target hormones haven't yet been discovered. Whether thyroid hormone activates any of the orphan receptors is currently unknown.

Hormonal Disruptors

Receptor sites can be blocked or activated by chemicals known as hormonal disruptors. Because of their ability to bind to foreign receptors, hormonal disruptors can be used therapeutically. When blockage of estrogen is desired, for example, a plant substance with mildly estrogenic effects such as red clover can be administered, minimizing estrogen stimulation. However, hormonal disruptors rarely act beneficially.

Numerous environmental hormonal disruptors have been identified. Although many hormonal disruptors, such as PCB and DDT, are no longer produced, they're still prevalent since they don't degrade well. The list of known and suspected hormonal disruptors includes organic pesticides, phthalates, heavy metals, plastics, phenolic compounds and styrene dimers and trimers.[25] The organ most affected by hormonal disruptors is the adrenal gland, which produces stress hormones, followed by the thyroid gland.[26]

When receptor sites of the thyroid cells are blocked, the intended hormonal message can't be relayed. When the wrong message or no message is sent, thyroid function is affected. In *Screaming To Be Heard, Hormonal Connections Women Suspect ... and Doctors Ignore*, Dr. Elizabeth Vliet explains how disruptors prevent thyroid hormone from exerting its effects. Consequently, laboratory values may stay normal for months or years while the patient is actually suffering from the effects of thyroid hormone deficiency.[27]

The Superfamily of Receptors

Cell receptors for steroid hormones, thyroid hormones, vitamin D and the retinoids (vitamin A and its derivatives) regulate the transcription of specific genes on the cells where they're located. These receptors are all part of a larger family of transcription factors regulated by similar chemical processes. The TSH receptor is a member of the family of G protein-coupled receptors and is structurally similar to the receptors for the pituitary hormones, luteinizing hormone (LH) and follicle-stimulating hormone (FSH), which are reproductive hormones capable of binding to each others' receptors.

Effects of Thyroid Hormone on Body Weight

In conditions of starvation or fasting, T3 levels are decreased. Whenever T3 isn't delivered in sufficient amounts, (for instance, in impaired conversion of T4 into T3) and when zinc stores are deficient, leptin levels are also decreased. Consequently, leptin becomes inefficient in enhancing metabolism, which causes increased food cravings and less efficient burning of calories. Thyroid hormone plays a central role in diet since it alters levels of various chemical transmitters such as beta-endorphins and serotonin, the molecules that regulate eating behavior. Thyroid hormone also directly affects appetite centers in the brain. Excess thyroid hormone, for instance, increases one's appetite for carbohydrates. Caloric restriction decreases TSH secretion despite a decline in T3 levels.

Synthesis of Thyroid Hormone

Synthesis of thyroid hormones requires that the mineral iodine organically binds to the amino acid tyrosine. Residues of tyrosine (tyrosol residues) are present in thyroglobulin. The ability to convert tyrosine into thyroxine is not a monopoly of thyroid tissue. Other tissues in the body can also synthesize thyroxine. Although they lack thyroids, plants and invertebrates can also combine iodine and protein to form compounds similar to thyroxine. Vertebrates, however, have thyroids that serve as the primary site of synthesis, with thyroid complexity and structure varying from species to species.

In man, essential raw materials, such as iodide, are trapped at the base of follicular cells by interfollicular capillaries. From there, they're transported to the follicular lumen and oxidized to reactive iodine. There, iodine reacts with the tyrosine present in thyroglobulin. Thyroid hormone synthesis involves the following steps as well as several intermediate steps. Various enzymes, amino acids, minerals, carbohydrates and vitamins are utilized during the process and are critical for proper thyroid hormone synthesis.

Steps in Thyroid Hormone Synthesis

1. In a process of organification, iodide ions are concentrated in the thyroid into organic iodine by hydrogen peroxide or oxygen, limited by available iodine stores.
2. The iodine taken up by the active thyroid cells binds (iodinates) with tyrosine resulting in the formation of monoiodotyrosine (MIT) and diiodotyrosine (DIT). The enzyme thyroid peroxidase (TPO, thyroperoxidase) is required for this reaction.

3. The coupling process: when two DIT residues couple, thyroxine (T4) is formed. Whereas when one DIT residue combines with one MIT residue, triiodothyronine (T3) is formed. The enzyme thyroid peroxidase is also required for this reaction.

Note: Deiodination of T4 into T3 within the thyroid gland itself liberates iodide ions that can be reused for further hormone synthesis. Deiodination in the thyroid gland requires an enzyme similar to the 5'deiodinase that catalyzes T4 to T3 in extrathyroidal tissue.[28]

5'deiodinase Enzymes and Deiodination (Conversion) of T4

Deiodination refers to the loss of one iodine atom from T4, which produces T3. This process typically occurs away from the thyroid (in peripheral tissue). Chemicals known as 5'deiodinase enzymes are necessary for this conversion. There are three types of 5' deiodinase (Type 1, 2 and 3, also known as D1, D2, D3); their specificity is determined by the different tissue in which they're found. These enzymes regulate the amount and type of T3 produced. D2 regulates the conversion to T4 to T3 in the pituitary and brain. Unlike other organs that can utilize circulating T3, the brain and pituitary rely on freshly converted T3.

Besides T3 and rT3, other intermediate compounds are produced and released during thyroid hormone synthesis and T4 deiodination. TETRAC, or tetraiodothyroacetic acid, is derived as a breakdown product of T4. Triiodothyropyruvic acid (TRIAC) is derived from the degradation of T3. Both TETRAC and TRIAC have been found in diet products. Their use as a dietary supplement may induce or aggravate Graves' disease.

Thyroid Hormone Release

Before thyroid hormones can be secreted into the circulation, they must be released or cleaved from thyroglobulin. Proteolysis is the process whereby the major thyroid hormones thyroxine and triiodothyronine are cleaved from thyroglobulin. Usually, thyroxine secretion predominates. Lysosomal enzymes help degrade thyroglobulin.

After their secretion into the blood, thyroid hormones attach to plasma proteins and circulate through the body. About 70 percent of circulating T4 is bound to a protein fraction known as thyroxine binding globulin (TBG), 10 to 15 percent to transthyretin (TTR), and 15 to 20 percent to albumin. Most of the circulating T3 is bound to TBG. However, T3 has less of an affinity for protein than T4 and is more freely disassociated.

Normally, a small amount of thyroid hormone remains unbound to

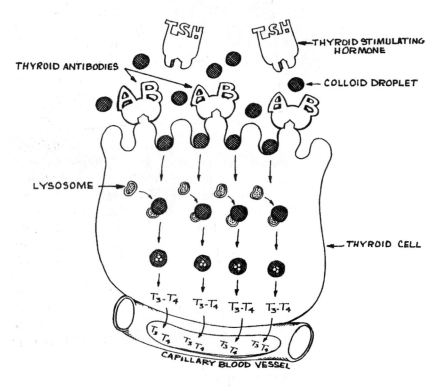

THE OVER STIMULATION OF THE THYROID CELL
BY THE THYROID ANTIBODIES LEADING TO THE
OVER PRODUCTION OF T₃ AND T₄

The Role of Antibodies in Graves' Disease

protein, with about 0.03 percent of T4 and 0.3 percent of T3 remaining free. It is the free fractions, Free T3 and Free T4, that presumably are the active hormonal forms.

T3/T4 Ratio in Graves' Disease

In Graves' disease, the proportion of unbound hormone (free T3/free T4) is increased due to a slight decrease in binding proteins and an increased level of circulating T4. Therefore, in GD, the ratio of T3 to T4 found in thyroglobulin is usually twice the normal ratio. Total daily production of T3 is disproportionately increased due to increased secretion of T3 from the thyroid gland and increased peripheral conversion of T4 to T3.

Consequently, blood levels may reflect an increased level of T3 while T4 remains in the normal range. This is known as T3 thyrotoxicosis and it may have a benevolent effect. Dr. P. Reed Larsen, et al., write, "Experience suggests that patients with T3 toxicosis are more likely to have a long-term remission after withdrawal of antithyroid drug therapy than patients with the usual form of thyrotoxicosis."[29]

Peripheral Conversion of T4 to T3

The majority of T3 (approximately 75 percent) present in the body originates from peripheral deiodination of T4. Peripheral sites include liver (responsible for 30 percent of peripheral deiodination), kidney, skeletal muscle, brain, pituitary, brown adipose tissue and several other organs. There are two distinct types of T3 produced (distinct from rT3), the particular type produced depending on the deiodinase enzyme present in the particular organ where conversion occurs. Recent studies suggest that one type of T3 is produced in the brain and pituitary, and the second type is produced in the other deiodination sites.

Approximately 35 percent of T4 is converted to T3. An additional 15 percent to 20 percent is changed to TETRAC or conjugated and excreted in urine or bile. The remainder of T4 is deiodinated to reverse T3. Further deiodination then occurs with T2 formed from both T3 and rT3.

Autoregulation

Autoregulation is a protective measure influenced by levels of iodine and thyroid hormone. As mentioned, excess iodine solution inhibits thyroid hormone's release from the thyroid. The body's autoregulatory mechanism causes an escape from this inhibition, thereby preventing blood levels of thyroid hormone from becoming critically low and causing goiter or hypothyroidism. Autoregulation serves to maintain a pool of organic iodine in the form of thyroid hormones and their immediate precursors. This system, rather like the concept of hibernation, serves as the first line of defense against fluctuations in the supply of iodine. Normally, when autoregulation is no longer capable of defending against low hormone levels, activation of the pituitary-hypothalamic-thyroid axis will ensue.

Strong iodine also causes a transient inhibition of thyroid hormone synthesis known as the Wolff-Chaikoff effect. The body has a natural regulatory mechanism known as the "escape from the Wolff-Chaikoff effect" that puts a halt to this effect after two days, preventing hypothyroidism from developing.

Thyroid Disorders

More than 200 million people in the world have some form of thyroid disease, and 20 million of these people reside in the United States.

The Colorado Thyroid Disease Prevalence Study released in February, 2000 reports that an additional 10 percent of the population, more than 13 million Americans, have undiagnosed thyroid disease. Overall, 2.7 percent of women and 0.23 percent of men have current Graves' disease or a history of it.[30]

Inflammatory Diseases and Thyroiditis

Inflammatory diseases of the thyroid are collectively the most commonly seen thyroid disorders. Individually, they range from the rare case of acute bacterial thyroiditis to the even rarer Riedel's thyroiditis. Thyroiditis, an inflammatory thyroid disorder often induced by a bacterial or viral infection, usually causes hypothyroidism, although it may occasionally result in hyperthyroidism.

Most commonly seen are the conditions of subacute thyroiditis, which include subacute granulomatous (also known as painful) thyroiditis and subacute lymphocytic (painless) thyroiditis. Dr. Peter Singer, in *The Medical Clinics of North America*, a guide for physicians, writes, "From a clinical standpoint, it is essential to differentiate subacute painless thyroiditis from Graves' disease, because these two disorders also may mimic each other, yet only Graves' disease requires specific therapy."[31] Most thyroid disorders are disorders of hypothyroidism (decreased thyroid hormone, its symptoms myxoedema or myxedema) or hyperthyroidism, its symptoms thyrotoxicosis.

Disorders of Thyrotoxicosis

Although thyrotoxicosis has many causes, the two predominating causes are GD and toxic solitary or multinodular goiter (Plummer's disease; thyroid adenoma is also called Plummer's disease).[32] Toxic multinodular goiter is also called Marine-Lenhart syndrome;[33] Marine-Lenhart syndrome is also called nodular Graves' disease.[34] Simple or nontoxic goiter refers to any thyroid enlargement not associated with hyperthyroidism and that doesn't result from inflammation or malignancy.

PLUMMER'S DISEASE

Plummer's disease results from one or more thyroid nodules trapping and organifying excess iodine and consequently secreting excess thyroid hormone independent of TSH regulation. Despite suppressed TSH levels, the nodules keep trapping iodine and forming thyroid hormone. Although Plummer's disease may be confused with GD, patients with Plummer's disease are usually older at the time of diagnosis and they don't experience the antibody involvement or the skin and eye disorders associated with GD. Recent studies indicate that that most "hot" or "autonomous" thyroid nodules result from TSH receptor mutations.[35] There are a number of other causes of thyrotoxicosis. Disorders of thyrotoxicosis are generally differentiated into three classes depending on the source responsible for excess thyroid hormone.[36]

CAUSES OF THYROTOXICOSIS

1. Most frequently seen are disorders caused by hyperfunction of the gland resulting from excess TSH (or by antibodies binding to the TSH receptor). This is seen in pituitary tumors, trophoblastic tumors, and in Graves' disease. This category also includes congenital hyperthyroidism due to a recently discovered mutation in the TSH receptor gene (identical to Graves' disease except for the absence of thyroid antibodies) and transient periods of Hashimoto's thyroiditis when stimulating TSH receptor antibodies predominate.

     Although Hashimoto's thyroiditis (HT) usually causes hypothyroidism, it may also cause sporadic releases of thyroid hormone, so-called silent thyrotoxicosis. HT causes a variety of syndromes that may occur either concomitantly or sequentially. In some instances, HT may evolve into a clinically pathological syndrome indistinguishable from Graves' disease or Graves' ophthalmophathy.

2. The second category results from an inflammatory process. It encompasses the thyrotoxic states associated with subacute thyroiditis and the syndrome termed chronic thyroiditis with spontaneously resolving thyrotoxicosis, which occurs when excess thyroid hormone leaks from the gland due to inflammation. The inflammatory disorders are transitory since the stores of preformed hormone present within the inflamed gland are finite. Thus, these disorders are self-limited. Causes include acute viral or bacterial thyroiditis and viral De Quervains thyroiditis.

3. The third category includes instances where the source of excess hormone is exogenous or outside of the body as in thyrotoxicosis facitia (patients willfully ingesting excess medication). This category also includes disorders related to accidental ingestion as in "hamburger thyrotoxicosis" and disorders caused by unintentionally ingesting substances adulterated or contaminated with thyroid hormone. In recent years, mini-epidemics of Graves' disease have been reported after the ingestion of thyroid contaminated meat in the Midwest ("hamburger toxicosis").[37] Certain diet pills containing thyroid hormone have caused similar problems in Japan.[38]

This category also includes various conditions resulting from circumstances unrelated to thyroid function. This includes TSH excess caused by the rare functioning metastatic thyroid carcinoma, solitary hyperfunctioning adenomas, radiation thyroiditis, excessive TSH stimulation, excessive iodine intake, or struma ovarii, a condition caused by an ovarian teratoma that contains hyperfunctional ectopic thyroid tissue. Such teratomas can also be found in locations other than the ovary. Struma ovarii rarely causes thyrotoxicosis and is usually diagnosed only during surgery for an ovarian tumor.[39]

Hyperthyroid vs. Nonhyperthyroid Thyrotoxicosis

Symptoms of thyrotoxicosis, including abnormal thyroid function tests, may occur even though the thyroid is normal. In these conditions, known as nonhyperthyoid thyrotoxic states, factors outside of the thyroid gland cause transient thyrotoxicosis.

In true hyperthyroidism, hyperfunction of the thyroid is reflected in increased radioiodine uptake (see imaging tests in chapter 5), whereas in the nonhyperthyroid thyrotoxic states (transient conditions of thyroiditis, iodine-induced hyperthyroidism, exogenous thyroid ingestion) thyroid function is subnormal and the radioiodine uptake is low. Treatment of thyrotoxicosis by decreasing hormone synthesis (antithyroid agents, surgery, or radioiodine) is appropriate in hyperthyroidism, but it's inappropriate and ineffective in other forms of thyrotoxicosis.[40] Antibiotics and anti-inflammatory medications are used to treat inflammatory disorders such as subacute thyroiditis.

Subclinical Hyperthyroidism

Subclinical hyperthyroidism refers to a condition in which serum TSH is decreased to levels below the normal range, and levels of FT3 and FT4 are normal. Subclinical hyperthyroidism may be caused by excessive thyroid replacement therapy or slight endogenous overproduction of thyroid hormone. Subclinical hyperthyroidism may also occur after extended periods of hyperthyroidism. In this instance, it may take many months before the TSH level reflects a normal pituitary response. Depressed TSH levels may also be caused by other conditions such as depression and severe nonthyroidal illness and by the use of certain medications such as glucocorticods or dopamine.

In patients undergoing treatment for GD, FT4 and FT3 are better indicators of thyroid status. Subclinical hyperthyroidism in this case is difficult to ascertain. There is debate regarding whether patients with subclincal hyperthyroidism should be treated since the risks for atrial fibrillation and decreased bone density that could result in osteoporosis may be increased. Since suppressed TSH levels are often transient, patients with subclinical hyperthyroidism are usually monitored for symptoms and later retested.

Hashitoxicosis

Hashitoxicosis is a disorder in which symptoms of thyrotoxicosis occur in patients with Hashimoto's thyroiditis, a hypothyroid disorder. In Hashitoxicosis, the stimulating TSH receptor antibodies of GD are more likely to be present than the thyroid peroxidase antibodies associated with HT. The presence of abundant lymphocytes and Askanazy cells in thyroid tissue confirms the diagnosis in patients with characteristic symptoms.[41]

4 Graves' Opthalmopathy, Dermopathy and Acropachy

Various thyroid on-line bulletin boards display a stream of posts regarding Graves' ophthalmopathy (GO; also known as thyroid eye disease) and Graves' dermopathy. Concerns include sudden loss of color, blurred or double vision, eye pain, and the swollen leathery skin of pretibial myxedema (PTM). In chapter 4, I describe the symptoms, signs and causes of Graves' ophthalmopathy and dermopathy, along with current treatment options.

Graves Ophthalmopathy

When the characteristic eye involvement associated with GD is present, but the patient is euthyroid (normal blood thyroid hormone levels), the term euthyroid Graves' disease is used. Most patients who initially appear to only have the eye disease, nevertheless, on careful exam, have been found to have evidence of thyroid autoimmunity.

The characteristic eye disorder seen in Graves' disease is called Graves' ophthalmopathy (GO) or thyroid eye disease (TED). GO is also known as Graves' eye disease, endocrine ophthalmopathy, dysthyroid orbitopathy and immune exophthalmos.

GO is an autoimmune disorder independent of GD, although 33 percent to 50 percent of GO cases are seen in association with the thyroid disturbances characteristic of GD. GO is also seen concomitantly with approximately 10 percent of cases of HT and in other conditions of thyroiditis. It may also be seen after long-term lithium therapy.[1] There are two distinct manifestations of GO, a congestive infiltrative process and a spastic disorder.

Congestive Orbital (Eye) Disease

The extraocular eye muscles appear to be the primary target in GO. The congestive process is characterized by white blood cells accumulating in (infiltrating) orbital fibroadipose and skeletal muscle tissue. This congestion may be associated with edema (fluid retention) and may eventually progress to fibrosis (an increase of fibrous tissue similar to scar tissue). The physical manifestations are enlargement of both the extraocular muscles and the connective tissue behind the globe.

As a result the globe is displaced anteriorly resulting in proptosis (protrusion of the eyeball; exophthalmos). Patients with congestive eye disease may have bilateral proptosis (proptosis occurring in both eyes), which can limit the range of eye movement. The enlarged and fibrotic extraocular and eyelid muscles are restricted in their motion, resulting in diplopia (double vision) and lid retraction.

Spastic Eye Symptoms

A more common, but less troublesome, eye disorder distinct from the mechanical or congestive infiltration is caused by the effects of excess catecholamine stimulation, caused by excess thyroid hormone. The clinical signs include spastic eye movement characterized by a staring expression. The extraocular muscle, in particular, is affected.

This condition is alleviated by drugs such as guanethidine and beta adrenergic blocking drugs (beta blockers). Symptoms are exacerbated (worsened) by ingesting drugs such as ephedrine or antihistamine compounds. While symptoms caused by excess thyroid hormone abate when thyrotoxicosis is relieved, congestive infiltration may follow an independent course and is reported to be seldom influenced by return to a euthyroid state.

Incidence of GO in Graves' Disease

Estimates of the number of patients with GD who also have GO vary depending on the sensitivity of the detection method. With sensitive techniques such as computed tomography (CT), nearly all GD patients will exhibit evidence of extraocular muscle involvement. Clinically evident GO occurs in 10 percent to 25 percent of GD patients if eyelid signs are excluded and 30 percent to 45 percent if eyelids changes are included. Fewer than 5 percent of GD patients experience severe GO. GO may develop before, concurrently with, or after the diagnosis of hyperthyroidism. More than 80 percent of thyroid patients who develop severe eye disease do so within 18 months of detection of hyperthyroidism.[2] Ten percent of these patients were initially hypothyroid, and another 10 percent appear to have no thyroid involvement.

Sex Related Differences and the Effects of Smoking

Gender bias has been demonstrated with men composing a relatively greater proportion of severe cases. The prevalence of cigarette smokers is higher in patients with GO and in patients with other thyroid disorders. The mechanisms underlying this finding remain unclear, although smokers are also more likely to develop goiter and higher levels of serum thyroglobulin, which suggests that thyroid damage may contribute to GO.[3]

Symptoms Associated with Graves' Ophthalmopathy

These include blurred or double vision (diplopia), redness or swelling, dryness, exophthalmy (protrusion, exophthalmos, proptosis), sensitivity to light (photophobia), excess tearing, decreased eye movement and discomfort.

Manifestations and Stages of GO

Patients with GO may complain of a gritty, sandy sensation in the eyes or of pressure. Lacrimation (tearing), photophobia, blurring of vision and double vision are common symptoms. Visual blurring may be caused by a decreased tear film on the surface of the cornea or minor extraocular muscle imbalance. This blurring clears when either eye is closed. Eye pain is related to severe corneal involvement or to inflammation. Eye pain is generally the first symptom to disappear after treatment. Occasionally the thin conjunctiva overlying the white portion of the eye may redden, giving the eyes a bloodshot appearance.

Of greater importance is the visual blurring that may continue for weeks and persists with one eye closed. It's often associated with a perceived reduction in color brightness, diminished visual acuity, loss of peripheral vision, or as an alteration in visual quality in one portion of the visual field. These symptoms suggest optic neuropathy.

Optic Neuropathy

Optic neuropathy is a disorder in which the optic nerve, which connects the eye to the brain, is compressed. Optic neuropathy is generally seen in patients with extremely enlarged extraocular muscles that squeeze the optic nerve deep within the eye socket. In rare patients, inflammation develops in the eye muscles and also the orbital fat in the rear portion of the orbit (the apex), causing a decrease in blood flow to the optic nerve.

Symptoms include blurred vision, decreased color vision, or shadows or holes in the field of vision. Sight loss can occur either on one side (unilateral) or both sides (bilateral) and may not be noticed unless vision in

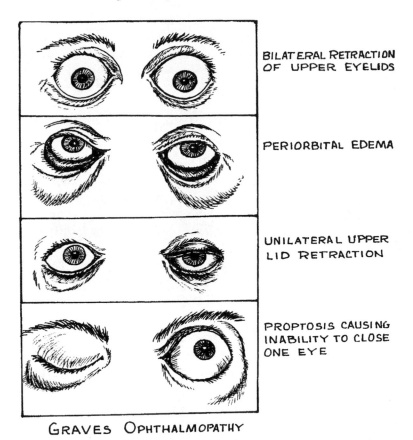

BILATERAL RETRACTION OF UPPER EYELIDS

PERIORBITAL EDEMA

UNILATERAL UPPER LID RETRACTION

PROPTOSIS CAUSING INABILITY TO CLOSE ONE EYE

GRAVES OPHTHALMOPATHY

Graves' Opthalmopathy (adapted from Werner and Ingbar's The Thyroid, a Fundamental and Clincal Text, *7th ed., edited by Lewis Braverman and Robert Utiger, Lippincott-Raven Publishing, 1996).*

each eye is assessed independently. Loss of color vision is one of the first symptoms of optic nerve involvement. The inability to distinguish the color red, in patients not previously diagnosed as color blind, is one of the first signs of color vision loss.

Symptoms Associated with Proptosis

Proptosis associated with lid retraction results in increased corneal exposure. This may lead to keratitis or corneal ulcer, with symptoms of tearing, general eye discomfort and blurred vision. Chemosis (conjunctival swelling and injection) and periorbital edema (swelling around the eye often manifested as pouches or bags under the eye) result from local inflammation and impaired orbital venous drainage.

Whether due to proptosis or to eyelid retraction, the exposed cornea tends to become dry and inflamed. It's important to protect the cornea by avoidance of smoke, air currents and other irritants. My friend Mary B found it necessary to lubricate her eyes constantly with artificial tears and wear tinted glasses year 'round during her course of GO.

Progressive and Malignant Exophthalamos and Exophthalmic Ophthalmoplegia

When exophthalmos progresses rapidly and becomes the major concern in GO, it is termed progressive exophthalmos, and, if severe, malignant exophthalmos. The term exophthalmic ophthalmoplegia refers to the ocular muscle weakness that results in impaired upward gaze. Other ocular manifestations include convergence and strabismus with varying degrees of diplopia.

Ophthalmoplegia usually affects one eye and may cause paralysis of the upward gaze. Exophthalmos may be unilateral in the early stage, but this condition usually progresses to bilateral involvement.

Causes of Diplopia

Diplopia (double vision) in GO is caused by restriction of antagonist muscles rather than weakness of agonist muscles. Restriction of eye movement occurs as a result of a build up of scar-like tissue or fibrosis within various eye muscles, generally in an uneven fashion. When inflamed, the eye muscles may work inefficiently, causing the eyes to move to different degrees, adding to the problem. Initially, diplopia may be persistent and present only early in the morning or when the patient is tired. As the condition progresses, images in double vision separate farther apart and the condition becomes persistent.

Diplopia may cause neck problems such as torticollis (also known as "wry neck," characterized by a stiff painful neck) as the patient tries to compensate for the ocular motility imbalance. Since diplopia may spontaneously resolve, general criteria for corrective surgery of diplopia is double vision in the front gaze that has been stable for at least six months. Success, which occurs in 90 percent of the surgical cases, is demonstrated by single vision in primary and reading positions.[4]

Staring

In euthyroid patients the staring appearance can be caused by severe proptosis or from fibrosis and scarring of the eyelid levator muscles. This symptom also results from excess thyroid hormone.

Eye Signs

Although there are more than 27 eponymic signs associated with thyroid eye disease (listed below), only bilateral (affecting both eyes) proptosis with eyelid retraction is virtually characteristic. Lid lag on downgaze (von Graefe's sign) is very typical, as is an increased intraocular pressure on upgaze.

Table of Eye Signs

Ballet's	Paralysis of one or more extraocular muscles
Boston's	Uneven jerky motion of the upper lid on inferior movement
Cowen's	Extensive "hippus" of the consensual pupillary light reflex
Dalrymple's	Upper lid retraction
Enroth's	Edema of the lower lid
Gellinek's	Abnormal pigmentation of the upper lid
Gifford's	Difficult eversion of the upper lid
Goffroy's	Absent creases in the forehead on superior gaze
Griffith's	Lower lid lag on upward gaze
Knie's	Uneven pupil dilation in dim light
Kocher's	Spasmatic retraction of the upper lid during fixation
Loewi's	Dilation of the pupil with 1/1000 epinephrine
Means'	Increased superior scleral show on upgaze
Möbius'	Deficient convergence
Payne/Trousseau	Dislocation of globe
Pochin's	Reduced amplitude of blinking
Riesman's	Bruit over eyelid
Rosenbach's	Tremor of the gently closed lids
Sainton's	Frontalis contraction after cessation of levator activity
Snellen/Donder's	Bruit over the eye
Suker's	Inability to maintain fixation on extreme lateral gaze
Stellwag's	Incomplete and infrequent blinking
Vigouroux's	Puffiness of the lids
Von Graefe's	Upper eyelid lag on downgaze
Wilder's	Jerking of eyes on movement from abduction to adduction[5]

From "The Ophthalmopathy of Graves' Disease" by Devron Char, M.D., in Medical Clinics of North America, The Thyroid, Vol. 75, No. 1, January, 1991, Edited by Francis Greenspan, M.D. Table reprinted by permission of the publisher, W.B. Saunders.

Pathology

Enlargement of the extraocular muscles is the predominant orbital abnormality in infiltrative GO. Chronic orbital inflammation is characterized by edema, excess mucopolysaccharides, especially glycosaminoglycan

(GAG) deposits, lymphocyte cell infiltration, fatty infiltration and orbital fibroblast (early eye tissue cell) proliferation. Muscle enlargement is due to muscle fiber separation caused by edema, fibrosis and lymphocytes. Although the muscles are enlarged, the muscle fibers are usually normal.

Extraocular Muscle

The extraocular muscles originate at Zinn's annulus, the fibrous periosteal (situated next to the bone) extension located at the apex (back) of the orbit that forms the posterior attachment site of the muscles. The visual axis and the axis of the orbit are not precisely parallel. Consequently, the superior rectus muscles elevate and rotate the eyes inwardly, while the inferior rector muscles lower and outwardly rotate the eyes.

Both oblique muscles run posteriorly to their attachment on the eye. Normally the superior oblique muscles depress, abduct and rotate the eyes inwardly. The inferior oblique muscles elevate, adduct and rotate the eyes outwardly. In contrast, the medial and lateral rectus muscles are straightforward abductors and adductors, respectively.

The extraocular muscles are encased by fibrous connective tissue that creates a boundary between the intraconal compartment and the extraconal space. Connective tissue, along with the limited flexibility of the extraocular muscles, restricts anterior motion of the eyes when retrobulbar pressure increases. While correcting diplopia, recession of the rectus muscle may occur, increasing proptosis.

Each orbital cavity holds an average volume of 26 ml. Normally, this cavity is occupied anteriorly by the globe and posteriorly by the extraocular muscles, connective tissue, vessels and nerves. The extent of orbital protrusion (protrusion, exophthalmos) is related to the extent which the orbital soft tissues fill the orbital cavity. An increase in orbital volume of only 4 ml is thought to result in 6 mm of proptosis. The normal range of extraocular muscle is 3.0 to 6.8 ml, and of retrobulbar fat and connective tissue from 8.2 to 14.0 ml. In patients with GO, muscle volume has been reported to be as high as 21.6 ml, and fat and connective tissue volume as high as 22.6 ml have been reported.[6]

The Genetic Component of GO

A recent study shows a correlation between GO and an allele of the cytotoxic T lymphocyte antigen-4 gene (CTLA-4). Although CTLA-4 has previously been linked with type 1 diabetes and GD, new research shows that the CTLA-4 gene confers a risk for GO development, and the strength of the association is related to the severity of the disease.[7]

The Autoimmune Element in GO

Researchers at Wright State University in Dayton, Ohio, have completed studies that suggest that TSH receptor protein is targeted in GO. This protein is found in both skin and orbital tissue of both normal and Graves' patients. In patients with GD, but not normal patients, messenger RNA (mRNA) is present, and the fibroblasts are activated suggesting that activated fibroblasts are distributed throughout the body in Graves' disease.[8]

It's suspected that stimulating thyrotropin receptor antibodies (TRAb) in the serum of Graves' patients, along with cytokines released in the immune process, are responsible for the differentiation of fibroblasts into adipocytes and for the production of GAG seen in GO and pretibial myxedema. Stimulating TRAb causes the fibroblasts to proliferate and differentiate into adipocytes, but the autoreactive T cells produced during the immune response keep the inflammatory process alive.

Cytokines such as interferon-gamma, which are released by T cells and macrophages, stimulate orbital fibroblasts to produce GAG. GAG is responsible for the edema, chemosis and proptosis of GO. Cytokines also cause the orbital fibroblasts to express HLA-DR (see chapter 7). HLA-DR is normally only expressed on lymphocytes, monocytes and endothelial cells. Its presence on fibroblasts is aberrant, allowing theses cells to present autoantigens to receptive T cells. This perpetuates the autoimmune inflammatory response.

Normal Progression of Graves' Ophthalmopathy

Most researchers agree that ophthalmopathy in Graves' disease is self-limiting. The course of GO characteristically worsens over an initial period of three to six months, followed by a lengthy plateau that may last several years. Many patients experience spontaneous improvement after a course of periodic flare-ups (exacerbations). GO usually occurs 0–18 months after the diagnosis of hyperthyroidism.

During the progressive phase of GO, vision threatening complications may arise, including optic neuropathy and corneal ulceration. Measures to reduce orbital inflammation have the greatest efficacy during this progressive or "hot" stage. During the resolution phase the extraocular muscles may heal by progressive fibrosis or scarring, resulting in fibrotic contractures and diplopia.

Once inflamed, GO may remain active for several months to as long as five years. After becoming inactive for six months, recurrence of eye disease is infrequent and may coincide with poor control of thyroid hormone levels.

Diagnosis of Graves' Ophthalmopathy

Diagnosis is straightforward in hyperthyroid patients. In euthyroid patients, a vigilant effort is generally made to detect an underlying thyroid disorder. On the other hand, some patients with thyrotoxicosis may have eye problems unrelated to thyroid disease. And some patients with GO remain euthyroid. Symptom that appears to be related to excess thyroid hormone are upper eyelid elevation and spastic signs.

Ocular findings are most specific for GO when they occur bilaterally and in certain combinations. The concurrence of bilateral lid retraction with proptosis and restrictive eye movement is virtually diagnostic. Markedly asymmetric or unilateral occurrence of most of these symptoms suggests a different origin for the ocular disease.

The Objective Eye Examination

The eye exam begins with an assessment of visual acuity in each eye. The pupillary responses to light are evaluated. When both a reduction in visual acuity and an afferent pupillary defect are present, optic neuropathy is likely and formal field testing is mandatory. The eyes are then inspected for periorbital edema, lid edema and lid lag. Diplopia field testing and the Lancaster or Hess screens are used to determine the degree of extraocular muscle impairment.

Ethnic changes from the normal range have been established. For instance, Asians have an upper limit of 18 mm of protrusion as measured from the lateral orbital rim, as compared with 20 mm for whites and 22 mm for blacks.[9]

Bilateral proptosis in itself is not diagnostic of GO. It may result as a consequence of shallow orbits as in Crouzon's disease, or be due to large globes (seen in severe myopia), or to retroocular fat accumulation as occurs in exogenous steroid administration. Other causes include Cushing's syndrome, obesity, lithium therapy, cirrhosis, orbital pseudotumor, Wegener's granulomatosus, lymphoma and metastatic tumors.[10]

Even though unilateral proptosis is less specific, GO is its single most common cause, representing 15 percent to 28 percent of cases. Axial proptosis, in which the eye is displaced in an anterior direction, is a frequent finding in GO. Other ocular deviations, such as those in which the eye position appears down and out, down and in, or elevated with proptosis, are typically seen in other pathologic processes.[11]

The eye signs of Graves' disease have been classified by the American Thyroid Association as a mnemonic system in which the first letters of each category constitute the term NOSPECS.

Class 0 — No physical signs or symptoms.

Class 1 — Only signs, no symptoms (signs limited to upper lid retraction, stare, lid lag, and proptosis to 22 mm).

Class 2 — Soft tissue involvement with periorbital edema, congestion or redness of the conjunctiva and swelling of the conjunctiva (chemosis).

Class 3 — Proptosis >22 mm as measured by Hertel exophthalmometry.

Class 4 — Extraocular muscle involvement, most commonly the inferior rectus with involvement impairing upward gaze.

Class 5 — Corneal involvement (keratitis).

Class 6 — Sight loss from optic nerve involvement.[12]

NOSPECS represents a useful system for evaluation. Objective measurements for each eye separately (as recommended) include documentation of maximus lid fissure width, assessment of exposure keratitis and extraocular muscle function, measurement of intraocular pressure, and measurements of visual acuity, fields and color vision.

However, some ophthalmologists do not rely on *NOSPECS* or any of its modifications for categorization or treatment decisions. Their reasoning is that patients often progress from one class to another without proceeding through the interval steps, awarding the system no prognostic value. Also, the separate components comprising GO may vary in their severity or not be equal in terms of visual or cosmetic debility.[13]

Although lid retraction and proptosis are most commonly associated with Graves' disease, they may also be seen in Hashimoto's thyroiditis and the autoimmune condition myasthenia gravis. Other causes of proptosis include the following.

Non-neoplastic Conditions That Can Simulate
Early Thyroid Changes of Lid Retraction
or Apparent Proptosis

Myopia	Hypokalemic periodic paralysis
Posterior commissure brain lesions (Parinaud's syndrome)	Cushing's syndrome
	Chronic obstructive lung disease
Congenital anomalies	Uremia
Cirrhosis	Superior vena cava syndrome
Medication (lithium, steroids, etc.) induced	Sympathomimetic drugs (some diet pills and antihistamines)
Contralateral ptosis	Nerve III lesions
Hydrocephalus	Status after lid surgery[14]

Table reprinted courtesy of W.B. Saunders from "The Ophthalmopathy of Graves' Disease" by Devron Char, M.D., in Medical Clinics of North America, *Vol. 75, No. 1,* The Thyroid, *Edited by Greenspan, Francis, M.D., W.B. Saunders Co., Jan., 1991, 97–99.*

Imaging Studies in GO

Not all patients with GO require imaging studies for diagnosis or treatment, especially if there is thyroid involvement, no apparent corneal staining and good vision. The primary indication for radiographic evaluation is to confirm the diagnosis when there is uncertainty. When imaging studies are required, magnetic resonance imaging (MRI), computed tomography (CT) and ultrasonography are the methods commonly employed.

Proptosis may be measured by a variety of instruments such as the Hertel exophthalmometer. However, the most sensitive measurements are made by high resolution orbital imaging. The typical imaging pattern in GO demonstrates enlarged recti muscles, usually with the tendons spared and varying amounts of orbital fat. In up to 30 percent of cases, only a single muscle is involved and occasionally the only abnormality is an increase in orbital fat. Both CT and MRI allow measurements of extraocular muscle thickness and provide good visualization in the critical area at the orbital apex. MRI using a 1.5 tesla unit and orbital surface coils provides optimal spatial resolution of the orbit.

A disadvantage to MRI is that image reformation in different planes is not always available. Also, it is more expensive and takes longer. An advantage is that is provides better anatomic detail, and, with a fat saturation-gadolinium-DTPA protocol, is unparalleled for delineation of subtle compressive optic neuropathy. MRI after gadolinium–DPTA administration can distinguish between muscles that are swollen due to fatty degeneration, fibrosis and edema. T2 weighted MRI images may also demonstrate active inflammation.

CT imaging may also be used to estimate the volume of extraocular muscle and retroocular fat tissue. Advantages to CT are that it is faster and less expensive. CT imaging, with axial and coronal views, is the preferred study due to its ability to provide bony detail. Ultrasonography, the first method in use for high resolution orbital imaging, is least applicable for determining visualization in the critical area of the orbital axis.

Factors Influencing GO Development

GD treatment may affect the natural course of GO. Because radioiodine therapy evokes transient increases in serum concentrations of stimulating TRAb, the cross-reaction of these antibodies to eye tissue is suspected to be a potential causative agent for GO. Radioiodine has been reported both to increase the likelihood of developing GO as well as to exacerbate the severity of disease in patients with preexisting symptoms. Similar changes have not been associated with other treatment options.[15]

A report released in 1998 involving a study of 443 Graves' patients having mild proptosis, intermittent diplopia, and mild conjunctival and periorbital inflammation but no optic neuropathy indicated that radioiodine ablation for hyperthyroidism may cause GO to develop or worsen. Patients treated with only methimazole did not exhibit worsening of GO. The study's authors did not see a worsening of symptoms of patients who were given corticosteroids in conjunction with radioiodine.[16]

Cigarette Smoking

It's long been known that both GO and GD are associated with smoking. One recent study reports that smoking is associated with decreased levels of interleukin-1α-receptor antagonist. From this, researchers postulate that "smoking may exacerbate inflammation in GO by lowering interleukin-1-α-receptor antagonists levels and increasing the relative activity of interleukin-1-α."[17] Interleukin-1-α stimulates GAG production.

In another recent study conducted by the Department of Ophthalmology at the University of South Florida, cultured orbital fibroblasts obtained from patients undergoing orbital decompression exposed to tar and nicotine alone failed to exhibit HLA-DR expression, which is associated with the autoimmune response. However, when interferon-gamma (500 U/ml) was added to either nicotine or tar before they were added to the cultured fibroblasts, HLA-DR was expressed. Research is focused on interventions to decrease the interactions between cigarette components, cytokines and orbital fibroblasts.[18]

Treatment of Graves' Ophthalmopathy

Treatment of GO depends on the patient's overall condition, specific eye symptoms and disease severity. Most patients have minor disturbances that can be treated with local protective measures such as tinted glasses, eye drops of 1 percent methylcullulose, prisms, protective eye patches, eye gels, artificial tear ointments and taping the eyelids shut at night. Patients with only minor eye signs such as stare and lid-lag or light sensitivity (photophobia) or excessive tearing (epiphora) are best treated with artificial tears or lubrication ointments to prevent or heal corneal surface injury.

Suze, a friend from Canada, reports that she was bothered by sore eyes until she began using Lacri-lube, a thick optical ointment. At night she applies a thick layer of the gel and tapes her eyes shut with two strips of micropore tape. She also reports finding relief using gelled eye masks that can be refrigerated before use. Mary B recommends using sterile methylcellulose drops. Although they are sold over the counter, she advises obtaining a prescription for the drops in order to get insurance compensation.

Non-Surgical Treatment Options

Current treatment options include the use of diuretics to decrease fluid content, corticosteroids to suppress the immune system and reduce inflammation, orbital radiation therapy to reduce soft tissue inflammation and proptosis and improve eye muscle function, prisms to reduce diplopia, 1 percent methylcellulose drops to prevent dryness and various types of ocular surgery. In some clinical trials plasmapheresis has resulted in improvement, and recently, the immunosuppressive drug cyclosporine has shown promising results.

PRISMS

Prism lenses worn on glasses are used to correct double vision. Prisms can be ground into lenses or pressed on with frunell press on prisms. Both work well and the eyes do not need to move in all directions for them to work. One patient, Jake, has used both types of prisms and explains that he could not look up for five years before he began using them. He reports that frunell prisms are usually used when the doctor is trying to determine what works, although the more expensive ground in prisms are considered superior. Jake also mentioned that a frunell prism lens is used in lighthouses to concentrate the light beam. Doctors found it worked to bend light and adapted it for use in correcting double vision.

OCREOTIDE

Ocreotide, a chemical that exerts pharmacologic actions similar to the natural hormone somatostatin, has proved effective in some individuals. Patients who have somatostatin receptors in their eye muscle and who have localization of nuclear isotopes on Octreoscan–111 scanning have shown improvement when treated with octreotide 300 mcg daily over 12 weeks.[19] However, side effects make its use prohibitive for most patients.

CORTICOSTEROIDS

Besides their anti-inflammatory and immunosuppresive effects, corticosteroids may directly inhibit GAG synthesis and also its release from fibroblasts. Corticosteroids relieve pain involved with soft tissue inflammation, reduce orbital swelling and edema, and ameliorate the pain of compressive optic neuropathy. Improvement in proptosis may occur but symptoms may be exacerbated after discontinuation of treatment.

Kelly Hale, president of the American Foundation of Thyroid Patients, reports that receiving a short course of corticosteroids before her radioiodine treatment prevented worsening of her mild thyroid eye disease. She later used a short course (7 to 10 days) of corticosteroids for a flare-up of her eye symptoms. The steroids worked effectively and she did not experience an exacerbation of symptoms after stopping steroid treatment. In her opinion, keeping the course of steroids short is the key to preventing a rebound effect.

Steroids are used in the early stages of GO before extensive fibrosis has occurred. Taken orally in doses up to 80 mg/day, prednisone proves effective in most patients. Side effects include high blood pressure, insomnia, weight gain, depression, relapse of eye symptoms after stopping treatment and incomplete reversal of the disease in some cases.

ORBITAL SUPERVOLTAGE RADIOTHERAPY

Conflicting reports of the efficacy occur because radiotherapy is often used in combination with steroids.[20] However, good responses have occurred in patients using radiotherapy with or without steroids. Some patients initially resistant to steroids improve after radiotherapy. Radiotherapy seems to work best in patients with a short history of eye disease and is not recommended for patients with coexisting diabetic retinopathy.[21]

In one recent study, the field of binocular single vision was enlarged in 11 of 17 patients after irradiation, compared with two of 15 patients in the control group.[22] Still, 75 percent of the patients receiving orbital irradiation later required strabismus surgery. The conclusion of this study indicated that in patients with moderately severe GO, radiotherapy is only effective at treating motility impairment.

At Stanford, physicians treat progressive GO by aiming a fine X-ray beam at the eye muscles. This technique, originally developed to treat cancer, uses a medical linear accelerator, a compact version of an atom smasher. This instrument uses pulses of microwave energy to excite electrons to near-light speed, then aims them against a gold-plated target. The resulting collision produces highly penetrative X-rays, which are emitted from the machine and targeted to the patient's orbital muscles.

Lymphocytes responsible for eye inflammation are particularly sensitive to radiation and are preferentially killed by low dose of X-rays. This allows connective tissue swelling to regress. Some radiation oncologists prefer to treat the disease while it is progressive, rather than waiting for it to stabilize, thereby preventing it from advancing, particularly if symptoms prevent patients from performing their jobs or cause undue discomfort.[23]

PLASMAPHERESIS

Plasmapheresis, a procedure using therapeutic phlebotomy (unit of blood is drawn and the cells returned to the patient) is another controversial method. The idea behind it is that circulating immunoglobulins in the plasma will be removed and their levels diminished. The drawbacks are that it is expensive and any improvement is transient since antibody production is an ongoing process.

Eye Surgeries

Patients with advanced soft tissue inflammation, ophthalmoplegia, moderate to severe proptosis or optic neuropathy often require surgery. Anticipated changes during the active phase of GD are often taken into consideration. Surgery is generally postponed until the active eye disease (the hot phase) has subsided unless there is progressive optic nerve involvement. A succession of surgeries may be required. One GD patient reports having had 17 separate surgeries. With the exception of orbital decompression, most of the surgeries discussed can be performed on an outpatient basis or as a same day surgery.

In an article describing surgical options in *Thyroid USA*, a newsletter published by the American Foundation of Thyroid Patients, ophthalmologists report that during the active (changing) phase of GO, the physician has three main jobs:

1. To be certain that eye changes are due only to GO and not some other simultaneous disease process. The authors report that this is a common occurrence that is frequently missed.
2. To carefully monitor eye health and quickly intervene if vision or eye comfort are threatened.
3. To help determine when the active phase of GO has passed and restorative intervention is appropriate.[24]

Surgical Protocol

The wide range of problems seen in GO is best managed by a team of physicians specializing in different aspects of GO. Such a team might include a neuro-ophthalmologist (specialist in ophthalmology and neurology), an eye muscle specialist (strabismologist), and an oculoplastic surgeon (specialist in GO and plastic surgery).[25]

Orbital decompression is the standard surgical approach for GO and is usually performed first, followed by extraocular muscle surgery or correction of double vision if indicated, which is, in turn, followed by eyelid surgery if indicated.

If this sequence is deviated from, the benefits of an operation may be lost either by the recurrence of the disease or by the effects of a later procedure. For instance, orbital decompression may influence the ocular motility and change the lid aperture. Adjustment or recession of the inferior rectus muscle may alter upper and lower lid retraction. Among the following list of surgeries there may be several customized variations.

EYE MUSCLE SURGERIES

Occasionally, eye muscle enlargement causes a decrease in mobility resulting in diplopia, which may improve spontaneously. If intervention is required, various procedures are available to realign the eyes. Usually, no skin incisions are required and outpatient surgery under general anesthesia is performed. Eye muscle surgery is generally performed after orbital decompression since this procedure may change eye muscle functions. Soreness following surgery is usually mild and lasts for one to three days.

EYELID SURGERIES

The eyelids in GO may become puffy and fluid filled (periorbital edema), and the skin below the eye may sag from stretching. Occasionally, the eyelids may retract away from the iris, exposing excess white sclera. Or the eyelids may droop, interfering with the visual range. Corrective surgery is usually performed under local anesthesia. Incisions are usually small and easily camouflaged. Pain is usually mild, lasting one day, although bruising may persist for up to 14 days. Ice cold compresses are used during the first two days post-op, followed by warm compresses for the duration until bruising is healed.[26]

ORBITAL DECOMPRESSION

The orbit refers to the bony chamber that houses the eye, the optic nerve and the eye muscles. In GO, enlarged orbital muscles and increased fat may cause orbital nerve compression or proptosis. Orbital decompression reduces the amount of tissue within the orbit or enlarges the orbit by removing some of the bony supporting walls and expanding the orbit into nearby spaces, most commonly the sinuses. Because patients with GO often have sinus problems, some physicians recommend having simultaneous sinus surgery. Furthermore, orbital decompression increases the risk of sinus disease, and sinus disease can lead to visual disturbances. [27]

Orbital decompression can be considered at any point in which expansion of the bony orbital volume is desired. A second variety of orbital decompression, used on patients with significant orbital fat, removes only orbital fat without removing any bone. This variety is used only after the eye disease has remained stable for at least six months.[28]

Several other surgeries for orbital decompression have evolved over the years, including one, two, three and four wall decompression. All varieties require a skin incision of 5–10 mm at the corner of the eye. There may be temporary discomfort (one to three days), although bruising may

persist for 14 days. Orbital decompression surgery is frequently compli-
cated by worsening of pre-existing diplopia regardless of the method
employed. Additional surgery is often required after an appropriate length
of time to allow for swelling to subside and stabilization of the myopathy.

EFFECTS OF ORBITAL DECOMPRESSION ON EYELID RETRACTION

Lower lid retraction may accompany proptosis, and it frequently
occurs after adjustment of the inferior rectus muscle and may be worsened by orbital decompression. One surgery used to correct lower lid
retraction involves placing a graft from the upper lid into the lower lid.
One surgical procedure used for upper lid retraction is eyelid lengthen-
ing, with or without removal of excess skin or fat deposits (dermatocha-
lasis). Alternately, plastic weights may be inserted in the eyelid and later
be removed if needed.

The Dermopathy of Graves' Disease

The skin conditions associated with Graves' disease may be related
to thyrotoxicosis or autoimmunity, or they may occur as a distinct pecu-
liarity of GD. The major dermopathy, pretibial myxedema (PTM), almost
always accompanies by GO.

Skin Changes Related to Thyrotoxicosis

Changes in metabolic rate due to GD may affect the skin and its
appendages (hair and nails). Many GD patients report increased acne,
which is caused by nutrient deficiencies as well as increased sebum production. Also, the epidermal and dermal tissues of the skin are target
organs since they have their own thyroid hormone receptors. Epidermal
cell division and breakdown (with results similar to exfoliation) are
increased in GD, which partially accounts for the youthful appearance
often seen in GD patients.

The skin in thyrotoxicosis is usually warm and moist with a velvety
texture. Episodic flushing may occur over the face and the throat, and
telangiectac vessels (spider veins and capillaries) may also develop in these
areas. The face, palms and elbows may appear ruddy. Milaria bumps (small
blister like bumps that usually appear on the forehead) may occur as a
result of increased sweating and poral occlusion. Pigment alterations (both
hyperpigmentation and hypopigmentation) sometimes occur in the skin
of patients with thyrotoxicosis. The hyperpigmentation, which is diffuse
and may occur in various parts of the body, may involve genitalia, body
creases and scars.

Hair Changes

Thyrotoxicosis causes increased hair growth by accelerating the growth cycle in hair follicles. However, moderate hair loss occurs in 20 percent to 40 percent of thyrotoxic patients with no relation to disease severity. Axillary hair may also decrease. The hair in thyrotoxicosis is usually fine and soft and is reported to hold a permanent wave poorly, probably because of changes in the protein content.

Almost 25 percent of patients with alopecia areata, a condition of hair loss and thinning, are reported to have thyroid hormone abnormalities or elevation of TPO antibody levels or both, suggesting that autoimmune disease may be associated with this condition.[29]

Fingernail changes

The fingernails in thyrotoxicosis become shiny, soft and brittle because of alterations in the keratin matrix and supporting dermal layers. The rate of nail growth is increased, and longitudinal striations associated with a flattening of the surface contour result in a scoop or shovel appearance. Many patients have onycholysis (distal separation from its underlying bed, also called Plummer's nails). The nail changes in GD resolve spontaneously as hyperthyroidism improves.

Pretibial Myxedema (PTM)

Pretibial myxedema (PTM), which is also known as infiltrative dermopathy and localized myxedema, is a skin disorder that typically affects the anterior surface skin of the lower legs in the pretibial area. PTM is usually confined to the pretibial area including the front of the lower legs, the top of the feet and the toes, although it may involve the arms, face, shoulders and trunk.

PTM, which occurs in about 2 percent to 3 percent of the patients with Graves' disease,[30] is almost always associated with GO, usually of severe degree. However, the condition can occur in patients without thyrotoxicosis, and it is also seen in patients with chronic autoimmune thyroiditis. Older patients are reported to be at more risk of developing pretibial myxedema, and pretibial myxedema frequently occurs in females in their 60s. Females are 3.5 times more likely to be affected than males. The onset of localized myxedema is most frequently seen 12 to 24 months after the diagnosis of thyrotoxicosis[31].

Approximately 5 percent of patients with clinically evident GO develop PTM, and 12 percent to 15 percent of patients with severe GO are affected. In one study, 88 percent of patients with PTM had proptosis.[32] Almost all patients with PTM have high concentrations of TSH receptor

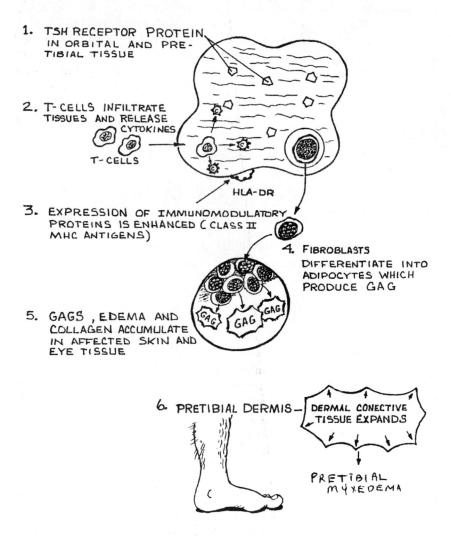

COMMON ANTIGEN THEORY
PRODUCTION OF GAG (GLYCOSAMINOGLYCAN) PRIMARILY HYALURONAN

1. TSH RECEPTOR PROTEIN IN ORBITAL AND PRE-TIBIAL TISSUE

2. T-CELLS INFILTRATE TISSUES AND RELEASE CYTOKINES

   T-CELLS

   HLA-DR

3. EXPRESSION OF IMMUNOMODULATORY PROTEINS IS ENHANCED (CLASS II MHC ANTIGENS)

4. FIBROBLASTS DIFFERENTIATE INTO ADIPOCYTES WHICH PRODUCE GAG

5. GAGS, EDEMA AND COLLAGEN ACCUMULATE IN AFFECTED SKIN AND EYE TISSUE

   GAG GAG GAG

6. PRETIBIAL DERMIS — DERMAL CONECTIVE TISSUE EXPANDS

   PRETIBIAL MYXEDEMA

Common Antigen Theory

antibodies and are reported to have more severe Graves' disease.[33] I'm an exception, having developed PTM after treatment despite having had mild GD and no clinically evident GO. About half of cases occur during the active stage of thyrotoxicosis. The condition can also occur independently of thyrotoxicosis and it may also be seen in patients with HT.

SYMPTOMS

PTM usually begins with raised waxy reddish-brown plaques and papules that develop on the front of the shin. The lesions are thought to be only of cosmetic importance, although large lesions can cause nerve entrapment. The affected area differs from normal skin by virtue of the skin being raised and thickened with a *peau d'orange* appearance that may be pruritic (itchy) and hyperpigmented.

The lesions of PTM are usually discrete with a sometimes waxy, nodular configuration, but in some instances they appear to have merged in with the normal tissue surface. The lesions and affected tissue have accumulations of GAG, the same substance found in the retroorbital tissue of patients with GO.

In PTM, GAG is diffusely dispersed in the reticular part of the dermis and rarely in the innermost papillary dermis. PTM is structurally similar to hypothyroid myxedema, but in PTM, hyperkeratosis (resulting in thicker, leathery skin), greater abundance of GAG (rendering a swollen appearance), and mononuclear cell infiltration are more typically seen.

The localized myxedema of GD may appear in several clinical forms: diffuse, nonpitting edema (most common occurrence), raised lesions on a background of nonpitting edema, sharply diffused nodular lesions, and the relatively rare elephantiasic form, consisting of nodular lesions mixed with lymphedema that do not ulcerate.

TREATMENT

Usually treatment isn't needed, but in severe cases, application of a high potency fluorinated corticosteroid cream offers improvement. Nightly application of this cream covered by cellophane or plastic film has been reported to reduce symptoms. Systemic corticosteroid therapy may also help.[34] Plasmapheresis has also helped extremely severe lesions transiently improve.[35] And in severe cases, intravenous immunoglobulins are sometimes used, although their effects are also transient and the procedure is costly.

Vitiligo

Vitiligo is a pigmentation disorder in which melanocytes (cells that manufacture pigment) in the skin, mucous membranes, and the retina are destroyed. Consequently, white patches of unpigmented skin appear, and hair growing on the affected area may turn white. An autoimmune disease, vitiligo is listed here because the incidence of vitiligo in GD is reported to be 7 percent.[36] Ninety-five percent of people with vitiligo develop it before they are 40. The disorder affects all races and sexes equally.

Researchers suspect that vitiligo is caused by antibodies that destroy

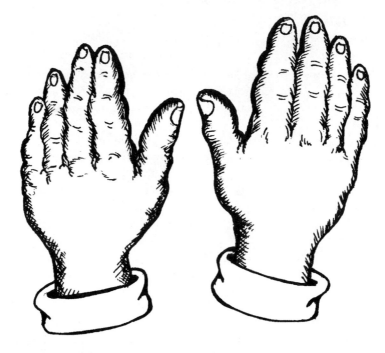

Acropachy: A dermatological condition seen in Graves' Disease which is character-
ized by soft connective tissue swelling.

melanocytes. Some patients have reported that a single event such as sun-
burn or stress triggered their condition. Vitiligo appears to be more common in people with certain autoimmune diseases, including GD, although
most people with vitiligo have no other autoimmune condition.

Current treatment options include medical, surgical and adjunctive
or complementary treatments. Psoralen photochemotherapy (psoralen and
ultraviolet A therapy or PUVA) is probably the most beneficial treatment
available today, although its use is time consuming.[37]

Thyroid Acropachy

Thyroid acropachy, a disorder characterized by soft tissue swelling
that usually affects the hands and feet, is the least common manifestation
of GD. Acropachy usually appears in combination with GO or PTM.
Although patients with acropachy usually have a history of thyrotoxicosis, the disorder may occur in euthyroid patients and in patients with
autoimmune hypothyroidism. Symptoms of acropachy are rarely the first
GD symptoms to occur. The usual order is thyroid dysfunction, followed
by GO, dermopathy and acropachy. Only 7 percent of patients with PTM

exhibit thyroid acropachy.[38] Acropachy represents the sole instance in GD in which males and females are affected equally. Although it usually occurs two to three years after symptoms of hyperthyroidism, acropachy can occur as late as 40 years after the onset of thyroid dysfunction.[39]

PATHOLOGY AND DIAGNOSIS

Acropachy typically causes asymmetric soft tissue swelling of the hands and feet, usually in association with clubbing of the fingers and toes, which is considered a different disorder. Although tissue swelling is pronounced, the joints remain unaffected. The skin is commonly pigmented and leathery with equal involvement of upper and lower extremities. Although it is generally considered painless, some patients with acropachy have lymphatic obstruction, extreme swelling, loss of function and considerable pain.

Imaging studies reveal fusiform soft tissue swelling of the digits along with subperiosteal bone formation. The metacarpals, the proximal and middle phalanges of the fingers, and the metatarsal and proximal phalanges of the toes are usually targeted, whereas the long bones of the extremities are rarely involved. The skin is similar to that seen in PTM with fibroblast activation and GAG deposits. The pathology of thyroid acropachy remains unclear but the disease process suggests that there is autoimmune activation of periosteal bone fibroblast cells.[40] Treatment consists of local corticosteroid therapy covered by occlusive compression dressings.

5 *The Diagnosis of Graves' Disease*

Chapter five discusses the physical signs and symptoms, the clues found in family history, and the laboratory and imaging test results which, when viewed together, lead to a diagnosis of Graves' disease. Also described are other medical conditions that may be confused with GD and often must be ruled out before a diagnosis of GD can be made.

Usually, GD is first suspected when patients complain to their doctor about certain symptoms such as an elevated heart rate or goiter. Laboratory tests for thyroid function confirm the diagnosis of hyperthyroidism, and thyroid antibody titers or radioiodine uptake scans confirm Graves' disease. For patients with mild or no symptoms, GD may be first suspected when routine laboratory tests are abnormal. Asymptomatic (without symptoms) patients who only have suppressed TSH levels are said to have subclinical Graves' disease.

Diagnostic Clues

In women between the ages of 20 to 50, or patients with a family history of autoimmune or thyroid disorders, GD should be suspected when several characteristic symptoms are present. However, even in patients with obvious symptoms, GD is often misdiagnosed, especially if one symptom skews the clinical picture. One young adult male reported that his employer and his doctor were both convinced that he was a drug addict because of his weight loss, flushed appearance and hand tremor. Subjected to several drug screens which proved negative, his diagnosis was delayed for six months. Meanwhile, he suffered undue anguish, stressed by the accusations and frightened by his symptoms.

Disorders Related to the Development of Graves' Disease

Conditions thought to increase the risk of autoimmune thyroid disease include Down's syndrome, Turner's syndrome (ovarian disorder), manic depression, and having a family history of Alzheimer's disease,[1] a disorder my mother had.

Development of GD After Treatment for Other Conditions

GD may occur after patients undergo treatment for other conditions. In one study, a patient developed GD after being treated with radioiodine for a thyroid adenoma.[2] In another study, one third of multiple sclerosis (MS) patients treated with a monoclonal antibody used to lower their white blood cell count developed GD within six months.[3] In yet another report, one MS patient developed GD after being treated with interferon beta-1b.[4]

Graves' disease and other AITDs are more prevalent in patients diagnosed with breast cancer.[5] In a recent review of breast cancer and thyroid disease conducted by Johns Hopkins University, a slight increase in breast cancer among GD patients was reported. This report concludes that the increased risk may result from treatment with I-131.[6]

Several studies report a disproportionate increase in dyslexia and left-handedness in patients with autoimmune diseases. Because so many dyslexics are male and left-handed, it has been postulated that in these instances autoimmunity may be related to the suppression of the thymus by testosterone. Since the thymus plays a significant role in the maturation of the immune system, its suppression by testosterone could be the link in males.[7]

Coexisting Autoimmune Conditions

The most important autoimmune endocrine disorders that coexist with both GD and HT include type 1 diabetes mellitus, Addison's disease, autoimmune oophritis (an ovarian disorder), and autoimmune hypoparathyroidism. The late John Fitzgerald Kennedy, Jr., was said to have Addison's disease, which his father had, as well as GD.[8]

In addition to the link with autoimmune endocrine diseases, a relation exists between GD and several non-endocrine autoimmune diseases arising from the same embryonic endoderm, including pernicious anemia, atrophic gastritis, myasthenia gravis, Sjögren's syndrome, chronic active hepatitis and primary biliary cirrhosis (see chapter 6).

The Diagnostic Exam

Once Graves' disease is suspected, the physical examination focuses on discerning characteristic symptoms such as goiter, tachycardia and exophthalmos. To check for goiter, the patient is seated with the neck moderately extended. The patient may be asked to drink a glass of water to facilitate swallowing. If a mass is present when the patient swallows, it is observed for movement. Goiterous masses exhibit movement unless the patient has a retrosternal goiter and the mass is obscured. The thyroid is palpated by the doctor placing light pressure on the neck with his fingers and probing the area for nodules. Vigorous palpation can exacerbate symptoms and is one of the causes of thyroid storm.

The thyroid gland, in severe cases of Graves' disease, may exhibit a noticeable "thrill" on palpation and an audible "bruit" (these terms respectively refer to the feel and sound of increased blood flow). A systolic or continuous bruit is commonly heard over the hyperplastic hyperactive thyroid gland associated with active GD.

Diseases Often Confused with Graves' Disease

Although GD is the most common cause of hyperthyroidism, it's important to differentiate it from other disorders or causes of hyperthyroidism since treatments vary. For instance, therapies for GD would not be effective for subacute bacterial thyroiditis.

Hereditary Hyperthyroidism

A distinct hereditary form of hyperthyroidism is often confused with GD. In hereditary hyperthyroidism, patients have a diffuse painless goiter, symptoms of thyrotoxicosis, accelerated bone maturation, and an elevated radioiodine uptake test. However, there are no signs of autoimmunity such as the thyroid autoantibodies typically seen in GD. Transmission appears to be autosomal dominant. Here, and also in the following three disorders, a negative thyroid antibody test helps confirm the diagnosis.

Hyperthyroidism Caused by
a Mutation to the TSH Receptor

Another condition resembling the hyperthyroidism of Graves' disease is caused by a mutation of one amino acid in the TSH receptor. This mutation occurs in the putative binding site region for TSH and TSH stimulating immunoglobulins. The mutation was found in the genomic DNA of the thyroid but not in the tongue, epidermis or lymphocytes. Therefore, it is not considered a polymorphism, but rather a somatic mutation.[9]

Fatigue

GD is most often misdiagnosed as anxiety. Similar to GD, anxiety disorders are characterized by symptoms of fatigue, heart palpitations, tachycardia, nervous irritability and insomnia. Fatigue differs in that the fatigued individual has no psychological desire to be active. Unlike most patients with GD, fatigued patients are often listless and often feel exhausted on awakening. Also, the pulse in fatigue is normal, whereas in GD, it frequently remains elevated even at rest. Also, the palms are cool and clammy in fatigue. In GD they are warm and moist. Reflexes are faster than normal in both conditions.

The laboratory helps distinguish GD from fatigue. In fatigue, laboratory thyroid function tests are normal unless there is an underlying disorder such as anorexia nervosa or endogenous depression that may cause a depressed TSH.

Chronic Obstructive Pulmonary Disease

Chronic obstructive pulmonary disease (COPD), a respiratory disorder, may lead to a warm, flushed skin, tremulousness and a bounding pulse, especially when in association with increased blood levels of carbon dioxide. Mild exophthalmos may occur in both disorders. And corticosteroids used to treat COPD may suppress TSH, causing low blood levels regardless of thyroid function, making diagnosis difficult. However, in COPD, levels of T4, or T3 or both are generally normal or low, whereas in GD, they're elevated.

Pheochromocytoma

Pheochromocytoma, a condition of excess catecholamines usually caused by a tumor, is characterized by tachycardia, increased sweating, hypermetabolism and hot flashes. Other similarities to GD include nervous irritability, eyelid retraction and tremulousness. Weight loss may occur despite a healthy appetite, and hyperglycemia can occur. However, in pheochromocytoma, thyroid function tests should be normal while blood and urine catecholamine levels are elevated. Also, diastolic hypertension is often present in pheochromocytoma whereas diastolic blood pressure is reduced in GD.

Familial Dysalbuminemic Hyperthyroxinemia

Familial dysalbuminemic hyperthyroxinemia is a condition characterized by increased levels of both total and free T4 caused by a hereditary protein defect. An abnormal type of albumin is present that causes increased thyroid hormone binding. The altered protein in this condition preferentially binds T4 but it doesn't bind T3. Thus, levels of T4 and FT4 are increased although T3, FT3 and TSH are normal.[10]

Laboratory Evaluation of Graves' Disease

In the routine physical exam, certain abnormal results detected in a chemistry profile may suggest thyrotoxicosis. These abnormalities include decreased cholesterol, high concentrations of alkaline phosphatase (a bone and liver enzyme) and increased calcium.

Laboratory thyroid function tests may include levels of:

1. Thyroid hormones, thyroxine (T4) and triiodothyronine (T3). Although total hormone determinations (total T4 or total T3) are still available, most doctors order free thyroid hormone levels (available to the body's cells), free T4 (FT4) and free T3 (FT3). Reverse T3 (rT3) is used to explain abnormal T3 results in non-thyroidal illness.
2. The pituitary hormone TSH (thyroid stimulating hormone), which is a valuable indicator of thyroid function
3. Thyroid antibodies
4. Thyroid proteins
5. Tests of dynamic thyroid function

Clinical Laboratory Picture in Graves' Disease

In active Graves' disease, TSH is suppressed, often to <0.01 mIU/L, and total and free T4 and/or T3 levels are high. Thyroid antibodies confirm AITD, with stimulating antibodies to the TSH receptor (TSI or stimulating TRAb) diagnostic for GD (a normal TSH and the absence of TSH receptor antibodies doesn't exclude GD when thyroid hormone levels are elevated). Thyroid proteins are used to further evaluate results when T4 and T3 levels are high despite a normal TSH and an absence of symptoms. Tests of dynamic thyroid function are used to evaluate TSH suppression in hypothyroidism.

Often, conversion of T4 to T3 is impaired, resulting in a normal T3 and an elevated FT4 (T4 toxicosis). Occasionally, the discrepancy between T4 and T3 levels may be exaggerated with T4 being normal and T3 alone being elevated (T3 toxicosis). In GD, T3 elevation is often proportionately higher than T4 elevation. In this instance, the RAI uptake test may be normal,[11] confusing diagnosis.

A Note About Reference Values

Reference values (normal ranges) and units of measurement vary depending on the method used. All results must be compared to the range employed by the testing laboratory. Units of measurement indicate the amount of a substance present in a known volume. Results given in mcg/ml, for example, indicate how many micrograms are present in one milliliter of serum. Reference values for the following tests are listed as general guidelines.

T4 (Thyroxine), Total

T4 is the major thyroid hormone with blood levels ten to 20 times that of T3. Total T4 reflects the thyroid's ability to secrete hormone. In blood, most T4 is bound (linked) to protein and unavailable to cells. Changes in binding proteins (due to certain physiological conditions or medications) alter the total T4 concentration but rarely affect the FT4.

Reference Range: Adults = 5.0–12.5 ug/dL or 0.8–1.5 ng/dL
0–4 days (neonates) = 5.9–15.0 ug/dL
21 weeks up to 20 years = 5.6–14.9 ug/dL

Interpretation: T4 levels are elevated in hyperthyroidism and when TBG and transthyretin levels and are increased (in estrogen therapy, pregnancy, certain drugs). T4 is decreased in pituitary TSH deficiency, primary hypothyroidism, hypothalamic TRH deficiency, nonthyroidal illness, and when levels of TBG are decreased. Other causes of altered T4 results include psychiatric disease, and medications including amiodarone, amphetamine, heparin, heroin, propranolol and iodine-containing radio-contrast media.[12]

Serious illness (non-thyroidal illness) such as trauma or surgery depresses T4 level in 25 percent of patients; consequently, in severely ill or hospitalized patients, the total T4 result may not accurately reflect thyroid status. In patients with normal TBG levels and no evidence of co-existing non-thyroidal illness, T4 is a good index of thyroid function.[13]

Free T4 (FT4, Free Thyroxine)

Free T4 or FT4 (approximately 0.03 percent of total T4) represents the T4 fraction which has been cleaved from its carrier protein and is available for use by the body's tissues. FT4 levels are controlled by a negative feedback mechanism causing constant levels of FT4 regardless of the binding protein concentration. Some immunoassays may provide falsely low results due to nonspecific reactions with reagent proteins. The most accurate determinations of FT4 employ dialysis methods.[14]

Reference Values: Non-dialysis methods: 0.8–1.5 ng/dL for adults
Non-dialysis methods: 0.8–2.0 ng/dL for ages 2 weeks up to 21 years
Direct dialysis methods: 0.8–2.7 ng/dL for ages 21–87 years

Interpretation: FT4 levels indicate the amount of thyroxine available for use by the tissues and cells in both hypothyroidism (low levels) and hyperthyroidism (high levels). TSH and FT4 are recommended as the initial step in evaluating patients with suspected thyroid disorders. In nonthyroidal illness, FT4 is usually normal or slightly elevated although it is true that 50 percent of severely ill hospitalized patients show decreased FT4 levels.

T3 (TRIIODOTHYRONINE), TOTAL

T3 is more metabolically active, but its effects are briefer. About 20 percent of T3 is produced in the thyroid gland, and 80 percent is produced by conversion from T4. T3 may be affected by increased binding proteins and is often low in sick or hospitalized patients.

Reference Values: 94–269 ng/dL for 1–9 years
80–213 ng/dL for 10–20 years
70–180 ng/dL for 21–87 years[15] or 0.6–1.8 ug/dL[16]

Interpretation: Elevated total T3 levels may occur in pregnancy, during estrogen therapy, and in infectious hepatitis. Depressed T3 levels occur in drug therapy with dexamethasone and glucocorticoids, and in iodine deficiency. T3 values >230 ng/dL are consistent with hyperthyroidism or increased binding proteins.[17] T3 levels are necessary to assess patients suspected of having thyrotoxicosis when TSH is decreased and the FT4 value is normal. In extremely sick hospitalized patients, T3 is decreased and reverse T3 is increased.

FREE T3 (FT3, FREE TRIIODOTHYRONINE)

Normally, T3 circulates tightly bound to thyroxine binding globulin (TBG) and albumin. Only 0.3 percent of the total T3 is unbound or free, and this portion is the active form since it reacts with the body's cells. Elevations in FT3 are associated with thyrotoxicosis or excess thyroid hormone therapy. FT3 is performed by dialysis or non-dialysis methods.

Reference Values: Adults
230–420 pg/dL or 2.3–4.2 pmol/L or 2.0–5.0 ng/L in non-dialysis assays
210–440 pg/dL or 2.1–4.4 pmol/L and 200–380 pg/dL in pregnancy in tracer dialysis assays

Interpretation: When increased plasma thyroxine binding globulin (TBG) concentration is suspected as the cause of an elevated total T3, the FT3 dialysis assay can differentiate this condition. FT3 is increased in GD, T3 thyrotoxicosis, thyroid hormone resistance and in functional thyroid adenoma. FT3 is decreased in nonthyroidal illness and hypothyroidism. FT3 and T3 may be superior to FT4 and T4 for the monitoring of patients receiving thyroid replacement therapy.[18]

REVERSE T3 (RT3)

Reverse T3, a thyroid hormone considered metabolically inactive, differs from T3 in the positions of its iodine atoms. Increased rT3 is produced at the expense of T3.[19] RT3 is formed in conditions where adequate T3 is not needed and where its effects might be harmful. Since the introduction of FT3 assays, reverse T3 levels are rarely ordered.

Reference Values:

Adults: 10–24 ng/dL or 0.18–0.51 nmol/L

1 month up to 20 years: 10–35 ng/dL

Cord Blood: 102–342 ng/dL

Interpretation: Reverse T3 is increased in the euthyroid sick syndrome seen in many chronically ill patients, the fetus and newborn, low T3 syndrome, hyperthyroidism, fasting, malnutrition, anorexia nervosa, poorly controlled diabetes mellitus, trauma, heat stroke, surgery and systemic illness. Reverse T3 is decreased in hypothyroidism.

THYROID STIMULATING HORMONE (TSH, THYROTROPIN)

Thyrotropin or TSH is a pituitary hormone that regulates levels of thyroid hormone in the blood. TSH is considered to be far more sensitive than FT4 in detecting changes in thyroid function, because small changes in FT4 away from the normal set-point cause large changes in TSH concentration. However, after ablative treatment, it may take many weeks to many months for TSH to adequately reflect thyroid function.

Reference Values: 0.4–5.0 mIU/L, Borderline Hypothyroid: 5.1–7.0 mIU/L

In screening for thyroid disorders, a TSH concentration between 0.3 and 5.0 mIU/L suggests euthyroidism. TSH levels <0.1 mIU/L suggest a diagnosis of hyperthyroidism and TSH concentrations >7.0 mIU/L suggest hypothyroidism.

Interpretation: In active GD, levels of TSH are low, often <0.01. In primary hypothyroidism, TSH is elevated. Typically, a minimum of six to eight weeks of lag time are required to achieve normal TSH levels upon initiation of thyroid hormone replacement therapy.[20]

Serum TSH concentrations begin to rise several hours before the onset of sleep, reaching maximal concentrations between 11 P.M. and 6 A.M., then declining with the lowest concentrations occurring at 11 A.M. The diurnal variation in TSH level approximates + 50 percent; consequently, time of day may influence the measured TSH concentration. Daytime TSH levels vary by less than 10 percent.[21] TSH values decline with surgical stress, caloric restriction, and certain psychological states such as anorexia nervosa and depression.[22] Dopamine, glucocorticoids and bromocriptine cause a transient suppression of TSH.

Increased TSH Sensitivity
(S-TSH and Third Generation Tests)

Today's fourth generation TSH assays, performed at most reference laboratories, detect levels as low as 0.001 mIu/L. However, most clinical laboratories use immunoassay methods sensitive to 0.03 mIu/ml. Fourth generation methods are recommended for monitoring T4 replacement or suppressive (used in cancer) therapy.

THYROXINE BINDING GLOBULIN (TBG)

TBG, a protein produced in the liver, binds both T4 and T3. Because TBG accounts for 75 percent of plasma protein thyroxine-binding activity, increased levels of TBG alter T4 and T3 concentrations. TBG levels are high at birth, peaking at about the fifth day.

Reference Values:	Females	Males
1–5 days	2.2–4.2 mg/dL	2.2–4.2 mg/dL
1–9 years	1.5–2.7 mg/dL	1.2–2.8 mg/dL
10–19 years	1.4–3.0 mg/dL	1.4–2.6 mg/dL
20–90 years	1.7–3.6 mg/dL	1.7–3.6 mg/dL

Interpretation: TBG concentration should be interpreted in conjunction with the T4 results. The T4/TBG ratio should be 0.25–0.60. Elevated ratios indicate hyperthyroidism and reduced ratios indicate hypothyroidism.[23] Certain diseases and medications alter serum TBG levels. TBG is increased by estrogen therapy, oral contraceptive agents, tamoxifen (despite being an estrogen antagonist), pregnancy and hepatitis. TBG may be decreased in cirrhosis, in the nephrotic syndrome and by androgens including anabolic steroids. The non-steroidal anti-inflammatory drugs fenclofenac, mefenamic acid, aspirin and salicylate compete with T4 for binding to TBG, with effects depending on the total drug concentration. Therapeutic doses of salicylate lower serum T4 by 40 percent and T3 by 30 percent.

THYROGLOBULIN (hTG)

Thyroglobulin is a large molecular weight protein produced by the thyroid gland. Normally hTG is found only in the thyroid. Thyroglobulin is released in certain conditions, particularly thyroid cancers, and in hyperthyroidism.

Reference Values: <59.4 ng/ml in patients with normal thyroids
<5 ng/ml in patients without thyroid glands

Interpretation: The serum thyroglobulin level reflects physical damage or inflammation of the thyroid gland as well as the magnitude of TSH stimulation. All forms of TSH dependent hyperthyroidism, including GD, toxic nodular goiter and thyroiditis cause elevated serum thyroglobulin.

The main uses of thyroglobulin levels are for post-operative monitoring of patients with thyroid cancers, differential diagnosis of hyperthyroidism due to exogenous causes (with excess replacement thyroid, thyroglobulin levels are low), and for determining in hypothyroid infants if there is any functional thyroid tissue present.

Cautions: Thyroglobulin autoantibodies interfere in this assay. Anti-thyroglobulin antibodies are measured in all samples.

T3 UPTAKE (TBG ASSESSMENT)

The T3 uptake test is used to assess the protein binding capacity of thyroxine (T4). Fluctuations in TBG concentrations lead to changes in T4 and T3 levels. The test is based on the ability of TBG to bind with T3 tracer and provides an indirect measurement of TBG.

Reference Values: 26 percent to 40 percent uptake

Interpretation: The T3 uptake test is increased in hyperthyroidism, renal failure and malnutrition and decreased in hypothyroidism, pregnancy and acute hepatitis.

Thyroid Autoantibodies

Although thyroglobulin and TPO autoantibodies confirm or rule out sutoimmune thyroid disease (AITD), the stimulating TRAb test (TSI, stimulating TRAb) is used to confirm GD. The absence of TSI, however, doesn't exclude a diagnosis of GD since antibodies may form circulating immune complexes (CICs) and thereby escape detection. Most patients with AITD have a combination of thyroid antibodies. TPO antibodies seen in 90 percent of patients with HT, and TSI antibodies are present in 70 percent of patients with GD. However, when antithyroglobulin antibodies are also tested in HT patients, and TBII and TGI are also tested in GD patients, test positivity increases to 95 percent and 90 percent, respectively.[24]

TSH (THYROTROPIN) RECEPTOR ANTIBODIES

There are three types of TSH receptor antibodies: stimulating, blocking and binding. In active GD, the characteristic TSH receptor antibody is a stimulating type (Stimulating TSH [thyrotropin] receptor antibody or TRAb, stimulating type, TSAb or thyroid stimulating immunoglobulin [TSI]). TSI acts as an agonist, mimicking TSH and causing excess thyroid hormone production. TSI are diagnostic for GD and the cause of Graves' hyperthyroidism. GD patients usually have a combination of TRAb, with TSI predominating. According to Specialty Laboratories, TSI are present in 95 percent of GD patients[25] (some TSI methods include measurement of TBII). Higher TSI titers are seen in patients with active

GD, large goiters, severe exophthalmos or pretibial myxedema. On occasion, TSI may be present years after ablative treatment.

The presence of thryrotropin receptor blocking antibodies (TRBAb, TSBAb) in patients with GD usually causes no symptoms, but when they predominate, they may cause hypothyroidism, especially after treatment when TSI levels decline and blocking antibodies appear.[26] Blocking antibodies inhibit TSH–generated cAMP in thyroid cells. In some laboratories, total TRAb is measured by TSI assay. Discrepancies usually are due to the presence of TRBAb.[27] TSBAb are more often seen in atrophic thyroiditis and severe hypothyroidism, but atrophic thyroiditis may occur in the absence of blocking antibodies. Blocking antibodies are seen in 59 percent of patients with nongoitrous autoimmune thyroiditis and 10 percent of patients with goitrous autoimmune thyroiditis.[28]

Thryotropin receptor binding inhibitory antibodies (TRAb, binding type, TBII) interfere with the binding of TSH to the receptor and are commonly seen in atrophic (condition where thyroid cells atrophy, leading to hypothyroidism) rather than goitrous thyroiditis. Assays for binding TRAb frequently reflect the presence of either or both the stimulatory and inhibitory immunoglobulin classes since both types bind to the TSH receptor. Thus, in some assays, a measure of TBII includes TSI.

TRAb Reference Ranges:
>   TRAb, stimulating type (TSAb, TSI) = <130 percent of basal activity
>   Indications: Increased in Graves' disease, Hashitoxicosis and neonatal thyrotoxicosis
>   TRAb, binding type (TBII or Thyrotropin-binding inhibitory immunoglobulin) = <10 percent inhibition
>   10 percent to 100 percent inhibition in Graves' disease
>   Indications: Increased in Graves' disease, atrophic thyroiditis, postpartum autoimmune thyroid disease, neonatal Graves' disease and transient neonatal hypothyroidism.
>   TRAb, blocking type (TBAb or Thyrotropin-blocking antibody) = <10 percent inhibition
>   Indications: Increased in atrophic thyroiditis, Hashimoto's thyroiditis, and transient congenital hypothyroidism

The Use of TSI Levels to Monitor Treatment

Jeannette, a marriage and family counselor, described the benefits of antibody titers in her own therapy. Her high TSI titer established a baseline for her immune dysfunction and confirmed her diagnosis. Midway through her course of antithyroid drug treatment, she had a second TSI titer which was much lower, indicating that she was responding to treatment and unlikely to have a relapse upon discontinuing treatment. She has currently been in remission for more than two years.

Jeannette also reported that shortly after her diagnosis of Graves' disease, her brother developed symptoms of GD. However, his negative thyroid antibody results indicated that he didn't have AITD. He was subsequently diagnosed with acute bacterial thyroiditis due to an infection he developed following sinus surgery.

Other Thyroid Autoantibodies Seen in Graves' Disease

The thyroid autoantibodies most frequently seen in GD, besides TSH receptor antibodies, are antibodies to thyroglobulin and thyroid peroxidase, and thyroid growth stimulating immunoglobulins (TGI). Antibodies to T4, T3 and TSH occasionally exist in patients with AITD but they're rarely tested. Using sensitive assays, about 25 percent of normal women and about 10 percent of normal men have autoantibodies to thyroid peroxidase (TPO) or thyroglobulin, making them less specific of an indicator.[29]

THYROID GROWTH STIMULATING IMMUNOGLOBULINS

Autoantibodies with the ability to increase DNA synthesis in thyrocytes (pituitary cells that produce thyrotropin) are termed thyroid growth stimulating immunoglobulins (TGI). TGI are seen in patients with GD, autoimmune thyroiditis and nonspecific goiter. When GD patients are tested for both TGI and TSI, nearly 100 percent of patients are positive for one or the other antibody.[30]

Reference Range <130 percent of basal activity

Interpretation: Used in the diagnosis of Graves' disease and for differential diagnosis of goiter. Increased in Graves' disease, autoimmune thyroiditis and nonspecific goiter.

ANTITHYROGLOBULIN ANTIBODIES (TGAB, ATG, ATA)

Antithyroglobulin antibodies (TgAb or ATG) were the first antibodies to be discovered. TgAb are seen in most patients with Hashimoto's thyroiditis and in 50 percent of patients with GD. The prevalence of TgAb in normal women is 18 percent, with higher frequencies in older women (30 percent). In men the prevalence is much lower (3 to 6 percent). In all cases the prevalence of TgAb increases with age.[31]

Reference Range = <2 IU/ml

Indications: Indicated for confirmation of autoimmune thyroid disease, screening before thyroglobulin assay. The test may be used to distinguish GD from toxic nodular goiter. Increased in HT, Graves' disease and postpartum thyroiditis.

Interferences: Antithyroglobulin antibodies interfere with measurement of thyroglobulin.

THYROID PEROXIDASE ANTIBODIES (TPO AB) AND ANTIMICROSOMAL ANTIBODIES

Thyroid microsomal antigen is a component of the carrier vesicles in which newly synthesized thyroglobulin is transferred to the follicular lumen for storage. The primary autoantigen (element eliciting an autoimmune response) in the microsomal particle is the enzyme thyroid peroxidase (TPO).

Thyroid peroxidase antibodies (TPO Ab) are a more sensitive determinator of the microsomal particle of thyroid cells. In the laboratory, TPO Ab have replaced anti-microsomal antibodies. When either antibody titer is ordered, the test for TPO Ab is usually performed. TPO Ab are present in the serum of almost all patients with HT and 57 to 88 percent of patients with GD. The highest titers are found in hypothyroid patients with HT. Low level antibody titers are found in 10 to 13 percent of normal women and 3 percent of normal men.[32]

Euthyroid patients with high titers of TPO antibodies and increasing levels of TSH are thought to have a 3 percent to 4 percent chance each year of developing hypothyroidism.

Reference Range = <2.0 Iu/ml

Interpretation: Indicated for confirmation of autoimmune thyroid disease.

Elevated in Hashimoto's thyroiditis, Primary hypothyroidism (due to HT), Graves' disease and postpartum thyroiditis.

ANTI-TSH AUTOANTIBODY

Patients with GD may rarely develop antibodies to TSH. Anti–TSH antibodies interfere with serum TSH assays. When a patient has low serum TSH and low free thyroid hormone concentrations, it is appropriate to determine if anti–TSH antibodies are present.

Reference Range = Negative

Indications: Indicated for evaluation of discordant serum TSH levels. Increased in autoimmune thyroid disease and other autoimmune disease states.

ANTI-T3 AUTOANTIBODY

Patients with AITD, including GD, may rarely develop antibodies to T3. Anti–T3 antibodies interfere with assay measurement of T3. When a patient has a serum T3 concentration that is discordant with other test results, e.g., elevated T3 with normal TSH, it may be appropriate to determine if anti–T3 antibodies are present.

Reference Range = Negative

Indications: Indicated for evaluation of discordant serum T3 levels. Elevated in autoimmune thyroid disease and other autoimmune disease states.

ANTI-T4 AUTOANTIBODY

Patients with AITD, including GD, may rarely develop antibodies to T4.

Reference Range = Negative

Indications: Indicated when a patient has a serum T4 concentration that is discordant with other test results, e.g. elevated serum T4 alone in the absence of TBG excess and presence of a detectable serum TSH concentration.

Tests of Dynamic Thyroid Function

THRYOTROPIN RELEASING HORMONE (TRH) STIMULATION TEST

The TRH stimulation test is used to assess pituitary thyrotropin (TSH) and prolactin reserves, to establish TSH suppression by thyroid hormone, to confirm endogenous hyperthyroidism, or to monitor thyroid hormone suppression therapy.

Procedure: Blood is drawn for a baseline TSH determination. With the patient recumbent, 200–500 ug (5–7 ug/kg in children) of TRH is administered as an intravenous bolus. For assessment of pituitary TSH reserve, samples are drawn at 30 minutes and 60 minutes after the dose. For evaluation of TRH suppression, a 30 minute sample is drawn.

Interpretation: Normally the serum TSH rises to 7–30 mU/L following TRH administration. A peak value between 0.1 and 7 mU/L is considered "blunted." The increase in TSH should be at least 6 m/L in males and in females younger than 40, and 1 mU/ml in males over 40. Simultaneous measurements of prolactin should show a two to three fold increase. Blunted TSH responses may occur in hypopituitarism, hyperthyroidism, nonthyroidal illness, depression and Cushing disease (an adrenal disorder).

An exaggerated TSH increase indicates low-grade hypothyroidism even if the basal TSH level is normal. When the thyroid gland is minimally failing, the pituitary gland contains greater amounts of TSH. In response to TRH administration, high amounts of TSH are released. When there is thyroid hormone excess, the thyroid contains little TSH.[33]

Cautions: Since TRH may cause transient hypertension or hypotension, this test is rarely used in the assessment of Graves' disease. It is more likely to be used in hypothyroid Graves' patients (after ablative treatment) who continue to have suppressed TSH levels.

Lab Test Interferences

Certain drugs directly interfere with thyroid laboratory tests because they cause changes in the absorption of thyroid hormone in the body, or in the body's ability to convert T4 into T3. Medications and other substances can cause markedly different results when blood samples are obtained shortly after ingestion of the interfering substance.

Abnormal thyroid function test results aren't always related to abnormal thyroid function. Besides interferences from medicines, the non-thyroidal sick state causes suppressed hormone levels. In evaluating lab results, the effects of interfering medications (along with the time of last dose and dietary influences) as well as the patient's condition and symptoms must be taken into consideration. The following medications and conditions can influence thyroid laboratory tests.

- Medications affecting liver function (acetaminophen, vitamin A derivatives) accelerate T4 metabolism causing disproportionately high levels of T3.
- Anticonvulsants: Both phenobarbital and phenytoin (Dilantin) inhibit TSH secretion in rats. At concentrations above the therapeutic range, phenytoin inhibits T4 binding to TBG and induces accelerated metabolism of T4 with increased conversion to T3. The net result is a 15-20 percent lowering of T4 and FT4. Phenytoin has been shown to interfere with binding of T3 to pituitary receptors. Carbamazepine (Tegretol) has similar effects.[34]
- Dopamine (L-dopa) and bromocriptine produce a prompt, transient suppression of TSH secretion and radioiodine uptake.
- Glucocorticoids, particularly in "stress" doses inhibit TSH secretion acutely, decrease serum TBG and impair the conversion of T4 to T3. The net effects are a low T4 and a slightly decreased FT4, a low or very low T3, and a low TSH. In patients with primary hypothyroidism, TSH may be suppressed into the normal range, confusing diagnosis.
- Androgens, including anabolic steroids, decrease TBG levels in the blood, thereby lowering T4 and T3 while leaving FT3 and FT4 unaffected.
- Estrogens, Tamoxifen, Methadone, and heroin increase the level of TBG and its binding in the blood, increasing T4 and T3 while leaving FT3 and FT4 unaffected.[35]
- Beta adrenergic receptor antagonists (propranolol, metoprolol) and calcium channel blocker drugs inhibit the conversion of T4 to T3 resulting in decreased T3 and FT3.

- Iron, aluminum and calcium may prevent the complete absorption of T4 if ingested within two hours of a therapeutic dose. Lithium causes decreased levels of both T4 and T3.
- Amphetamine abuse causes an increase in total T4 and FT4.[36]
- The non-steroidal anti-inflammatory drugs (NSAIDs) fenclofenac, mefenamic acid, aspirin and furosemide compete with T4 for binding to TBG. The effect depends on the total drug concentration. Therapeutic doses of salicylate (aspirin) lower serum total T4 by 40 percent and serum T3 by 30 percent. Naproxen lowers serum T3, but not T4, while TSH isn't altered. NSAIDs and free fatty acids have been shown to displace T3 from binding to nuclear receptors, diminishing the effects of T3.[37]
- Amiodarone contains 37 percent iodine. Thus, some effects occur while the drug slowly metabolizes. Amiodarone impedes the conversion of T4 to T3 with resulting decreases in T3 and rT3. Because metabolism is lowered, levels of T4 and FT4 are increased.
- Sertaline (Zoloft) is associated with elevated TSH levels in patients treated with thyroxine, indicating a decrease in the effectiveness of their thyroxine.[38]
- A transient elevation of FT4 occurs in acute psychosis, estrogen withdrawal, iodine administration, the onset of T4 therapy (until levels stabilize), gallbladder contrast agents, initial response to high altitude exposure and selenium deficiency due to decreased peripheral conversion of T4.[39]

Imaging Tests

Although ultrasonography is occasionally used to determine thyroid volume or size or to detect nodules, the test most often used diagnostically is the radioiodine uptake scan (RAI-U). Except in cases of excess iodine ingestion or transient bacterial thyroiditis, radioiodine uptake is elevated in most all instances of hyperthyroidism.

Radioiodine Uptake Scan (RAI-U)

The radioiodine uptake (RAI-U) test is the only direct test of thyroid function. Laboratory tests are indirect, measuring hormones that may be affected by pituitary function. RAI-U usually employs the radioisotope I-123, as a tag for I-127, the body's stable form of iodine. RAI-U reflects the thyroid gland's clearance of iodine. This test is not relied on as much as previously because of improved laboratory tests. The diagnostic accuracy of the RAI-U does not approach that of measuring TSH plus FT4 or FT3 levels to determine hyperthyroidism, followed by a TSI determination to confirm GD.[40]

However, a recent article in *Postgraduate Medicine* advises that RAI uptake measure is essential for differentiating between GD and conditions causing low uptake such as subacute or granulomatous goiter, silent and postpartum thyroiditis, exogenous thyroid hormone supplementation and iodine induced hyperthyroidism. Measurement of TRAb, the article states, is indicted only for patients with euthyroid Graves' ophthalmopathy, and in pregnant women with a history of Graves' disease who have had thyroid ablation.[41]

The major advantage of RAI-U over antibody testing is that it can be performed locally, generating faster results. Also, RAI-U has value in excluding thyrotoxicosis not caused by conditions of a hyper-functioning thyroid such as ectopic thyroid tissue, or iodine induced thyrotoxicosis and before surgery as an imaging tool.[42] However, because of dietary changes contributing to an increased iodine intake, the normal RAI-U range among the U.S. population has significantly increased since RAI-U first came into use, making it not as significant of an indicator as in the past.[43]

RAI-U PRINCIPLE

The principle of the radioiodine uptake scan is simple. External X or gamma irradiation is capable of uniformly penetrating the entire thyroid gland within seconds to minutes following a given dose. Just as the thyroid takes up iodine, it takes up radioiodine without recognizing the difference. Radioiodines are absorbed and incorporated into the thyroid follicle. Here they remain while undergoing radioactive decay.

Localized in the gland, the distribution of radiation from radioiodines depends on the type and energy of the emissions, the follicle size and the distribution of iodine within the follicle. The mean range of particles in the thyroid is variable. It's much shorter for non-beta emitters such as I-123 than for beta emitters such as I-131, I-132 and I-133.

RAI-U PROCEDURE

The procedure involves the oral administration of radioiodine, usually I-123 taken in a drink or as a capsule. The residual radioiodine is later measured. RAI-U measures the amount of iodine taken up by the thyroid in a given length of time varying from two to 24 hours. RAI-U is dependent on the activity of the thyroid's iodine trapping mechanism, the rate of organic binding of iodine within the gland, and the rate of iodine release.

In a hyperthyroid patient with a minimal endogenous iodine and a fast turnover rate, the RAI-U measured at an earlier time is usually elevated, although at 24 hours it may fall within the normal range. Thus an earlier time, generally six hours, is recommended for the uptake scan. A high concentration of dietary iodine will interfere with the uptake of radioiodine. If the scan is to be performed within four hours of the dose, the patient is advised to fast. Any medications and recent radiographs with contrast agents need to be mentioned. RAI-U is contraindicated in patients who are pregnant or breast feeding.

NORMAL RAI-U RANGE

The normal RAI-U varies from one geographical region to another. Each testing facility determines a normal range dependent on the time interval between dose and scan. Normal ranges are usually about 2 percent to 12 percent at two hours, 5 percent to 15 percent at six hours, and 8 percent to 35 percent at 24 hours. RAI-U is increased in hyperthyroidism, iodine deficiency, pregnancy, hydatidiform mole, recovery phase of subacute thyroiditis, rebound after TSH suppression or following withdrawal of strong iodine or ATDs if TSH is elevated, therapeutic lithium, chronic thyroiditis if TSH elevated and inborn errors of thyroid synthesis.

RAI-U can also be increased in disorders in which iodine accumulation is normal but hormone secretion is impaired, such as in patients with abnormal thyroglobulin synthesis. RAI-U is also increased in dietary insufficiency, soybean ingestion since it binds T4 in the gut, nephrotic syndrome and chronic diarrheal states.

RAI-U is decreased in primary and central hypothyroidism, status post-thyroidectomy, post-radioiodine ablation, thyroid hormone administration, destructive or active phase of subacute thyroiditis, postpartum or sporadic lymphocytic (painless) thyroiditis, iodine excess and the ingestion of thionamides, sulfonamides, perchlorate, thiocyanate, amiodarone, glucocorticoid therapy and salicylates at levels >5 g/d. Drugs having minor effects include phenybutazone, resorcinol and sulfonylureas.

SOURCES OF ERROR

Exposure to excess iodine is the most common cause of a decreased RAI-U. Special offenders are organic iodinated dyes used as X-ray contrast media and the heart medication amiodarone. Depending on the contrast dye used, the RAI-U may be falsely suppressed for up to several months. A single large dose of iodide can depress the test for several days, and chronic iodide ingestion may affect the results for many weeks. Because it's stored in fat, amiodarone may interfere with test results for as long as several months.

RAI-U AND SCAN IN GRAVES' DISEASE

Most patients with hyperthyroidism caused by GD have an elevated RAI-U. However, in elderly patients, the RAI-U is less likely to show elevated levels. RAI-U in subacute, silent or postpartum thyroiditis and

exogenous thyroid administration is usually low. In severe thyrotoxicosis, GD patients may rarely take up and dissipate their oral dose of I-125
so quickly that the uptake is decreased by the time the measurement is
made.[44]

The RAI-U may be scanned (RAI-U scan) to determine its pattern of
distribution. If scintiscan is performed, the thyroid in GD appears diffusely
(predominantly even distribution of radioiodine) enlarged. In contrast,
hot nodules will take up more radioiodine than surrounding tissue and
cold nodules will take up less. However, the thyroid doesn't function as a
single homogeneous unit. Radioautographic studies reveal variations
among different areas of the gland and in different follicles. In fact, there
may be iodine pools in the thyroid that are cleared at different rates.

HAZARDS OF RADIOIODINE IN DIAGNOSTIC TESTS

According to Dr. John Gofman, a physician and doctor of nuclear
and physical chemistry, radioiodines that deliver beta particles provide the
same effects as external X-rays, provided the same quantity of ionizing
radiation energy is delivered to a specific tissue or organ when administered at a comparable age. While evaluating the effects of ionizing radiation on chromosomes for the Atomic Energy Commission, Dr. Gofman
found that because cell division proceeds slowly in the thyroid, the effects
of ionizing radiation may take more than 30 years to emerge. This is particularly true, he reports, for adults exposed to low doses at low dose rates.[45]

Because of the ability of the thyroid gland to concentrate up to 12
grams of radioiodine, it is said to be uniquely susceptible to the biologic
effects of radioiodine exposure. Results may vary from no discernible clinical effects to metabolically important processes such as acute radiation thyroiditis and to the induction of both benign and malignant neoplasms.
Furthermore, there are no available long-term studies of irradiated pop-
ulations followed to the completion of their life spans.[46]

Radioiodine Isotopes

The isotopes of iodine in current use are produced by irradiation in
nuclear reactors, cyclotron-charged particle irradiation, or in a process
that separates them from nuclear fission products. The shorter half life of
I-123 makes it preferable for measuring RAI-U because the radiation delivered to the thyroid per amount of administered I-123 is only about one
hundredth of that delivered by I-131, which is used in ablation.

IODINE-131

I-131 is used for the diagnosis and treatment of thyroid disorders. Its
gamma ray emissions are useful diagnostically, and its beta particle emissions are useful in therapy. At one time, I-131 was the only isotope used

medically. It is no longer considered ideal for RAI-U because of its high level of beta emissions.

IODINE-123

I-123 is considered ideal for thyroid function studies. The half-life is 13.3 hours and it has no beta emissions. An accurate radioiodine uptake scan can be performed 20 minutes after an intravenous dose or one to 24 hours following an oral dose. Using oral doses in the range of 100–300μCi, a precise scan be made six hours after the dose.[47]

TECHNETIUM-99M

Technetium-99m is used for diagnostic studies of thyroid structure because its emissions are favorable, and the material is readily available from a generator system. The half life of technetium-99m is six hours and it doesn't produce beta emissions. Although the material is actively trapped in the thyroid much like iodine, it doesn't undergo organification. A technetium pertechnetate thyroid scan has the ability to differentiate between GD or nodular thyroid disease since it provides better anatomical definition.[48]

Ultrasonography

Ultrasonography is based on the principle that body tissues have a property called acoustic impedance. Sound waves entering tissue can be either transmitted through the tissue or reflected (echoed). The ease of distinguishing cystic from solid lesions in tissue is based on the different properties of acoustic impedance. For example, tissue that is calcified has a much higher impedance than other tissue. Ultrasound is very sensitive in its ability to detect thyroid lesions and in distinguishing solid lesions from simple and complex cysts. That it is unable to distinguish between malignant and benign lesions is a drawback.

In GD, the thyroid is usually enlarged. Its echo pattern is inhomogeneous and normal to low in intensity compared to normal glands, which have a more uniform echo texture. Using color flow Doppler equipment, the intense vascularity of the thyroid in GD can be easily demonstrated.[49] This technique also offers an ideal measurement of thyroid volume. The intensity of the flow pattern, however, is not correlated to disease severity. Since a diminishment of thyroid volume is one of the first indicators of response to therapy in GD, ultrasonography is sometimes used during the course of antithyroid drug therapy.

Computed Tomography

Differences as small as 0.5 percent in the density of soft tissues can be determined using computed tomography (CT). Easily visualized because of its high iodine content, the thyroid can be viewed as a three-dimensional image in relation to the trachea, esophagus and surrounding structures. The radiation dose used is small and there is minimal exposure to other areas of the body.

The procedure requires the patient to remain supine with his neck hyperextended. This position provides elevation of the thyroid in the neck and prevents interferences from the shoulders. A frontal scan is taken to locate the landmarks of the neck. Scanning then begins at the level of the vocal chords. During each scan, which takes one to three seconds, the patient is directed not to swallow.

In GD, CT demonstrates thyroid enlargement with homogeneous density. Total iodine content is increased, but the iodine concentration is decreased, which results in a decreased CT density. In GD the density is usually 50 percent to 70 percent of the normal value.

Magnetic Resonance Imaging (MRI)

MRI is a noninvasive technique of imaging tissues based on their magnetic properties. Improvements in soft tissue contrast permit superior definition of many anatomic structures of the neck in multiple planes with thinner sections, higher resolution, and shorter scanning times. Limitations include sensitivity to physiologic tissue that affects imaging quality and the inability of MRI to identify calcification as readily as CT.

In GD, the thyroid is enlarged, occasionally lobulated, with a slightly heterogeneous, diffusely increased signal on both T1 and T2 weighted images. The intensity on T2 weighted images often exceeds that of fat. The thyroid to muscle signal ratio is linearly related to both the serum thyroxine (T4) concentration and the 24 hour radioiodine uptake scan. Following radioiodine ablation, the signal ratio falls proportionately in response to changes in the serum T4 and radioactive iodine uptake. Changes may reflect differences in tissue water content, thyroglobulin content, blood flow or vascularity of the thyroid. This is only seen in Graves' disease.[50]

6 *Autoantibodies and Autoimmune Diseases Associated with GD*

Because other autoimmune diseases may accompany Graves' disease, when symptoms associated with another autoimmune disease occur, physicians often test for the autoantibodies associated with the suspected disorder. Since many symptoms such as joint pain are seen in both thyroid and non-thyroid related conditions, antibody tests help to diagnose or rule out other autoimmune disorders that may co-exist with GD.

Autoantibodies in Graves' Disease

Although thyroid autoantibodies predominate in GD, antibodies directed toward other organs may also be present. Anti-parietal antibodies and acetylcholine receptor antibodies are the ones most often seen in GD. As previously mentioned, the presence of autoantibodies doesn't indicate that the associated disease is present or that it will develop. For instance, GD patients with acetylcholine receptor antibodies may or may not develop myasthenia gravis, and thyroglobulin antibodies are seen in 30 percent of normal older women.

GD patients have also been reported to have antibodies to the thyroidal iodide symporter (involved in the mechanism by which thyroid cells take up iodine), the adrenal steroidogenic enzymes and ovarian components of the pituitary. Approximately 25 percent of patients with active GD also have low level titers of anti–DNA antibodies and also antibodies to liver mitochondria and to islet cells in the pancreas.

Autoantibodies and Specific Autoimmune Disorders

In this chapter, I describe various autoantibodies and autoimmune disorders that may co-exist with GD. Often, the value in testing for them is in establishing baseline levels for future comparison. Autoimmune disorders most commonly associated with GD include HT, SLE, Sjögren's disease, antiphospholipid syndrome, primary biliary cirrhosis, mixed connective tissue disease, chronic active hepatitis, rheumatoid arthritis, scleroderma, pernicious anemia (PA), Type 1 diabetes, myasthenia gravis, gluten sensitivity enteropathy (GSE, celiac disease), multiple sclerosis and idiopathic thrombocytopenic purpura.

Acetylcholine Receptor Antibodies and Myasthenia Gravis

Acetylcholine (Ach) receptor antibodies (AChR Ab), including the blocking and modulating nicotinic varieties, are found in high concentrations in 90 percent of patients with autoimmune myasthenia gravis (MG) or thymoma (tumor of the thymus) with MG, and in 71 percent of patients with ocular MG. AChR antibodies in a patient's serum supports the diagnosis of autoimmune MG, a disease primarily affecting the neuromuscular junction.

In MG, the normal transmission between nerve and muscle cells is impaired due to blockage or dysfunction of the acetylcholine receptor. Ach is released both spontaneously at a constant rate, and in response to nerve impulses that release larger amounts. Drugs such as curare work to immobilize muscle by blocking the acetylcholine receptor, producing symptoms similar to those of AChR Ab.

AChR Ab are not found in congenital forms of MG and are rare in neurologic conditions other than acquired MG. AChR Ab are also seen in subclinical MG, in recipients of D–penicillamine, and in patients with thymoma without clinical evidence of MG. Significant AChR Ab titers are frequently present in autoimmune liver disease and are occasionally seen in GD, thyroiditis, and amyotrophic lateral sclerosis (ALS).

Reference Range = Values >0.02 nmol/L are consistent with a diagnosis of acquired MG. Lower values (0.03–1.0 nmol/L) are seen in ocular MG.

Myasthenia Gravis is characterized by weakness and easy fatiguability that results from an autoantibody-mediated loss of functional acetylcholine receptors in the muscle postsynaptic membrane. Symptoms include muscle weakness that may cause paralysis of affected muscles, facial weakness, speech difficulties, difficulty with chewing, swallowing and breathing, and inability to support the trunk, head or neck. In patients with concurrent hyperthyroidism or hypothyroidism, symptoms may be exaggerated. About 80 percent of patients with MG have thymic hyperplasia, which is also associated with GD.

Antiparietal Cell Antibodies, and Pernicious Anemia and Type A Chronic Gastritis

Antiparietal cell autoantibodies (PCA), along with intrinsic factor autoantibodies, are typically found in patients with pernicious anemia (PA) and in atrophic gastritis. Approximately 50 percent of patients with PA have thyroid autoantibodies and 30 percent of patients with autoimmune thyroid disease have PCA. In chronic gastritis, loss of intrinsic factor and the ability to secrete acid may lead to PA. PCA are found in 1 percent to 2 percent of normal subjects, and the frequency of detection increases with age.

Reference Range = Negative (Titer <20)

Elevated in atrophic gastritis, pernicious anemia, polyglandular autoimmune disease. Present in 30 percent of patients with autoimmune thyroid disease including GD.

Pernicious Anemia is a disease characterized by type A chronic gastritis and is associated with achlorhydria (deficient stomach acid), hypergastrinemia (elevated gastrin level),Vitamin B 12 malabsorption and immunoglobulin A (IgA) deficiency.

Chronic Type A Gastritis, an inflammation of the stomach including atrophy and the development of ulcers, can be divided into two separate subtypes. Type B, which is more often associated with the gastric mucosa, is usually due to an infection of h*elicobacter pylori.* Type A gastritis is associated with autoimmunity and PA.

Anti-Gliadin Ab and Gluten Sensitivity Enteropathy (GSE)

Anti-gliadin antibodies, antibodies to gliadin, produced in response to gluten, the protein component of wheat, barley, rye and oats, are associated with gluten sensitivity enteropathy (GSE), an autoimmune disease that often accompanies GD.

Reference Values: <0.9 GIV= Negative; >3.0 GIV= Strongly Positive (my level, despite only having vague symptoms, was 6.1 GIV)

Gluten sensitivity enteropathy (GSE) or celiac disease, also known as sprue, is characterized by inflammation of the small intestinal mucosa and ulceration caused by an abnormal immunologic response to gluten. Tissue changes include edema and swelling, coarsening of tissue fibers and chronic inflammation. Late stages of the disease are characterized by excessive collagen deposits and are associated with anti-epithelial cell antibodies and an atrophy of stomach villi. Recent studies show that six months on a gluten free diet reduces both thyroid and gliadin antibodies in patients with both GSE and AITD.

Insulin Antibodies, Islet Cell Antibodies and Diabetes Mellitus

In Type 1 or insulin dependent diabetes mellitus (IDDM), the insulin secreting beta cells of the pancreatic islets become destroyed by antibodies. IDDM primarily originates in childhood, although in the sixth to seventh decades, another period of peak incidence occurs.

Insulin Antibodies are present in up to 80 percent of patients with IDDM, and they have also been reported in other autoimmune disorders, including Graves' disease.[1]

Reference Range = Negative or <1.1 percent

Indications: Used to assess insulin autoantibodies in prediabetic subjects and patients with other autoimmune disorders.

Islet Cell Antibodies (ICA): Cytoplasmic islet cell antibodies or ICA are directed against pancreatic islet cells. Although ICA attack all pancreatic islet cells, cell destruction appears to be restricted to insulin producing pancreatic cells known as beta cell, causing insulin deficiency.

Reference Range = Negative

Indications: Indicated as a market of autoimmune pancreatic disease and an early indicator of type 1 diabetes.

Insulin dependent diabetes mellitus may cause chronic complications including retinopathy, nephropathy and neuropathy. Environmental triggers include infectious agents, including vaccines. Approximately 39 percent of children with rubella develop AITD or IDDM later in life.[2] In several studies, insulin and islet cell autoantibodies have been found in 5 percent to 10 percent of newly diagnosed patients with Graves' diseases.[3]

Antinuclear Antibodies, DNA Antibodies and Systemic Lupus Erythematosus

Antinuclear antibodies (ANA): ANA directed against many different tissue components are positive in patients with a variety of autoimmune diseases, especially the systemic rheumatic diseases. Elevated values are found in nearly all cases of SLE and in most patients with other connective tissue disorders. ANA are found in many types of liver disease, including 60 percent of patients with chronic active hepatitis. Normal elderly patients with no hint of disease may have low titers of ANA (usually <160). Certain patterns of fluorescent nuclear staining (such as speckled or diffuse) have been found to correspond to certain nuclear components, but there is controversy regarding the usefulness of patterns.

Reference: None detected

Indications: Used as a primary screening test for SLE and other connective tissue disorders.

Anti-DNA antibodies: antibodies to both single and double stranded DNA are seen in more than 70 percent of patients with SLE. Although double stranded dsDNA antibodies are considered a marker for SLE, the test is not specific because these antibodies also occur in a significant number of patients with drug-induced SLE, Sjögren's syndrome patients, and patients with RA (Rheumatoid Arthritis). Some studies report that dsDNA antibodies are seen in 25 percent of patients with Graves' disease. Single stranded ss DNA antibodies and ANA are see in drug related lupus.

Reference: None detected

Systemic Lupus Erythematosus (SLE): SLE is an autoimmune disease involving multiple organs, including the kidney and lungs. Patients with SLE and discoid lupus often have a butterfly shaped rash that occurs on the cheeks. Autoantibodies found in SLE include ANA, antibodies to ss and ds DNA, extractable nuclear antigens and anti-cardiolipin antibodies.

Drug Related Lupus (DRL): Drug related lupus (DRL), a syndrome much like SLE, although the kidneys are rarely involved, is associated with nearly 100 different medicines. DRL develops in up to about 30 percent of patients on long-term procainamide therapy. DRL is also associated with antithyroid drugs and beta blocking agents, both of which are used for GD therapy.[4]

Although DRL usually occurs within four months of drug use, one 16-year-old GD patient developed DRL after being on the antithyroid drug propylthiouracil (PTU) for four years. Her symptoms resolved within a month or two of discontinuance of the medicine.

Liver Membrane Antibodies, Smooth Muscle Antibodies and Chronic Active Autoimmune Hepatitis

Chronic autoimmune hepatitis, which has two subtypes, is a rare liver disease primarily affecting women. This disease, characterized by cirrhosis, plasma cell infiltration of the liver and increased serum gamma globulin levels, is linked to the same HLA genes associated with GD. Tests for viral hepatitis are negative although autoimmune liver disease may later occur in patients with hepatitis C.

Anti-Smooth Muscle Antibodies (SMA): Used to evaluate patients suspected of having autoimmune chronic active hepatitis. Positive SMA results may occur in patients with active hepatitis caused by toxins so it is not specific for autoimmune hepatitis.

Reference Range: Negative

Liver Membrane Antibodies: liver/kidney microsome (LKM-1) antibodies occur in a subset of patients with chronic active hepatitis, predominantly children.

Reference Range: Negative

Chronic Active Autoimmune Hepatitis, although associated with a high degree of mortality when left untreated, shows a very favorable response to corticosteroids. It is seen in approximately eight times as many women as men, and its usual victims belong to two groups, young women between age 10 and 30, and older women aged 50 to 70. Autoimmune hepatitis has a predilection for individuals of northern European descent and is rare in southern Europeans, Africans and Asians.[5] Symptoms include easy fatiguability, menstrual disturbances, jaundice, nausea, vomiting and abdominal pain.

Anti-Mitochondrial Antibodies and Primary Biliary Cirrhosis

Primary biliary cirrhosis (PBC) is an autoimmune disorder that primarily causes inflammation and tissue destruction of the bile ducts of the liver. Chronic inflammation causes scar tissue to form in the bile ducts, interfering with the necessary excretion of bile. PBC affects nine times as many women as men, and targets middle-aged women. It's estimated that 84 percent of cases of PBC have one other associated autoimmune diseases, and 40 percent of cases have two or more other autoimmune diseases.[6]

Anti-Mitochondrial M2 Antibodies have been reported to be present in 79 percent to 94 percent of patients with primary biliary cirrhosis.

Reference Range: <1.0 units is considered negative; 1.0–1.3 units is inconclusive; >1.3 units = positive

Primary Biliary Cirrhosis has four characteristic stages that may overlap. Early stages include inflammation of bile ducts and lymphocytic infiltration causing an accumulation of acids and cholesterol in the blood. Late stages include high levels of copper in the liver, destruction of intrahepatic bile ducts and tissue cell destruction (necrosis). PBC is often seen in conjunction with keratoconjunctivitis sicca, characterized by dry eyes with a gritty sensation, and autoimmune thyroid disease, including GD.

Anti-Cardiolipin (Phospholipid) Antibodies and Antiphospholipid Disease (APL)

In antiphospholipid disease (APL), patients produce antibodies against phospholipid, a body fat found in every cell wall of the body. APL causes blood clotting which may initiate stroke, miscarriages and migraine headaches. APL has also been indicated as a causative factor in cardiovascular disease in women.

Anti-cardiolipin antibodies, IgG, IgM are moderately elevated (most patients have IgG or both IgG and IgM) in antiphospholipid antibody syndrome and APL.

Reference Range = IgG values of <15 GPL are considered negative
IgM values of <12 MPL are considered negative

Indications: Useful for prognostic assessment of pregnant patients with a history of recurrent, spontaneous fetal loss. Elevated values are seen in APL, SLE, spontaneous thromboses, and in patients with connective tissue disease.

Antiphospholipid disease occurs alone or it may accompany other autoimmune diseases as a disorder known as antiphospholipid antibody syndrome. APL is a significant cause of strokes in women under 35 and it is also associated with recurrent miscarriages. The American Autoimmune Related Diseases Association reports that although this disease is easily treated with aspirin, women with autoimmune diseases are rarely screened for this order or identified until after they have had a stroke or miscarriage.

Platelet Antibodies and Autoimmune (Idiopathic) Thrombocytopenic Purpura (ITP)

Platelets are blood components, distinct from red and white cells, critical for the normal clotting mechanism, particularly after vascular injury. Patients with insufficient platelets bruise easily. Slight pressure may cause tiny bruises known as petechiae. Patients may bleed profusely from minor injuries, especially those involving the nasal or oral areas.

Platelet Antibodies: This test is designed to detect antibodies to platelet glycoprotiens as well as antibodies to HLA class I antigens (HLA-A-B). Although HLA class I antibodies do not cause thrombocytopenia (decreased platelets), they're associated with refractoriness to platelet transfusions.

Reference Values: Negative for HLA alloantibodies and platelet specific antibodies.

Autoimmune thrombocytopenic purpura is a disorder characterized by thrombocytopenia (reduced platelet counts) and clotting disorders. Since many drugs and conditions are associated with thrombocytopenia, other causes are usually ruled out before the patient is tested for antiplatelet antibodies and a diagnosis of idiopathic thyrobocytopenic purpura (ITP) is made.

Recent reports of decreased platelet counts in patients with Graves' disease have linked GD to autoimmune thrombocytopenic purpura. According to one study, this condition reversed after treatment with the antithyroid medication carbimazole.[7] When it occurs in patients with AITD, ITP is generally mild and doesn't cause clinical symptoms.

Sjögren's Syndrome and Ro and La Antibodies

Sjögren's syndrome is a disease in which lymphocytes, cytokines and autoantibodies invade the exocrine glands, primarily the salivary and lacrimal glands, damaging them and inhibiting their ability to produce moisture. Middle aged women are the primary target. Xerophthalmia, an eye condition characterized by reduced tear flow, and xerostomia, which causes reduced salivary flow and mouth dryness, are the primary symptoms. According to a recent article in *The Female Patient*, this disorder often goes unrecognized and the typical patient is not diagnosed for 3.5 years.[8]

In primary Sjögren's syndrome, ocular and oral symptoms are part of a systemic pattern which may also include gynecological, renal, neurological and respiratory symptoms and arthritic and gastrointestinal disturbances. Secondary Sjögren's syndrome accompanies another autoimmune disease such as SLE.

Extractable nuclear antigen (ENA) antibodies include antibodies to the extractable nuclear antigens, Smith, RNP, sclerodoma, SSA and SSB. In Sjögren's syndrome, SSA and SSB, which are both small RNA protein complexes, are diagnostic.

SSA (Ro) antibodies are seen in 70 percent to 75 percent of Sjögren's patients, 30 percent to 40 percent of SLE patients, and 5 percent to 10 percent of patients with progressive systemic sclerosis (PSS).

SSB (La) antibodies are seen in 50 percent to 60 percent of Sjögren's patients and is diagnostic if it's the only ENA antibody present; seen in 15 percent to 20 percent of patients with SLE and 5 percent to 10 percent of patients with PSS.

Reference Range (Ro and La): <20 Units = None detected; 20–39 Units = Inconclusive; 40–80 Units = positive; >80 Units = Strongly positive[9]

Rheumatoid (RF) Factor is the antibody associated with rheumatoid arthritis and it's also seen in nearly all patients with Sjögren's syndrome.

Reference Range: <20 IU/ml = None detected

ANA — see section on ANA and SLE earlier in this chapter; most Sjögren's patients have moderate to high titers of ANA.

Sjögren's syndrome is suggested when patients complain of symptoms associated with oral dryness and ocular dyrness. Patients may also have salivary gland enlargement, esophageal muscle dysfunction, nasal dryness, nephritis and neurological manifestations. A sicca syndrome similar to that seen in Sjögren's syndrome may occur in GD patients following radioiodine ablation.

Chronic Autoimmune Thyroiditis and Autoimmune Polyglandular Syndrome

Chronic autoimmune thyroiditis eventually develops in approximately 20 percent of patients with GD who are treated with antithyroid drugs and the majority of ablated patients. Blocking TRAb contribute to the hypothyroidism in about one-third of cases.[10]

A clear cut association has been established between chronic autoimmune thyroiditis and primary B-cell lymphoma of the thyroid. Although the risk of thyroid lymphoma is increased 60 fold in Hashimoto's thyroiditis, lymphoma is still a rare occurrence. It's suspected that the prolonged stimulation of intrathyroidal B cells eventually produces a malignant clone.[11] Riedel's thyroiditis, a sclerosing thyroiditis that primarily occurs in middle aged women, has also been suggested to have an autoimmune etiology because many Riedel's patients have thyroid antibodies along with a lymphocytic infiltration.

Polyglandular autoimmune syndromes are clusters of diseases that have a tendency to coexist. The organs involved in these syndromes are characterized by organ specific mononuclear cell infiltration. For instance, in Addison's disease, the adrenal cortex shows marked infiltration while the adrenal medulla remains unaffected. Eventually, all affected organs undergo fibrosis and atrophy as all of their functional cells are destroyed.

Chronic Autoimmune Thyroiditis and Type 2 and 3 Autoimmune Polyglandular Syndrome

Chronic autoimmune thyroiditis always occurs in type 2 and type 3 autoimmune polyglandular syndrome. Besides its role in the polyglandular syndromes, chronic autoimmune thyroiditis is also likely to coexist with a number of other autoimmune diseases, including rheumatoid arthritis, SLE, Sjögren's syndrome, polymyalgia rheumatica, temporal arteritis, relapsing polychondritis, systemic sclerosis, chronic active hepatitis, primary biliary cirrhosis and dermatitis herpetiformins.

Type 1 Autoimmune Polyglandular (Polyendocrine) Syndrome (Type 1 APS)

Type 1 autoimmune polyglandular syndrome is associated with hypoparathyroidism, adrenal insufficiency and candidiasis (yeast infection).

It usually begins by age 10 although it may develop in adulthood and is manifested as a skin disorder. Typically, hypoparathyroidism develops next, followed by Addison's disease a few years later. Most conditions are familial although there is no HLA gene involvement.

Type 2 Autoimmune Polyglandular (Polyendocrine) Syndrome (Type 2 APS or Schmidt's Syndrome)

Type 2 autoimmune polyglandular syndrome is a syndrome characterized by adrenal insufficiency with either autoimmune thyroid disease or type 1 diabetes (insulin dependent, diabetes mellitus). Other conditions that may be associated include premature ovarian failure, myasthenia gravis, celiac disease, alopecia, hypophysitis, vitiligo, serositis and pernicious anemia.

Type 3 Autoimmune Polyglandular (Polyendocrine) Syndrome (Type 3 APS)

Type 3 autoimmune polyglandular syndrome involves autoimmune thyroid disease and at least two other autoimmune diseases, excluding Addison's disease. Most commonly seen with thyroiditis are IDDM, PA, and another organ specific autoimmune disease such as myasthenia gravis.

7 *Why Me? Genetic and Non-Genetic Influences*

The reason why only some of us develop autoimmune disease is influenced by hereditary and environmental factors. Having certain genes makes one genetically susceptible to developing certain autoimmune diseases. Why did I develop Graves' disease when my twin didn't? As a fraternal twin, his chance of developing GD is 30 percent. And besides our genetic differences, non-genetic influences likely played a role. Birth weight, for example, is known to correlate inversely with the prevalence of thyroid autoantibodies in women.[1] At birth, I weighed four pounds while he weighed six.

And although many GD patients initially suspect that they're the only one in their family with an autoimmune disorder, careful sleuthing often shows that a distant cousin has juvenile diabetes or a great grandmother had myasthenia gravis. In this chapter, I describe the major histocompatibility (MHC) genes, the genes that link these seemingly unrelated disorders. I also explain how MHC and other genes regulate autoimmunity and I describe the environmental factors that contribute to the development of autoimmune disease.

Polygenetic Component of GD

Several genes are involved in GD. These include thyroid specific genes such as the TSH receptor gene, immune system genes, protein transporter genes, cytokine genes, T cell receptor genes and genes that determine the structure of our immunoglobulins.

Genes inherited as pairs known as haplotypes are also associated with certain diseases. For instance, there is an increased frequency of the immune system genes HLA B8 and DR3 appearing together in white patients who develop GD.[2] And some genes are considered protective since their presence is associated with not developing a certain disorder. For instance, having the HLA DR 7 gene is thought to prevent GD development.

Genes and DNA

Cells are the building blocks of organisms. Each of the 10 trillion cells in the human body (except blood cells) contains the entire human genome — all the information needed to build a human being. This information is encoded in six billion base pairs, subunits of DNA are present in the cell nucleus and mitochondria.

Chromosomes are constructed of deoxyribonucleic acid (DNA). DNA is made from the nitrogen-containing amino acid bases thymine, cytosine, adenine and guanine. To each base is added a molecule of the sugar deoxyribose, which forms a nucleoside, and a molecule of phosphoric acid, which makes the compound a nucleotide.

Depending on how the sugar and phosphate attach to carbons in the base, different nucleotides are formed. Paired nucleotides, each nucleoside component linked through a phosphate bridge, form the double-stranded helix shaped molecule of DNA. The twist or helix of the molecule is a natural outcome of its composition. DNA follows strict base-pairing rules. For example, adenine will only pair with thymine, and cytosine with guanine. If the DNA language gets garbled or a misspelling occurs in the code, the cell may make a wrong protein or the wrong amount of the correct one. These glitches may cause diseases, including GD, when protein changes lead to the production of autoantibodies.

Functions of DNA

DNA has two functions, self-replication and the production of proteins. The information contained or encoded in DNA is processed into proteins. Like DNA, proteins are linear compounds, but instead of being composed of nucleic acids, proteins are composed of amino acids. The hormonal or endocrine disruptors mentioned in chapter 3, chemicals such as the polyaromatic hydrocarbons (PAHs) from petroleum products, are capable of binding with DNA, causing changes or mutations that may lead to cancer.

Chromosomes and Genes

The cell nucleus is composed of long, thin strands (approximately six feet) of DNA packed into 23 pairs of chromosomes. Each human chromosome contains the DNA for thousands of individual genes arranged like beads on a string. Genes are short pieces of DNA that tell the cell what proteins to produce and thereby how to act.

As cells divide, the chromosome material is usually duplicated by the dividing cell. Then it is equally divided by the two identical cells (progeny) produced in a process known as mitosis. In animal reproduction, however, the ovum and sperm do not duplicate their chromosomes. Instead, they unite to form a zygote with one chromosome derived from each parent. The display of a person's chromosomes is called a karyotype.

Alleles

Alleles are differing forms of the same gene that can occupy a given locus or position on a chromosome. The existence of allelic forms (as in Mendel's experimental smooth and wrinkled peas) is referred to as polymorphism. Of two alleles for a given gene, there is one dominant and one recessive gene that determine specific outcomes.

RNA and Protein Synthesis

Like DNA, RNA is a nucleotide composed of the same bases as DNA except that uracil replaces thymine. The sugar molecule in RNA is ribose, a compound recently introduced in the health food industry as a performance enhancer for athletes.

There are four species or RNA subtypes, each with defined functions: messenger RNA (mRNA), ribosomal RNA (rRNA), transfer RNA (tRNA) and small nuclear RNA (SnRNA). Messenger RNA is the molecule from which the protein is made, ribosomal RNA is the major constituent of ribosomes (the structure on which proteins are made), transfer RNA is the molecule that brings the proper amino acid into place as the protein is constructed, and small nuclear RNA splice small sections of mRNA.

All four species are derived from the information encoded in the DNA. The process in which RNA is made is known as transcription. Messenger RNA is then translated into a particular sequence of amino acids forming protein according to the genetic code.

The Major Histocompatibility Complex and Its Genes

Molecules that mark a cell as being "self" or part of the body are encoded by a group of genes located on the short arm of chromosome six called the major histocompatibility complex (MHC). The prefix histo refers to tissue. This system was first discovered when attempts were made to find compatible tissue donors for organ transplants. It was discovered that the MHC genes and the molecules they encode vary from one person to another and control the immune response.

Human Leukocyte Antigens

In humans, the MHC is called the human leukocyte antigen or HLA system. The genes expressed on the body's cells are HLA antigens. In organ transplants, a certain number of HLA genes in the donor and the transplant patient must match for the organ to be compatible. Otherwise, the body's immune system cells would recognize the foreign gene as non-self or foreign and react to it, initiating a syndrome leading to organ rejection.

The MHC complex consists of a series of genes that code for proteins expressed on the cell surface of all nucleated cells, particularly lymphocytes. Their principal function is to protect the body from disease by controlling the immune response system. These genes are located within the HLA region on the short arm of chromosome 6 in man.

Within the MHC complex, there are three subsets known as Class I, Class II, and Class III antigens or genes, which are described in the following two sections. In the immune reaction, certain events are limited to antigens expressed in only one particular subset. Although Class II antigens are generally associated with GD, other MHC genes, such as those encoding the tumor necrosis factor, also have an association.

Gene Locus and Haplotypes

The MHC loci (positions of genes on chromosome, singular = locus) are closely linked. The complex of linked genes that are inherited as a group on the same chromosome are known as haplotypes. (For instance, the allele B8 and the allele D3 are often inherited as a couple.) Each individual inherits two MHC haplotypes, one from each parent, and has two alleles for each of the loci. Thus there are four possible MHC genes in the offspring of ab and cd, known as ac, ad, bc and bd.

Linkage Disequilibrium

Linkage disequilibrium refers to the tendency for certain alleles at two linked loci to occur together as haplotypes significantly more often than what would be expected based on chance (for example, if all the children of ab/cd parents were ac). Haplotypes seen in certain disease often occur more often than expected, especially in certain ethnic groups.

Regulation in the MHC

The immune system is regulated by MHC markers that determine which particular antigens an individual can respond to and how strongly.

MHC markers also allow immune cells (macrophages, B cells and T cells) to communicate with one another.

In an infection, the invading microorganism infects cells or is engulfed by immune cells such as monocytes. Inside the cell, MHC Class I antigens alert T cells to the presence of body cells which have been detrimentally altered by infection or mutation.

Class II molecules, which are found on many immune system cells, act as receptors for antigen fragments. Once these fragments have bound to the MHC molecules and have been translocated to the cell surface, the MHC Class II complex alerts the helper T cells. Receptors on T cells interact with the antigen MHC complex, triggering both humoral (antibody producing) and cellular (cell, particularly T cell initiated) immune responses.

Specifically, the Ia (immune response associated) molecules are encoded by the HLA-D region and are called HLA-DR (d related) antigens. The activated B lymphocyte discussed in chapter 2 presents antigens through these HLA-DR molecules to T or B cells.

Class I molecules are coded by three loci of chromosome 6, the HLA-A, B and C regions that are expressed on most nucleated cells of the body and also platelets. The central function of Class I molecules is to recognize and oust virally infected or tumor cells. Class II are the Ia molecules (HLA-DR, HLA-DQ, and HLA-DP, DC/MB, SB subregions) and are expressed on macrophages, B lymphocytes and activated T lymphocytes. Class III includes the MHC linked complement components, (C2, C4 and BF), 21-hydroxylase (21OH), and tumor necrosis factor (TNF).

Antigenic Recognition

Immune system genes only react with specific antigens. Peptide antigens presented by MHC molecules are derived from two distinct sources:

1. Exogenously (originating outside the body) derived antigens, such as bacteria, that are taken into cells and ultimately presented by Class II MHC molecules to CD4 T helper cells (see antibody production in chapter 2). Here, they capture, process and present antigens for future use in delayed hypersensitivity reactions or the production of antibodies.

2. Endogenous antigens that originate in the internal environment of the cell. Endogenous peptides may include peptides from self-antigens or peptide fragments derived from early viral proteins produced in a virus-infected cells. These peptides are presented primarily by Class I MHC molecules and are recognized by CD8 positive T suppressor cells.

Thyroid Cell Antigens

Normally, thyroid epithelial cells don't express Class II antigens. However, they're expressed in thyroids of patients with GD. It's suspected that a local viral infection of the thyroid gland could cause production of interferon or other cytokines in the thyroid, which in turn would induce Class II expression, inducing step 2 of T cell activation.

HLA Genes Associated with GD

HLA-DR3 and HLA-B8 genes are linked to GD. The relative risks (likeliness of developing a disease) are highest for HLA-D and DR alleles, because the Class II HLA-DR3 molecule appears to be a stronger link. The association between GD and HLA-B8 and HLA-DR3 genes is seen in Caucasians as well as South African blacks.

However, GD is associated with different Class I and II HLA antigens in other ethnic groups, and within different ethnic groups there are sometimes subsets. For instance, the prevalence of HLA-BW46 is increased in Chinese men (but not women) with GD, and the relative risk for this allele is higher in men with early onset disease (age 10–19) than in men overall. The genetic focus seems to be on antibody production rather than disease production.

Haplotypes Associated with Autoimmune Disease

The most striking set of types that occur together as a marker for disease is HLA-A1, B8, DRw3/DR3. The frequency of this set is increased among patients with juvenile onset or type 1 diabetes, gluten sensitivity enteropathy, GD, dermatitis herpetiformis, chronic active hepatitis and several other diseases.

CTL Genes

Recently, another gene associated with the immune response, the cytotoxic lymphocyte CTLA-4, was found to be related to the propensity to develop GD and GO, especially in males. Its role appears to be associated with the second signal needed to invoke a progressive immune response provided by one of the adhesion molecules that exist on the antigen presenting cell. One of the most important adhesion molecules is B7. CTLA4 recognizes and interacts with the subset B7.2, giving a negative signal.

Familial Predisposition to GD

There is a distinct familial predisposition to Graves' disease. In GD family members, there is a tendency for the development of Hashimoto's disease, primary thyrotropic hypothyroidism, pernicious anemia, insulin dependent diabetes mellitus (IDDM), Sjögren's syndrome, lupus erythematosus, rheumatoid arthritis and idiopathic thyrombocytopenic purpura.[3]

In some patients, Graves' disease may change to Hashimoto's disease or primary autoimmune myxedema (see chapter 11) or vice versa. On rare occasions some patients with primary myxedema later become hyperthyroid.[4]

Genetic Susceptibility and GD

The presence of HLA B8 and HLA DR3 is related to a higher relative risk (approximately four times) of developing Graves' disease.[5] The importance of genetic factors is suggested by the clustering of GD within families. Also, GD occurs in both twins in 50 percent of identical twins while only 30 percent of fraternal twins can boast of this distinction.

About 15 percent of patients with GD have a close relative with the same disorder, and about 50 percent of first degree relatives of patients with GD have circulating thyroid autoantibodies and go on to develop overt thyroid disease. However, recent studies indicate that the role of heredity in AITD is not as significant as it had been previously considered.[6]

Some HLA-D/DR associated autoimmune diseases are due to altered or suppressed immune responses. In particular, juvenile onset insulin dependent diabetes mellitus (IDDM), GD, atrophic thyroiditis (primary myxedema) myasthenia gravis, pernicious anemia, celiac disease, Sjögren's syndrome and SLE are all linked with Dw3 and DR3 in Caucasians. DR genes are associated with a decreased number of T suppressor cells.

Non-MHC Genes

While HLA genes contribute to the development of GD, they aren't diagnostic markers. Although most GD patients are never tested for HLA genetic markers, studies indicate that the percentage of patients having these genes borders on 50 percent. Clearly, there are other genes involved, particularly those governing the TSH receptor on chromosome 14 as well as genes influencing immunoglobulin production, and others still to be discovered.

The Human Biologic Data Interchange (HBDI) Information Center in Philadelphia, Pa., which maintains an international database of information on families with GD, is conducting a survey. Both GD and HT are of particular interest to Dr. Yaron Tomer, assistant professor of medicine at Mount Sinai School of Medicine in New York, whose research for the HBDI study focuses on finding the genes responsible for GD and HT. Dr. Tomer has found several markers linked to GD, one of which is on the X chromosome, suggesting a cause for the increased incidence of GD seen in women.[7]

Good Stock Genes and Endocrine Disruptors

Since the discovery of DNA, researchers have regarded genes as the harbingers of health and disease. Phrases like "from good stock" conjure definite images. However, genes can be altered. Certain chemicals and viruses cripple DNA, causing genetic mutations that result in disease. And even if someone has good genes, hormonal disruptions can result in disease. And as previously mentioned, many chemicals are hormonal disruptors.

Until recently, tests to assess product toxicity were based on the substance's ability to cause genetic changes in exposed animals. For many years, it was assumed that the absence of genetic alterations confirmed product safety. And until researchers discovered the truth about the synthetic estrogen, diethylstilbesterol (DES), which waits a generation to show effects, researchers never even considered the possibility of a delayed response.

Besides neglecting to assess second generation gene mutations, earlier researchers neglected to evaluate products for endocrine effects. Theo Colborn and John Myers began studying sterility and birth defects in animals after observing peculiar reproductive changes, including female birds nesting together. They also found increased mortality, defective egg shells and progeny with birth defects. Alarmed, they began an evaluation of endocrine changes and realized certain environmental chemicals were the cause.

Their search then focused on which environmental chemicals caused hormonal changes. Once they pinpointed the responsible compounds, they began to study hormonal disruption in humans and found the same things. By opening the floodgates, Colborn et al. taught us that environmental hazards cause far greater effects on the second generation, including autoimmune thyroid disease.

Theories Regarding Autoimmunity

Autoimmune disease is associated with a loss of tolerance to "self" tissue antigens. Although a deficiency of T suppressor cells is often blamed, another popular theory proposes that, in GD, genetically controlled B cell hyperactivity, rather than a defect in the T cells, is the cause of disease. It's speculated that the immune system, given the job of watching out for foreign antigens, is deprived of its role when vaccinations and antibiotics step in.

Without antigens to fight, the immune system becomes more vigilant in its efforts to find antigens and form antibodies and mistakenly recognizes the thyroid as foreign.[8]

Potential Causes of Autoimmunity

1. Alterations of normal host components by type C viruses (oncovirus group such as California encephalitis virus) and retroviruses. Researchers at Tulane University in New Orleans, La., have identified a human intracisternal type A retroviral particle (HIAP) in more than 85 percent of patients with Graves' disease that are not present in control subjects.[9]
2. Haptens (immunogenic part of an antigen) or antigens such as androgens or endocrine disruptors that may complex to tissue proteins.
3. Immunity caused by a foreign antigen cross-reacting with tissue components and confusing the immune system is known as molecular mimicry. Involvement of HLA molecules in antigen presentation was observed as long ago as the early 1970s. It was also noted that CTLs generated against specific virus-infected cells only killed virus-infected cells bearing MHC antigens shared by the original infected cell. This phenomenon is referred to as MHC–restricted response. Molecules capable of masquerading as MHC antigens might bypass this restriction.

In one recent study, bacteria that cause food poisoning are shown to trigger autoimmune arthritis. Researchers found that immune system cells that fight bacteria may also affect normal cells that happen to carry a protein that resembles a bacterial protein. "Other so-called 'innocent bystander' cells, which may have been stressed by radiation, environmental toxins, or the body's own stress chemicals, can also fall victim."[10]

4. Depression of suppressor T cell activity. It has been postulated that in certain cases HLA gene products may resemble or be closely related in structure to an antigen of an ineffective agent, with the system becoming unresponsive due to cross-tolerance with the similar familiar agent.
5. The concept of cryptic antigenic epitopes (determinant or reactive areas of the antigen). T cell tolerance depends on self-antigens being seen in sufficient amounts to initiate the normal mechanisms for deleting autoreactive cells. However, few self-antigens are seen in sufficient concentrations to cause autoreactive T cell removal. It's proposed that these antigens contain what are called cryptic epitopes. T cells specific for these cryptic epitopes may be present in normal immune repertoires and become autoaggressive only if the concentration of such an epitope is increased.[11]
6. Genetic causes. Certain HLA-DR haplotypes confer reduced

suppressor T cell function. For example, normal people with HLA-DR3 haplotypes have reduced T cell suppressor activity compared to non–DR 3 subjects.[12] It's also suspected that HLA antigens may serve as receptors for pathogens, and that autoimmune disease susceptibility may be due to gene mutations.

Environmental Triggers of Thyroid Autoimmunity

Besides the mechanisms discussed above that are suspected to cause the production of autoantibodies in genetically susceptible individuals, there are other mechanisms suspected of goading the process on and triggering the development of Graves' disease. The following environmental causes have been implicated as causative factors.

1. DIETARY IODINE AND EXOGENOUS THYROID HORMONE
Both GD and HT are more prevalent in geographic locations with ample iodine. Both conditions are aggravated when iodine is added to the diet.[13] Graves' disease is also associated with the ingestion of dietary preparations containing kelp, high iodine sources such as certain iodine contrast media, or thyroid hormone precursors such as TRIAC.

Dr. Noel Rose and his team at the Department of Molecular Microbiology and Immunology at Johns Hopkins have demonstrated that T cells from patients with chronic lymphocytic thyroiditis proliferate in the presence of iodinated, but not non-iodinated, human thyroglobulin. The primary mechanism is the loss of certain antigenic determinants and the appearance of others, most importantly the thyroxine molecule.[14]

2. STRESS
In 1825, Parry described a patient who fell down stairs while in a wheelchair shortly before developing symptoms of GD. Also, refugees in Nazi prison camps had a higher incidence of thyrotoxicosis than seen in the general population. A higher incidence of Graves' disease has also been found in the inhabitants of countries engaged in war.

Both acute and chronic stress have been demonstrated to depress the immune system perhaps secondary to the cortisol release and disturbances in cytokine levels seen with stress. Stress induced immune suppression is presumably followed by a compensatory period of immune system hyperactivity. This could precipitate autoimmune thyroid disease, as in postpartum, GD which occurs three to nine months post-delivery.

3. SUPERANTIGENS, ALLERGENS AND INFECTIONS
Superantigens are potent T cell stimulatory molecules that bind to MHC class II molecules. The complex is recognized by particular T cells that are then activated and possibly deleted. Superantigens may be extrin-

sic or intrinsic, although no intrinsic superantigens have yet been detected in man. Extrinsic superantigens include a group of bacterial toxins (staphylococcal, streptococcal and mycoplasmal). The bacteria *Yersinia enterocolitica* has been demonstrated to mimic the TSH receptor antibody in patients with Graves' disease and between retroviral sequences and the TSH receptor.

The idea of an allergic response being a probable GD trigger is suggested in a recent Japanese study that reports elevations of immunoglobulin E (IgE) in the serum of one third of Graves' disease patients. Patients with higher levels of IgE were less likely to experience a reduction in TSH receptor antibodies after treatment with ATDs when compared to patients without IgE. The study's authors propose that the course of GD may be different in these groups. IgE is thought to stimulate the production of TRAb due to a contributing effect of interleukin (IL)-13 found in both allergies and GD.[15]

4. INTERFERONS, INTERLEUKINS AND LITHIUM

Numerous studies show that interferons and interleukins used in the treatment of other conditions contribute to the development of GD. Lithium used therapeutically is associated with the development of GD, perhaps due to its modulation of T cell function.[16]

5. HEAT SHOCK PROTEINS

Heat shock proteins are produced by heat shock and other stressful stimuli including exposure to oxidative radicals, alcohol, plant lectins, heavy metals (mercury, bismuth, lead, etc.) anoxia and infections. Heat shock proteins are immunogenic. In fact, bacterial infection can cause antibody production and T cell response. These antibodies and T cells can cross react with self-cellular heat shock proteins containing conserved epitopes. Heat shock protein 72 has recently been demonstrated to be expressed in thyroid tissue from patients with Graves' disease but not from normal subjects, which suggests that GD is associated with an autoimmune response to certain specific heat shock proteins.[17]

6. SEX STEROIDS

Estrogens have been implicated in the development of GD because GD occurs more frequently in women and rarely develops before puberty. In instances where the onset of GD occurs before puberty, males and females are at equal risk. The synthetic estrogen DES has been shown to cause permanent changes in T lymphocytes and NK cells that contribute to autoimmunity.[18] Endocrine disruptors may trick the body into thinking there is excess thyroid hormone. Endocrine disruptors include a large number of chemicals including PCBs, dioxin and furans, all of which are related to thyroid dysfunction.[19]

Furthermore, the normal suppression of T and B cells during pregnancy followed by the sudden flood of estrogen may account for the incidence of postpartum GD that occurs in 5 percent to 6 percent of women after delivery. Also, estrogen is known to affect antibody formation due to its influence over B cells. In general, circulating autoantibodies and the natural disease course tend to improve in pregnancy and worsen in the postpartum period.[20]

7. EXOGENOUS SUBSTANCES, STARVATION AND THYROID INJURY

Sunlight, drugs or certain viral infections may trigger a prominent autoimmune response by T cell activation or some other mechanism. Several reports have related the development of GD subsequent to states of starvation, both voluntarily by dieting or anorexia or involuntarily in concentration camps. Several women have reported developing Graves' after being on diets with severe calorie restriction.

Certain types of injury to the thyroid are followed by the development of thyroid autoantibodies and the development of GD. Injuries include radiation to the thyroid or neck for Hodgkin's disease and ethanol injection for the cure of toxic thyroid cancer. In certain instances, excessive palpation of the gland itself has been known to induce GD.

Metals, including cadmium, mercury, beryllium salts, tin, titanium dioxide and silica are capable of inducing autoimmunity. Formaldehyde, which is used in the medical laboratory to preserve tissue specimens, is associated with autoimmunity because it causes enhanced resistance to bacterial challenge. Formaldehyde is found in cigarette smoke, another substance highly associated with AITD and GO. Formaldehyde is also found in auto exhaust, smog, biomedical research, insulation, industrial processes and as a breakdown product of the artificial sweetener aspartame.

8 *Allopathic Treatment of Graves' Disease*

A competitive edge has wedged its way into mainstream medicine. In today's economically driven medical Olympics, where advertising campaigns are scrutinized as closely as capital equipment budgets, savvy marketing managers have thrown patient satisfaction into the competition arena. In several recent studies, patients were asked to describe their level of satisfaction following conventional treatment for Graves' disease.

In one study in which patients received thorough explanations regarding treatment and were then allowed to choose their own treatment options, most patients expressed satisfaction regardless of the treatment used.[1] Let this study be your guide. Learn what each treatment option entails, choose what works best for you, and find a practitioner who will closely monitor your progress and guide you through both side effects and after effects.

In this chapter, I describe conventional treatment options, and I describe studies that assess long-term treatment outcome.

Conventional Treatment Goals and Options

There is no cure for Graves' disease. Conventional allopathic treatment is merely palliative, designed to relieve symptoms by reducing available thyroid hormone.

Reducing the amount of thyroid hormone released into the blood is accomplished in conventional medicine either by using (1) chemical agents or medications such as antithyroid drugs (ATDs) that interfere with hormone synthesis or (2) surgical removal (thyroidectomy), or (3) radioiodine ablation. The first option inhibits the amount of thyroid hormone the body produces. The other options work by reducing the amount of functional thyroid tissue that can produce thyroid hormone.

There is no worldwide consensus among endocrinologists or patients regarding the best therapy. The major thyroid associations in the United States can't even agree. And no one treatment satisfies the special needs of all patients. Many factors must be considered, including the patient's age, sex, initial thyroid volume, severity of symptoms, personal philosophy, accessibility to medical treatment, economic status and general health status. And ultimately, patients should be allowed to choose their own treatment after considering the lifelong as well as the immediate consequences of the various approaches.

In the United States, radioiodine, generally the least expensive option, is most often recommended, although many endocrinologists advise that its use be restricted to patients older than 30 or 40. In most other countries, antithyroid drugs are the method of choice, and radioiodine is rarely used. In discussing treatment, Dr. P. Reed Larsen, chief of Harvard University Medical School's Thyroid Division, writes:

> One approach to the therapy in adults is to initiate treatment with antithyroid drugs in all patients to produce a euthyroid state before reaching a final decision regarding a definitive therapeutic strategy. This allows the patients to return to a euthyroid status as rapidly as possible and provides an estimate of the antithyroid drug dose requirements. The magnitude of the drug requirement and the size of the thyroid gland are factors considered in the evaluation of the patient with regard to the likelihood of a remission. The three options for treatment are explained to the patient during these first months of contact, and individual recommendations are then formulated.[2]

Spontaneous Remission

Although spontaneous remisssion is likely to occur in nearly a third of patients with GD, most doctors feel that because serious complications might arise, all patients should be treated aggressively. However, some doctors advise that patients with mild symptoms be monitored before starting treatment since for them spontaneous remission is likely.

Multiple Treatment Considerations

Patients do not necessarily use only their treatment of choice. Sometimes they don't respond adequately, or they may exhibit adverse reactions. Also, if symptoms re-occur after a patient achieves remission, different treatment may be recommended. However, if the previous treatment had worked reasonably well, it is usually used again. Regardless, it's wise to become familiar with all available options including alternative medical methods, used either alone or as a complementary therapy prescribed by integrative medical practitioners.

Antithyroid Drugs

Introduced in the mid–1940s, antithyroid drugs (ATDs) are an integral component of GD treatment. ATDs are used to diminish symptoms until a spontaneous remission occurs. The duration of treatment varies, ranging from several weeks to many years. ATDs are not effective in hyperthyroidism due to other causes besides GD.

The rate of remission (defined as being euthyroid for at least one year) has been reported as 20 percent to 40 percent in the U.S.[3] The likelihood of some treated patients being misdiagnosed and not actually having GD is thought to be responsible for the lower remission rates seen in some studies. The typical well iodized American diet works against ATDs and also contributes to the lower rates. In Europe, where ATDs are used as long as needed, the remission rate is much higher with nearly all patients achieving remission. Alternately, ATDs may be used to achieve a euthyroid state before ablation or surgery. Outside of the U.S., ATDs are the treatment of choice, especially in Europe and Japan.

Antithyroid Drug Choices

The antithyroid drugs most frequently used today are thioureylenes, chemicals that belong to the thionamide family and include propylthiouracil (6-propyl-2-thiouracil; PTU) and methimazole (1-methyl 2-mercaptoimidazole or MMMI; Tapazole), which is used in North America and Japan. In Great Britain and Europe, carbimazole (Neo-Mercazole), a derivative of methimazole, is used. (Carbimazole is metabolized to methimazole, which accounts for its antithyroid effect. Thus the effects of methimazole and carbimazole result from the same active ingredient.)

Aniline derivatives such as sulfonamides and polyhydric phenols such as resorcinol are also antithyroid drugs, but they are rarely used. Other compounds that act as antithyroid drugs include thionamides, iodide, lithium salts, thiouracil derivatives, oral cholecystographic agents, amiodarone, some anticonvulsant drugs and the iodide transport (ionic) inhibitors described later in this chapter. Of interest, topical resorcinol used on abraded skin has been found to cause symptoms of hypothyroidism such as goiter.[4]

Mode of Action (Pharmacodynamics)

Thionamides inhibit thyroid hormone secretion by effects that are either intrathyroidal (occur inside the thyroid) or extrathyroidal, for example, within the liver. Intrathyroidal effects include the inhibition of iodine oxidation, organification and iodotyrosine coupling, and alterations in thyroglobulin synthesis and structure. Trapped in the thyroid after ingestion in a mechanism similar to that of iodine transport, ATDs compete with tyrosine for available oxidized iodine. Consequently, iodine, which would normally bind with tyrosine to form thyroid hormone, is diverted. Extrathyroidal effects, which are seen with PTU but not methimazole, include inhibition of the enzyme thyroid peroxidase (TPO) needed to convert T4 to the more potent T3 in the peripheral tissues.

Effects on Autoimmunity

Patients treated with ATDs experience a decrease in their levels of stimulating TRAb. This immunosuppressive action occurs within the thyroid, the site of ATD concentration. ATDs also cause a decrease in thyroid antigen expression in thyroid cells and reduce the amount of prostglandins and cytokines released by thyroid cells. These phenomena cause a subsequent impairment or relaxation of the autoimmune response.

Thionamides also inhibit the generation of oxygen radicals in T and B cells and in antigen presenting cells. This may contribute to the decline seen in autoantibody titers of patients using ATDs.[5] Also, patients prepared before surgery with ATDs demonstrate thyroid glands that are depleted of lymphocytes compared to control patients.

Effectiveness After the Latent Period

ATDs are very (at least 90 percent) effective in controlling the symptoms of GD.[6] However, the effects aren't immediate. Although new thyroid hormone synthesis is inhibited when ATDs are initiated, the thyroid gland still has a large store of thyroid hormone. Until these hormone stores are depleted, the effects of ATDs are limited. This is considered the latent period. Its duration depends on the amount of stored hormone, its rate of release, and the patient's innate response to the ATD, with larger initial ATD doses decreasing the latent period. In general, euthyroidism is achieved within about six weeks.[7]

Dosage and Dosage Adjustments

The standard recommended dosages for ATDs are listed in the following sections with the individual drugs. However, adjustments are commonly made based on the patient's weight, size of goiter and severity of symptoms. Patients on ATDs must be on the alert for changes in thyroid status as well as adverse effects caused by the medication.

Within the first two weeks of starting treatment, improvement is demonstrated by decreased nervousness and palpitations, increased strength and weight gain reflecting a decreased metabolic rate. The time for peak effects depends on the specific drug used.

Dosage Adjustment

Once improvement is observed, the dosage is often substantially reduced in an effort to maintain a normal metabolic state. Occasionally, however, patients are prescribed a hefty dose of ATDs and told to return for a follow-up visit in two or three months. This may lead to pronounced hypothyroidism. Patient response can be so variable that the initial use of ATDs requires constant vigilance on the part of the patient and the doctor.

Goiter Changes and Treatment Response

In one-third to one-half of patients undergoing ATD treatment, the thyroid gland decreases in size. In the remaining patients, the thyroid may remain unchanged or it may become enlarged. An increase in goiter size may be due to a naturally occurring progression of the disease in which case the dosage of ATDs must be increased, or it may be a sign of hypothyroidism and due to excessive TSH secretion. This can be differentiated by checking for other clinical signs of thyroid dysfunction or by T4 and T3 levels. The serum TSH level is not helpful at this time as it may not yet reflect the changes in thyroid hormone and may remain subnormal or suppressed for many months after the T4 and T3 have changed. Even when the patient becomes euthyroid, it may take three or four months for TSH to rise.[8]

Criteria thought to be predictive of a sustained remission include a decrease in goiter size, control of symptoms with low doses after the initial period, T3 and reduced levels of serum stimulating TRAb.

Propylthiouracil

Discovered five years before methimazole, propylthiouracil (PTU) is used twice as often. PTU has a shorter plasma half-life (75 minutes) so it acts faster, stays in the circulation for a shorter period of time, and hence, must be taken more often. A 100 mg dose begins to wane in two to three hours. Although both PTU and methimazole cross the placenta and are found in breast milk, PTU does so to a lesser degree and is the drug of choice in pregnancy (see chapter 10). Its metabolism is not affected by kidney or liver disease.

The usual starting dose for PTU is 100 mg every eight hours or 150 mg every twelve hours. In some patients, daily doses as high as 1,200 mg are required. Resistance to doses as high as 2,000 mg are thought to be attributed to poor compliance. Doses larger than 300 mg should be divided and given every four to six hours. When large doses are required for control, remission is considered unlikely.[9]

PRECAUTIONS

A 1998 report by the U.S. Department of Health and Human Services indicates that there is sufficient evidence that PTU (same classification as estrogen) is reasonably anticipated to be a human carcinogen.[10] See side effects of ATDs later in this chapter.

Methimazole (Tapazole; Active Metabolite of Carbimazole)

Methimazole (MMMI) has a half life of four to six hours and is said to be ten to 50 times as potent as PTU, although its effects are not as consistent. Its peak serum concentrations occur one to two hours after ingestion. The intrathyroidal metabolism of methimazole is slow, with drug concentrations measured 17 to 20 hours after ingestion similar to those measured three to six hours after ingestion.

A dose as low as 0.5 mg may have an effect, but a dose of 10 to 15 mg is needed if effects are to last for 24 hours. Methimazole can be given once daily because of its longer half-life and its long duration of action. Drug metabolism is not affected by renal (kidney) disease although it is prolonged in patients with hepatic (liver) disease. Methimazole is the drug of choice in patients with GO as it appears to offer a protective effect.

PRECAUTIONS

Methimazole readily crosses the placental membranes and can cause fetal harm if used during pregnancy. Effects of subsequent hypothyroidism include goiter and cretinism in the developing fetus as well as rare instances of aplasia cutis, which causes scalp defects. It's recommended that postpartum patients receiving methimazole not nurse their babies.

Block and Replace ATD Protocol

In the block and replace protocol, a small dose of thyroxine is given in conjunction with ATDs. The rationale in adding thyroxine is to prevent the patient from becoming hypothyroid. Ideally, this would lead to fewer office visits and a prompt remission. However, some patients I know were kept on high doses of ATDs and low doses of thyroxine until they became severely hypothyroid. This protocol initially requires frequent monitoring, and the patient's individual disease course must be taken into consideration.

Originating in Japan where it yielded remission rates as high as 96 percent, the block and replace protocol hasn't yet met with the same success in the United States. Some researchers feel that the normal American diet with its high iodine content is to blame for the discrepancy. Another reason is that guidelines to determine remission are rarely used.

ADVANTAGES OF BLOCK AND REPLACE

A recent article in *Thyroid USA*, a newsletter published by the American Foundation of Thyroid Patients, described a recent study in which GD patients were treated with a low dose of methimazole in conjunction with thyroxine. Compared to the control group, which used only methimazole, patients on block and replace therapy achieved identical relapse rates, although relapse was delayed in the group using combination therapy. This was attributed to the fact that the thyroxine had to be gradually tapered down. The potential advantage to the combined therapy is a more stable thyroid status during treatment that may or not be found in patients using ATDs alone.[11]

PROTOCOL WITH HIGHER REMISSIONS

The markedly higher remission rates (96 percent) reported in the early Japanese studies appear to be directly related to the use of tangible guidelines such as T3 suppression tests to determine when remission has taken place. Initially, patients were given 300 to 450 mg daily of PTU or 30 to 45 mg of MMI until they became euthyroid. Then 1 ug/kg of body weight of T3 was added to the regimen.

At six month intervals, the patients were given a 20 minute RAI-U scan (T3 suppression test). When uptake results reached 10 percent, or 10 percent to 15 percent on two consecutive readings, the drugs were discontinued (normal RAI-U is about 25 percent). The time for suppression to occur ranged between 12 and 111 months with a mean of four years. The patients were then monitored at six month intervals for thyroid hormone levels. Of the patients who eventually relapsed, most of them had achieved early remissions (within one or two years). No patients who went into remission after 40 months of treatment had relapses.[12]

Advantages and Disadvantages of ATDs

As with any treatment, the benefits must outweigh the risks. Although regular monitoring is required, patients treated with ATDs are more likely to remain euthyroid after remission than in other conventional treatment options. Following remission, only 20 percent of GD patients treated with ATDs eventually become hypothyroid after 20 years.[13]

SIDE EFFECTS OF ATD TREATMENT

Both PTU and methimazole have rare side effects, which include agranulocytosis (decrease in granulocytic white blood cells seen in approximately 0.2 percent to 0.5 percent of treated patients) and liver problems that may be severe. Signs of infection, including fever or sore throat, should be reported immediately. A white blood cell count is then usually measured. If agranulocytosis occurs, the ATD is discontinued and the patient is treated for infection. A low white blood cell count is often seen in GD; thus, any blood cell counts determined subsequent to therapy must be compared to pre-treatment baseline determinations. These adverse reactions usually emerge within the first few weeks of therapy.

Approximately 5 percent to 10 percent of patients using ATDs report developing a mild rash that is manifested in different forms including hives. (Note: many GD patients not on ATDs develop hives.) Most patients who develop rashes continue on their ATDs using appropriate antihistamine treatment if indicated, although the symptoms rarely completely disappear. Exfoliative dermatitis, with symptoms of cracking and peeling skin, should be reported and the drug discontinued. Thiouracils prevent the conversion of dietary carotene into usable Vitamin A. Thus, additional Vitamin A may be needed to correct dermatitis. If thyroid supplement is given (see block and replacement protocol), it overcomes the vitamin antagonists, allowing dietary conversion to Vitamin A.[14]

Other rare reactions include arthralgia (neuralgic pain in one or more joints), myalgia (muscle pain), neuritis, fever, hepatitis (with PTU) or cholestatic jaundice (with methimazole), hepatocellular (liver cell) toxicity and rare liver necrosis, decreased platelets, hair loss, abnormal hair pigmentation, loss of taste sensation, lymph node or salivary gland enlargement, lupus-like syndrome, edema and toxic psychoses. Although agranulocytosis occurs equally with both drugs, the other side effects are seen more often with PTU,[15] suggesting that Vitamin A deficiency is a probable cause. Many of these symptoms are also seen in GD, making it difficult to determine the exact cause.

Allergies to ATDs may occur, usually showing up two to four weeks after therapy is initiated. In cases of allergy, patients are generally switched to another drug. Patients are rarely allergic to both PTU and methimazole. Patients on high doses of ATDs may become temporarily hypothyroid, especially if they aren't frequently monitored.

MONITORING TREATMENT

Once treatment begins, thyroid function tests including levels of FT4 and FT3 should be performed every two to four months. Once euthyroidism is established, patients should be monitored at four to six month intervals. Treatment response is associated with a decrease in goiter size. If the goiter increases, hypothyroidism has probably occurred, although lab tests may be necessary to distinguish hypothyroidism from hyperthyroidism caused by the natural progression of the disease.[16] Since hypothyroidism may have adverse effects on pre-existing GO,[17] it's important that the treatment is frequently monitored.

DISCONTINUING ANTITHYROID DRUGS

Debate surrounds the duration of ATD therapy, and with the normal variability of GD patients, an absolute time frame defies logic. Higher remission rates are associated with low antibody titers, small goiters, initial T3 toxicosis, milder symptoms and older patients since they frequently exhibit milder symptoms. One study described in chapter 9 reports higher remission rates using ATDs in conjunction with traditional Chinese medicine. The longer the course of therapy, the more likely it is to reduce antibody titers. Thus, most physicians feel therapy should be continued for six to 12 months. Initial T3 toxicosis and a small thyroid at the time of diagnosis, and achieving normal TSH levels during treatment, are both associated with a likely remission.[18]

Most patients report that their doses are gradually decreased prior to withdrawal of the drug. Some patients report decreasing their dose by small increments and taking low doses every other day before ATDs are completely withdrawn. Several patients report that they ended up having an additional short course of antithyroid drugs a year or so after their initial course of ATDs before they achieved permanent remission.

RELAPSE

Relapse most often occurs within three to six months after therapy is discontinued. Relapse is characteristically associated with a rise in serum T3 concentration preceding a rise in T4, and relapse is more likely in the postpartum period.[19] Because relapse can occur at any time, lifelong follow-up is required for all patients who achieve remission following the use of ATDs.

Surgery (Thyroidectomy)

Surgery is recommended for young patients, patients with GO, pregnant patients, patients with large goiters and patients also having suspicious thyroid nodules or multinodular goiters. Because it produces rapid effects, surgery is also recommended for patients who initially present with very large goiters and severe thyrotoxicosis since there is a higher failure rate with radioiodine in these individuals.[20]

Having access to advanced imaging studies, today's surgeons can study the thyroid's anatomy and density beforehand, and they can predetermine the thyroid gland's relationship to the parathyroid glands and other adjacent structures. Also, fine precision surgical tools facilitate identification of the laryngeal nerves. The current success of thyroidectomies can also be attributed to the implementation of pretreatment protocols that render the patient euthyroid before surgery and prepare the tissue to facilitate cutting.

Pretreatment

Before surgery, the patient is first made euthyroid with ATDs (takes about six weeks), which are continued until the day of surgery. Strong iodine solution (three drops of Lugol's solution or five drops SSKI used twice daily) is given for seven to ten days before surgery to prepare the tissue. Iodine makes the thyroid tissue less vascular (firmer), which facilitates surgery. Patients who are allergic to ATDs or noncompliant can be made euthyroid by treatment with iopanoic acid, dexamethasone and propranolol for five to seven days prior to surgery. All of these drugs should be discontinued before surgery.

Surgical Procedure

Surgical procedures for GD include subtotal, near-total, or total thyroidectomy. The most commonly used procedure is the bilateral subtotal thyroidectomy in which 1 to 2 grams of thyroid tissue is left on both sides. This is also considered the safest procedure. Debate surrounds the amount of tissue which should be removed, with most surgeons leaving 2 to 3 grams of tissue on either side of the neck.

Alternately, the surgeon may perform a procedure known as a Hartley-Dunhill procedure in which a total lobectomy is performed on one side and a subtotal thyroidectomy is performed on the other side, leaving about 4 to 5 grams of thyroid tissue. In patients with coexisting eye disease, total thyroidectomy is recommended because it is associated with a decreased level of stimulating TSH receptor antibodies.

Advantages and Disadvantages of Surgery

Surgery offers a prompt relief of symptoms with a decreased incidence of hypothyroidism when compared to radioiodine therapy. In addition, surgery requires less outpatient visits and the surgeon is able to detect and remove an existing thyroid carcinoma during surgery if one happens to be present.

Disadvantages include the rare possibility (approximately 1 percent)[21] of recurrent laryngeal nerve injury that can result in permanent vocal chord injury, and hypoparathyroidism (transient in 13 percent of patients and permanent in 1 percent).[22] The earliest symptoms of hypoparathyroidism, which may appear from one to seven days after surgery, include anxiety and depression, followed by heightened neuromuscular excitability and spasm. Usually, hypoparathyroidism is transient and can be treated with calcium, although at the onset it is impossible to predict if the condition is temporary or permanent.

Following surgery, the patient's serum calcium level is temporarily decreased and the phosphorus level increased. This decrease in blood calcium level, known as hypocalcemia, is independent of hypoparathyroidism and thought to be caused by the bone's retention of calcium. It is frequently accompanied by a transient increase in the level of serum alkaline phosphatase, an enzyme related to both bone and liver function, which is commonly elevated in hyperthyroidism and decreased in hypothyroidism.

MORTALITY

Mortality from thyroid surgery is rare today. The hazards of surgery are said to be inversely related to the experience of the surgical team, which makes it difficult to generalize about the rate of complications. It's wise to choose a surgeon and surgical team who perform many successful thyroidectomies. Bleeding onto the operative site, the most serious postoperative complication, can rapidly cause death by asphyxia. Also, if the laryngeal nerve is damaged bilaterally, the airway can be obstructed, requiring an emergency tracheostomy.

POST SURGICAL HYPOTHYROIDISM

Permanent hypothyroidism occurs in 4 percent to 40 percent of surgical patients.[23] Long-term studies indicate that the incidence of developing hypothyroidism after surgery increases over time, which may be due to the natural progression of the disease with the process possibly being accelerated by the surgical destruction of thyroid tissue. This is similar to the cumulative incidence of hypothyroidism over time seen after radioiodine treatment, but it's not as severe. The frequency of recurrence as well as the incidence of hypothyroidism appear to be related to the amount of thyroid tissue left.

RADIOIODINE ABLATION

In the United States, the majority of adult hyperthyroid patients are treated with radioiodine. Radioiodine is rarely used in children, however, because children treated with radioiodine have an increased risk of developing hyperparathyroidism.[24] In addition, the developing thyroid is more susceptible to the mutagenic effects of radiation. Radioiodine therapy is also contraindicated in women who are pregnant or breast-feeding. Other relative contraindications include progressive ophthalmopathy and the presence of isolated nodules. In Europe, radioiodine is used infrequently and rarely on women younger than 40. Although radioiodine is frequently recommended for elderly patients, some physicians feel that the increased risk of thyroid storm in the elderly puts them at too much risk.[25]

Effects of Ionizing Radiation

Dr. John Pacer, a Ph.D. physical chemist in Allentown, Pa., explained that ionizing radiation in the form of radioisotopes is a natural occurrence that works to maintain homeostasis.[26] In a process known as natural selection, radioisotopes destroy the weakest cells and spare the healthiest. Acting on cellular DNA, radioisotopes can destroy cells or cause mutations. Radioisotopes, Dr. Pacer added, are found in certain foods, particularly fruits such as bananas and tomatoes and in several types of wood. In medical treatment, radioisotopes aim to destroy cells, and cell mutations are a side effect.

Ionizing radiation includes particulate radiation (mainly alpha and beta particles) and electromagnetic radiation (including gamma and X-rays), which have extremely high frequency and short wavelengths. Radioiodine releases alpha and beta particles and gamma rays and each has their own rate of decay.

Iodine in its natural state has a molecular weight of 127. The isotopes of iodine in current use are produced by irradiation in nuclear reactors, cyclotron-charged particle irradiation, or in a process that separates them from nuclear fission products. Ionizing radiation is emitted when radioactive isotopes decay. Ionizing radiation disrupts the atoms and molecules of the tissues through which it passes. Because living tissue is composed of atoms joined into molecules, it is vulnerable to ionizing radiation. The molecular disruptions caused by irradiation produce ions and free radicals that can cause further biochemical damage including cell death, reproductive effects and cancer.[27]

The Question of Linear Energy Transfer

As radiation impinges on matter and bombards ions, it releases energy in a process known as linear energy transfer (LET). Estimation of the cumulative dose over time is known as dosimetry and the absorbed dose is defined as the energy absorbed per unit mass in joules per kilogram (gray or Gy; 1 Gy = 1 joule/kg of tissue) or in ergs per gram (rad).

The principle target for radiation induced cell killing is DNA, although it's not the only target. Although it was originally thought that effects were proportional to dose, the National Research Council lists several deviations from this rule, including the type of tissue targeted, the growth stage of the cells, cell sensitivity and the dose rate.[28]

Recent studies indicate that the energy transfer of radioisotopes may not be linear. Despite popular and universal application for a half century, this concept has yet to be validated or disproved. In studies of cell damage from Nagasaki bomb survivors, a purely cubic model, not a linear model, was found to fit the data best.[29]

Historical Overview

Radioiodine was first produced in 1937, and by 1950 when I-131 was made available, it evolved as a standard treatment for hyperthyroidism. Initially the use of radioiodine was limited because of the controversy surrounding radiation, already under criticism for being indiscriminately used in treating acne, thymus enlargement, tonsillitis, hemangioma (birthmark) and pertussis (whooping cough).

When radioiodine was being considered as a treatment for hyperthyroidism in the mid–1950s, physicians were alarmed by the results of a 1950 study in which ten of 28 patients with thyroid cancer had undergone previous irradiation. Subsequent studies showed an increased tumor risk with low doses of irradiation.

However, the Cooperative Thyrotoxicosis Therapy Study, comparing surgery, antithyroid drugs and radioiodine ablation, which was conducted at 26 institutions and involved tens of thousands of patients, concluded that radioiodine is safe treatment for hyperthyroidism. With publication of these results, radioiodine wended its way to the center stage of the treatment arena in the U.S. However, the debate regarding the safety of radiation continues to this day and is discussed later in this chapter.

Biological Effects of Radioiodine

When localized in the gland, the distribution of radiation depends on the type of radiation and the energy of the emissions, with 73 percent to 96 percent of the total radiation dose from radioiodines attributed to particulate irradiations. The mean particle range is highly variable although it is known to be longer for beta emitters such as I-131. Although I-131 emits both gamma and beta irradiation, beta particles, which have a path length of 1 to 2 mm, are responsible for the destruction seen in thyroid cells. Since their path length exceeds the diameter of thyroid cells, the cells are irradiated even if they haven't trapped radioiodine.

Determining an optimal ablative dose is difficult because of individual sensitivity and the varying size of the individual thyroid follicles. At the usual ablative doses, biological effects are primarily on thyroid function. Following ablation, radioiodine particles lodge in the thyroid follicle and remain while undergoing radioactive decay. The effective half-life of I-131 ranges from two to eight days, with a mean of 5.5 days.

The half-life denotes the time for the original dose to be reduced by 50 percent. The amount remaining will be further reduced by 50 percent every 5.5 days. For radioiodine, usually eight to ten half-life cycles are required for the entire dose to be reduced (44 to 55 days). Dr. Pacer reports that the actual time for radioiodine to leave the body depends on the dose.

Since atoms are being reduced, with an initial dose of one trillion atoms, when reduced by half each 5.5 days, it will take considerable time for the total RAI dose to be reduced.

Because the rate of cell division in the normal thyroid is quite slow, sublethal radiation effects such as the development of both benign and malignant neoplasms may take many years to become clinically apparent, especially at low doses.[30] When higher doses are used, most of the thyroid tissue is destroyed and the incidence of neoplasms is lower. To date, no irradiated population has been adequately studied through their life span. What studies have been done focus on mortality only. Studies indicate that internally used I-131 causes fewer biological effects on a rad for rad basis than external radiation given at a high, uniformly distributed dose, but its long term consequences are still uncertain.

TESTING FOR CELL DAMAGE

Dr. Joseph Gong, a cell biologist at the State University of New York at Buffalo, has studied the effects of ionizing radiation for the Atomic Energy Commission for many years. His lifelong passion has been to quantify these effects. Cellular effects of radiation, he has found, include prolonged increase of red cell precursors known as normoblasts in the bone marrow and the presence of a subpopulation of erythrocyte (red cells) with transferrin (involved in iron uptake) receptors. By measuring the percentage of erythrocytes with transferrin receptors present in a blood sample, Dr. Gong can assess radiation injury.

Dr. Gong has studied the effects of external radiation on humans and is able to measure the lifelong cumulative effects. In a series of personal communications, Dr. Gong said a study of irradiated Graves' patients would shed light on the effects of radioiodine.[31]

Chromosomal Damage

Although several studies have shown leukocyte (white blood cell) chromosomal abnormalities in patients treated with radioiodine, the clinical importance is unclear. As described in chapter 5, the whole body is exposed to radiation following radioiodine therapy. The Nuclear Regulatory Commission reports that a whole body dose as low as 0.1 Gy or 10 rad in 100,000 persons would cause 800 additional deaths from cancer.[32]

Gonadal irradiation is of particular concern because radioiodine is ultimately excreted in the urinary bladder. The estimated gonadal dose is thought to be similar to that of other common radiographic procedures such as barium enema and intravenous pyelography. Although little data is available, several studies of offspring of patients treated with radioiodine show no evidence of health effects.

One recent study showed that ionizing radiation is carcinogenic even without hitting the cell nucleus, an event that was previously thought necessary for mutations. Study results indicate that genetic damage at low dose radiation exposures is likely to be more significant than previously thought. Apparently, irradiation of the cytoplasm by alpha particles creates highly reactive free radicals that migrate to the cell nucleus and mutate the DNA.[33]

RAI Pretreatment

Some physicians use ATDs to deplete thyroid hormone stores prior to RAI to help prevent post ablation thyroid storm. However, pretreated patients often require a larger RAI dose, and some studies indicate that pretreatment renders the patient "radio-protective" or resistant to therapy. For this reason, it's recommended that patients stop ATDs for two to three weeks before ablation to allow adequate uptake of radioiodine by the thyroid.

However, recent studies indicate that the initial size of the thyroid, not the use of ATDs, may account for relapse. Radioisotopes, after all, destroy tissue at the end of their path length. That thyroid volume is a factor is suggested by reports showing that resistance to therapy is more often seen in men and in patients having larger thyroids. Thus resistance to RAI may be more of a result of underestimating thyroid volume than pretreatment. Some endocrinologists recommend using ultrasonography rather than the RAI-U to determine thyroid volume so that an appropriate ablative dose can be determined.

Radioiodine Procedure and Mode of Action

Patients are advised to avoid ingesting excess iodine for two weeks prior to ablation, and iodine contrast dyes are to be avoided. Excess iodine may interfere with the body's uptake of radioiodine. Strong iodine solution (see chapter 9) should not be used for the first three days after radioiodine treatment. However, it may be started on the 4th day to relieve symptoms of thyrotoxicosis until the I-131 becomes effective.[34]

Radioiodine treatment is usually administered in the form of a drink of I-131, commonly referred to as a radioactive cocktail. Taken orally, I-131 is dissolved in water or swallowed as a capsule. Since it is perceived by the body as iodine, I-131 is dissolved in water or swallowed as a capsule. Since it is perceived by the body as iodine, I-131 is rapidly absorbed and quickly concentrated, oxidized and organified by thyroid follicular cells.

I-131 is the standard isotope used for radioiodine ablation. An optimal dosage would render the patient euthyroid and stop short of hypothyroidism, but there is no general agreement on what constitutes an optimal dose. The methods of calculating the dose are controversial although most systems consider the RAI-U results (see chapter 5) and the size and density of the thyroid.

Radioiodine therapy is generally designed to deliver 5,000 to 10,000 rads to the thyroid tissue. This can usually be achieved by a dose of approximately 7.5 mCi. Many clinics have settled on an arbitrary dose calculated to result in the delivery of 185 to 222 Mbq (5 to 7 mCi) of I-131 to the thyroid gland 24 hours after administration. The standard dose has also been listed as 5.9 Mbq (160 uCi) per gram of estimated gland weight, which leads to a higher incidence of hypothyroidism. Thus, some physicians using this method administer prophylactic doses of thyroxine.

Efforts are being made to use doses that render the patient euthyroid rather than hypothyroid. A recent study in Hungary advised that there is no need to use doses greater than 10,000 rads if no ATD pretreatment is used. Six months after receiving doses of 7,000 rads of I-131, 81 percent of the patients in this study with small to moderate sized thyroids were cured of their symptoms. Sixty-two percent of patients became euthyroid and 19 percent hypothyroid. In patients with large thyroids similar results were achieved using 10,000 rads of I-131.[35]

Radiation Safety

Today, radiologists are required to explain the biological risks to the patient before RAI is administered.[36] The consent form the patient must sign follows guidelines directed by the Nuclear Regulatory Commission and is designed to ensure that the patient has been informed of other available treatment options, the spontaneous progression to hypothyroidism that occurs in GD and the potential risks of radiation.

Following ablation, the patient is instructed to avoid intimate contact, including kissing, for at least 24 hours. Because the thyroid glands of infants and young children are most susceptible to radiation, patients are instructed to avoid carrying infants on the shoulder and to avoid hugging children where thyroid to thyroid contact might occur. Since radioiodine is excreted via the urine, the toilet should be flushed two to three times after use, and the hands should be thoroughly washed. Pregnancy is not advised for three months after ablation, although some doctors recommend a delay of six months to a year.

In Europe, patients are quarantined following ablation for five days. Today, some, but not all, hospitals in the U.S. measure the patient's level of radioactive emissions before they're dismissed.

Advantages, Disadvantages and
Long Term Risks of RAI

The advantages of radioiodine ablation are that it is quickly administered, generally effective, relatively inexpensive and initially painless. It requires little in the way of initial follow-up office visits until hypothyroidism develops. The disadvantages of radioiodine are that it invariably causes permanent hypothyroidism, and it may affect other organs such as the salivary glands, the gastric glands, the parathyroid glands and the gonads. The difficulties in determining in optimal dose cause nearly 30 percent to 70 percent of patients to require a second ablation.[37] RAI is known to significantly induce or exacerbate GO and PTM.

Worsening of GO is reported to not occur in patients using corticosteroids with RAI (see chapter 4). One regimen involves using 0.4 to 0.5 mg/kg of prednisone for one month prior to radioiodine ablation with a gradual tapering over three to four months.[38] Although worsening of GO is not associated with surgery or the use of ATDs, the development of hypothyroidism, if not promptly diagnosed and treated, has an adverse effect on GO. Some endocrinologists advise avoiding radioiodine in patients with severe orbitopathy.[39]

Controversy also surrounds the cancer risk associated with radioiodine. Although most mortality studies report that radioiodine poses no increased cancer risk, a recent study in the British medical journal *Lancet* involving 7,417 patients treated between 1950 and 1991 in Birmingham, United Kingdom, indicates that although the overall risk of cancer is low, there is a significant increase in cancers of the thyroid and small bowel following radioiodine ablation. The authors of this study suggest that the increased relative risk for these cancers indicates a need for long-term vigilance in those receiving radioiodine.[40]

Another provocative study of roughly the same United Kingdom cohort reports that among hyperthyroid patients treated with radioiodine, mortality from all causes and mortality due to thyroid disease, cardiovascular and cerebrovascular disease (stroke) and fracture are increased. The highest incidence of mortality occurred in the first year following treatment and was observed primarily in women. The overall risk was confined to patients who were older than 49 at the time of treatment. The overall risk of fracture was confined to patients who were older than 59 at the time of treatment, which put them in the age range typically associated with increased fracture at the time of the study. Mortality from all causes increased with increasing cumulative doses of radioiodine.[41]

Although this study has been criticized, with critics saying that the causes of death were related to age more than to RAI, many GD patients

criticize the fact that there are no studies indicating the incidence of cancer apart from that associated with mortality.

A recent report of the Cooperative Thyrotoxicosis Therapy Follow-
up Study Group indicates that radioiodine does not increase total cancer
deaths, although it poses a significantly increased risk of death from thyroid cancer. Thyroid cancer risk is reported to possibly be a result of the
original thyroid disease, although this increased risk is not seen in patients
treated with ATDs or surgery.[42]

In addition, long-term studies of children and adolescents treated
with internal doses of radioiodine are difficult to find, and short term
studies have yielded variable results.[43] Thus, most endocrinologists refrain
from using radioiodine in children.

Radiation Thyroiditis and Hypoparathyroidism

Radiation thyroiditis develops within the first few weeks of treatment
and may lead to an exacerbation of symptoms resulting in serious consequences such as thyroid storm (see chapter 1). This is thought to be due
to the release of stored hormone from ruptured thyroid follicles. Milder
side effects include a sore throat and pain on swallowing, which are associated with thyroidal inflammation and tenderness.

On the cellular level symptoms include thyroid epithelial cell swelling
and necrosis, disruption of follicular cells, edema and infiltration with
leukocytes. After this acute phase, the thyroid is marred by fibrosis, vascular narrowing and lymphocytic infiltration. These changes are associated with a reduction in thyroid volume, which reflects thyroid damage.
These cellular effects, along with the release of stored hormone and antibodies from dying cells, are responsible for the early symptoms following
radioiodine ablation.

Used for hyperthyroidism, radioiodine reduces symptoms by destroying thyroid tissue, preferentially the active follicular cells. Biological effects
of I-131 include impaired replication of intact follicular cells, atrophy,
fibrosis and a chronic inflammatory response that may ultimately result
in permanent thyroid failure.[44] The parathyroid glands are exposed to
radiation and parathyroid reserve may be diminished in some patients.
However, development of overt hypoparathyroidism is thought to be
rare.[45]

Other Organ Involvement

Thyroid cells take up radioiodine in the same manner in which they
take up iodine, since they aren't able to distinguish between these isotopes. However, the nucleus of a radioactive iodine molecule has excess
energy. Therefore, it emits radiation that affects all of the cells that concen-

trate it. Besides the thyroid gland, radioiodine is taken up by the gonads, gastric glands, parathyroid glands, salivary glands, the skin, skeletal muscle, the adrenal gland and the pituitary gland. The effects of radioiodine on non-thyroidal tissues that concentrate iodide has received little attention.[46]

One study on the localization of radioiodine in the tissues of swine reported that radioiodine concentration was also evident in the lung, muscle, liver, pancreas, intestinal mucosa, thymus and spleen as well as the striated border of duodenal epithelial cells.[47] A recent CAT scan I had showed that my pancreas is "somewhat atrophied."

There was also a marked concentration in the collecting ducts of the submandibular gland and a lesser concentration in the secretory parenchyma of this gland. The highest concentration of radioactivity was found in the follicular epithelial cells of the thyroid gland, and this was consistently higher than that of thyroid connective tissue.[48]

In a recent report from the Cooperative Thyrotoxicosis Follow-up Study Group, the average dose of I-131 delivered to 17 different organs was evaluated. Besides the thyroid, the stomach, bladder and small intestine received the largest average dose (>100 mGy). The bone marrow, salivary glands, colon, rectum, liver, esophagus, kidney and breast were also listed as being affected by RAI.[49]

Hypothyroidism

When radioiodine was first introduced as a treatment for hyperthyroidism, the incidence of hypothyroidism was thought to be low. With the passage of time it became apparent that although the incidence of hypothyroidism is greatest during the first two years following treatment, with 25 percent to 50 percent of patients becoming hypothyroid within the first year,[50] the incidence increases at a rate of approximately 5 percent with each successive year.[51]

Rates vary with most studies showing the incidence of hypothyroidism following ablation to be as high as 90 percent. The sudden onset of hypothyroidism in a previously thyrotoxic patient may result in severe muscle cramps, especially in large muscle groups such as the trapezius or latissimus dorsi or the proximal muscles of the extremities. These symptoms may develop even when the thyroid hormone levels have only dropped to the low normal range and before the TSH has begun to rise.[52]

The development of hypothyroidism and thyroid failure is related to the increasingly high titers of stimulating TSH receptor antibodies seen following ablation. This contributes to the difficulty in determining an optimal ablative dose. A dose capable of causing immediate effects is associated with a high incidence of hypothyroidism, while a dose yielding gradual symptom reduction often results in a recurrence of hyperthyroidism.

Relapse Following Radioiodine

Relapse following radioiodine is most often seen in patients having larger pre-treatment thyroid volumes and higher pre-treatment levels of stimulating TSH receptor antibodies. Relapse is also associated with the volume of the thyroid remaining after treatment with larger volumes associated with relapse, except in the case of transient enlargement due to the inflammatory response.

Usually, euthyroidism and goiter shrinkage are evident within six to eight weeks after radioiodine therapy. Overall, more than 80 percent of patients become hypothyroid after one dose of radioiodine. Twenty-five to fifty percent of patients are hypothyroid within one year of ablation, and hypothyroidism occurs in the others at a rate of about 5 percent each subsequent year.[53] However, there is a current trend of administering a second dose within a few months if results aren't forthcoming. Thirty to 70 percent of ablated patients are reported as having a second dose and in fewer than 10 percent of cases, a third dose is used.[54]

Ionic Transport Inhibitors and Dexamethasone

Ionic inhibitors are substances that interfere with the thyroid's ability to concentrate iodide into iodine. These substances are monovalent hydrated ions that resemble iodine. Thus, they are able to displace it, inhibiting thyroid hormone synthesis.

One of the first ionic inhibitors discovered is the heart medication thiocyanate. Its natural ability to block thyroid hormone synthesis led researchers to develop compounds with similar modes of action. Certain plant compounds metabolize into thiocyanate after they are ingested and are known as goitrogens (see chapters 3 and 9).

Perchlorate is ten times as active as thiocyanate. Years ago, perchlorate was routinely used to treat hyperthyroidism using doses of 2 to 3 grams. At such excessive doses, perchlorate was found to cause aplastic anemia, which can be fatal. Since early 1990, perchlorate treatment has seen a revival using lower doses, 750 mg (0.75 grams). Perchlorate is currently being used to treat the thyrotoxicosis of GD and also amiodarone induced hyperthyroidism.[55] Present in concentrations of up to 1 percent in many fertilizers and as an atmospheric byproduct of solid fuel propellant used in rockets, missiles and fireworks, environmental perchlorate is suspected of causing hypothyroidism in children.

Other ionic inhibitors include lithium, which is used in the treatment of manic depression, fluoride, bromide, chlorine and iodinated radiographic contrast agents such as sodium iopanoate and sodium ipodate. These compounds have side effects that for the most part make them undesirable treatment agents, although lithium is sometimes used in severe thyrotoxicosis in place of strong iodine solution in patients who are allergic to iodine.

Lithium carbonate inhibits thyroid hormone secretion with the advantage that it doesn't interfere with radioiodine uptake. Lithium is generally used at a dose of 300 to 450 mg given every eight hours resulting in a serum concentration of 1 mEq/L, which is appropriate for the general therapeutic use of lithium, the range being 0.5 to 1.5 mEq/L. The fluoride compound fluoborate is considered as effective as perchlorate.

Ipodate used in doses of 1 gram daily causes a prompt reduction of serum T4 and T3 in hyperthyroid patients. The effects of ipodate include iodine release and inhibition of T4's conversion to T3. As with strong iodine solution, withdrawal of ipodate may result in an exacerbation of symptoms.

Dexamethasone administered as a 2 mg dose every six hours inhibits thyroid hormone secretion and the peripheral conversion of T4 to T3. Dexamethasone also has an immunosuppressive effect and is sometimes used along with beta adrenergic blocking agents and strong iodine solution to provide rapid relief in cases of severe thyrotoxicosis.[56]

The major advantage of these compounds is that they do not generally produce hypothyroidism, yet they effectively relieve symptoms of thyrotoxicosis. The disadvantage is the frequency of recurrence.

Beta Adrenergic Blocking Agents

Beta adrenergic receptor antagonists (beta blockers) are routinely prescribed to relieve symptoms of GD that result from excessive catecholamine stimulation. The major effects of beta blockers are on the cardiovascular system (slowing the heart and decreasing its contractions). Beta blockers decrease tremulousness, palpitations, tachycardia, excessive sweating, heat intolerance, nervousness, anxiety, eyelid retraction and the Graves' stare, but they do not normalize the metabolic rate. Beta blockers also reduce blood pressure in hypertensive patients but have no effect in patients with normal blood pressure. Beta blockers pose risks for pregnant patients. Those risks are described in chapter 10.

PROPRANOLOL

Propranolol is the drug usually prescribed (except in patients with bronchial disorders, chronic obstructive pulmonary disease or asthma since propranolol aggravates bronchospasm) because it has a slight diminishing effect on the conversion of T4 to T3. The dose initially prescribed is 20 to 40 mg of propranolol to be taken up to four times daily or 50 to 100 mg of atenolol or metoprolol, which can be taken once daily due to its longer half-life. For patients with severe symptoms, propranolol or esmolol can be given intravenously. For patients with congestive heart failure beta blockers should be avoided.

Many patients with mild to moderate symptoms report that they are instructed to take the medications as needed (without exceeding the maximum dose) with the precaution that beta blockers can cause sluggishness in some patients when used at higher doses. As the patient moves toward euthyroidism, the dosage is generally decreased, and discontinued when the patient becomes euthyroid. After continuous long term treatment, beta adrenergic antagonists should not be discontinued abruptly, as this can exacerbate angina and pose a risk of sudden death. Increased sensitivity to catecholamine stimulation may persist for one week. Therefore, when taken regularly, the drug should be tapered and withdrawn slowly.

SIDE EFFECTS OF BETA ADRENERGIC ANTAGONISTS

Side effects of beta blockers include decreased plasma potassium, decreased intraocular pressure, light-headedness, depression, lassitude, weakness, fatigue, visual disturbances, vivid dreams, an acute reversible syndrome characterized by disorientation for time and place, short term memory loss, nausea, vomiting, thrombocytopenic purpura, agranulocytosis and rare occurrences of drug related lupus.

Beta blockers may mask symptoms of thyrotoxicosis, and an abrupt withdrawal of the drug may be followed by an exacerbation of hyperthyroid symptoms, including the potential progression to thyroid storm.[57] Beta blockers are not recommended as the sole pretreatment agent before surgery since this situation is associated with thyroid storm.

Comparing Treatment Outcomes

The particular type of treatment, by virtue of its characteristic immune system effects, can significantly alter the course of Graves' disease. Of the three major conventional treatment methods, ATDs have the most beneficial immune system influence. There are significant changes in both the number and types of antibodies present after each of the different therapies. Stimulating TRAb are associated with thyrotoxicosis and GO while blocking TSH receptor antibodies are associated with hypothyroidism.

Antithyroid Drugs

Antithyroid drugs are generally associated with significant decreases in stimulating antibodies, although there is no change in binding antibodies.[58] A decrease in stimulating antibodies is predictive of remission. In one study a decrease was also seen in HLADR+T lymphocytes six months after treatment with methimazole.[59]

Another study demonstrated the development of transient hypothyroidism related to a transient increase in blocking TSH receptor antibodies three years after successful remission in a patient who had become euthyroid after one year of ATD treatment. Another patient developed permanent hypothyroidism associated with persistent blocking TSH receptor antibodies.[60]

Radioiodine Ablation

Following radioiodine ablation, most patients experience a significant increase in stimulating antibodies due to their release from dying follicular cells. Symptoms of hyperthyroidism peak two to four days after ablation and continue for several weeks to several months. Eventually, however, as cells continue being destroyed the mean thyroid volume is reduced to <8 ml, which prevents symptoms of hyperthyroidism from occurring.

However, the increase in stimulating antibodies in the presence of destroyed thyroid cells is thought to be responsible for the eventual development of hypothyroidism. In one study, 75 percent of RAI treated patients continued to have increased stimulating TSH receptor antibodies one year after treatment.[61] Following the eventual disappearance of stimulating antibodies, a minority of patients develop blocking TRAb, which are thought to also contribute to the occurrence of thyroid failure occasionally seen after RAI.

Another recent study conducted in Japan showed a reduction in RAI induced thyroid autoantibodies when methimazole was given to patients after radioiodine ablation. In patients treated with RAI alone, a maximum increase in thyroglobulin, thyroid peroxidase and TBII were seen three months after ablation. This response was blunted in patients receiving ATDs after ablation. One year after ablation, 80 percent of patients treated only with radioiodine were euthyroid or hypothyroid. Of the patients treated with methimazole after their ablations, only 22 percent were euthyroid or hypothyroid. This study showed that antithyroid drugs competed with radioiodine in a manner similar to its competition with iodine. Thus, administering ATDs after I-131 reduced I-131-induced thyroid damage as well as the efficacy of treatment and the titers of thyroid autantibodies.[62]

Surgery's Effect on Immunity

Following surgery, levels of TBII are reduced. In one study, four to five years after subtotal thyroidectomy, 76.8 percent of patients still in remission had TBII less than 20 percent. Immunologic remission correlated with hormonal remission in most instances.[63]

Treatment Outcome Studies

In one Swedish study involving 174 GD patients, younger patients (20 to 34 years) were treated with their choice of surgery or ATDs in conjunction with thyroxine (block and replace approach), while older patients were given the added option of radioiodine ablation. Two years after treatment, most patients recommended their treatment to others. In patients with GO, 20 percent reported that the eye problems were much more troublesome than the thyroid problems. The costs of treatment, with surgery being most expensive, were not as significantly different when relapses were taken into consideration.[64]

In another study conducted in Chile over a period of 30 years, Graves' patients treated with surgery, PTU or radioiodine were compared to determine the efficacy of achieving euthyroidism. Surgery resulted in euthyroidism in 70.2 percent of patients. I-131 accounted for the highest rate of hypothyroidism (72.1 percent) regardless of the ablative dose used. PTU used alone achieved remission in only 26.4 percent of patients. However, when PTU was combined with T4, the success rose to 62.5 percent. In the block and replace protocol designed by Yamamoto described earlier in this chapter, which is guided by RAI uptake suppression tests, 87.5 percent of patients achieved long-standing euthyroidism. The authors of this study recommend using PTU as a first approach and assessing the RAI-U or TRAb levels after six months. If improvement is seen, T4 is added to the regimen. If there is no improvement at this time, it's recommended that I-131 or surgery be used.[65]

9 *The Alternative Medical Approach to Treating Graves' Disease*

Crediting alternative medicine for her remission, Mary B likes telling people how Julie U and I saved her thyroid. In truth, we inspired Mary. Bemoaning the sad fate of our own thyroids, Julie and I merely urged Mary to choose treatment wisely. We wanted her to make a fully informed, independent decision based on information from a wide variety of sources, something both Julie and I had neglected to do.

When I first encountered Mary, a dynamic mother in her mid–30s who had recently completed her doctorate, she had been forced to discontinue PTU after experiencing liver problems. In the meantime, a racing heart was wearing her down, and she'd developed moderate GO. Anxious for her symptoms to resolve, she'd consulted a surgeon and set a tentative date. Before her scheduled surgery, I suggested Mary weigh the benefits against the risks for her situation. Attempting to curb Mary's tendency to rush, Julie reminded her that she didn't need to hurry unless her symptoms worsened since she'd been prescribed beta adrenergic blocking drugs to help manage her symptoms. Several other patients suggested that Mary wait until she weaned her daughter since they had experienced a reduction of symptoms after they stopped nursing.

Realizing that she could always opt for more aggressive measures if results weren't forthcoming, Mary cancelled her surgery and embraced alternative medicine. Now, she is one of a rising number of GD patients with a holistic healing story to tell (see chapter 12). In this chapter, I

describe some of the healing elements Mary employed along with a number of other time honored natural healing options used to treat Graves'
disease.

Alternative Treatment Goals

Alternative and allopathic medicine have identical primary goals for
treating GD. They both aim to reduce the amount of thyroid hormone
available to the body's cells. However, alternative medicine differs in that
its methods work subtly while taking the underlying causes of GD into
account. In addition, alternative medicine promotes the body's own natural healing ability. In alternative medicine, a combination of diet and
herbs are often used to reduce available thyroid hormone. Similar to the
effects of PTU, certain herbs also inhibit the enzyme responsible for the
peripheral conversion of T4 to the more potent T3. Energy healing, environmental concerns and stress reduction protocols address the underlying environmental causes or triggers of Graves' disease.

Alternative Healing Philosophy

Alternative medicine is shaped by our own cultural context as well as
Eastern tradition, and it employs a variety of options, varying between the
simplicity of attending a weekly yoga class to a life plan completely adhering to holistic guidelines. Alternative medicine recognizes that each of us
has an inherently unique physical and psychological profile or constitution resulting from predisposed hereditary, social and environmental factors. Also, each of us has an inherent life force.

This vital life force is called chi or qi in China, and kundalini in
ancient India. For optimal health, this vital force must be in balance, and
its flow must not be blocked. Its polar opposites are the yin and yang of
traditional Chinese medicine, the kyo and jitsu of Japanese shiatsu, and
the Ayurvedic doshas. Holistic medicine focuses on correcting these imbalances. Thus, five patients with similar symptoms would likely all be prescribed different treatments tailored to their unique constitution and flow
of vital energy.

Yin and Yang

Yin and yang refer to the opposing polarities, such as hot and cold,
which govern man as well as the universe. Yin and yang relationships are
apparent in the relationship of the sympathetic to the parasympathetic
divisions of the autonomous nervous system. Overactivity of the sympathetic nervous system results in excess yang ailments. Overactivity of the
parasympathetic system produces excess yin disorders.[1]

Opinions on the cause and treatment of disease may differ depending on the background of the herbalist or practitioner. Chinese medicine generally blames environmental factors as the cause of disease, whereas Ayurvedic medicine credits digestive problems for most diseases related to qi imbalance.

Advantages and Disadvantages
of Alternative Medicine

Alternative medicine may be insufficient used initially as the sole treatment for GD patients with moderate to severe symptoms. Many patients use alternative medicine alone after first becoming euthyroid by using a short course of ATDs. Because of the unpredictable nature of GD, all patients require the guidance of a trained practitioner. Even seemingly innocuous substances may cause harm if used inappropriately.

Alternative healing protocols include individual elements or procedures working in conjunction with one another. Options include strong iodine solution, herbs, diet, dietary supplements, homeopathic preparations, acupuncture and other forms of energy healing, yoga, Ayurvedic medicine, traditional Chinese medicine, Japanese Kampo, neural therapy, massage, anointing oils and stress reduction techniques.

Strong Iodine Solution

Strong iodine solution is the oldest therapeutic agent known for treating hyperthyroidism. However, iodine is also one of the most controversial substances used because of its paradoxical nature, especially at low doses. Complicating matters, most Graves' patients are extraordinarily sensitive to iodine, and a slight excess can aggravate or induce hyperthyroidism, whereas a saturated solution of potassium iodine (SSKI) can make these same patients hypothyroid. Most problems arising from the use of iodine involve kelp and other low dose iodine compounds described later in this chapter.

Before ATDs were discovered, strong potassium iodide (KI) solution was the only substance available to control the symptoms of hyperthyroidism. Its primary benefit is its ability to stop thyroid hormone release from the thyroid. This quickly reduces the amount of hormone present in the circulation. SSKI also decreases iodide transport into the cell and inhibits the synthesis of thyroid hormone (Wolff-Chaikoff effect). This transient (two-day) inhibition only occurs above critical concentrations of intracellular rather than extracellular iodide, as is seen in hyperthyroidism.[2] Strong iodine also causes thyroid cells to shrink and reaccumulate colloid in their follicles. These changes are similar to what would be expected if the excess glandular stimulus (autoantibodies in this case) was removed.

Dosage

Although larger doses are often used, the minimum dose needed to control thyrotoxicosis is 6 mg or 6,000 mcg given as one eighth of a drop of SSKI containing 1 gram of KI per ml. Or eight tenths of a drop of Lugol's solution (8 mg/drop) may be used. Patients with mild symptoms have been controlled for prolonged periods using up to one drop of SSKI three times daily, or three to five drops of Lugol's solution three times daily.[3] The usual doses in severe thyrotoxicosis are higher with five drops of Lugol's solution given every eight hours.[4] The effects of SSKI are rapid, and the effect on basal metabolism rate is comparable to that following thyroidectomy. The maximal effect is obtained after 10 to 15 days of continuous therapy.[5]

Regulatory Mechanism

Despite iodine's amazing power over thyroid function, the human body (with the exception of the fetus and neonate) has an innate protective regulatory system. This system overrides or halts iodine's inhibitory effect on thyroid hormone release before goiter has a chance to develop (similar to the escape from the Wolff-Chaikoff effect). The time frame for this escape from inhibition is variable, usually occurring after two to three weeks. During this escape from inhibition, excess iodine may exacerbate thyrotoxicosis. This may also occur if strong iodine solution is abruptly withdrawn during its inhibitory phase.

Disadvantages

Although side effects are rare, SSKI administered long-term can cause symptoms of toxicity. Symptoms include burning of the mouth or throat, severe headache, soreness of teeth and gums, eye irritation with swelling of eyelids, increased salivation and skin disorders. SSKI may also exacerbate thyrotoxicosis in patients with toxic nodular goiter. Allergy to iodine may rarely occur, causing acneiform eruptions (iodism), sialoadenitis (salivary gland inflammation) and vasculitis (inflammation of a blood or lymph vessel).[6]

Dietary Iodine and Kelp

Amounts of iodine greater than 150 mcg can exacerbate or induce hyperthyroidism in susceptible individuals. One kelp tablet contains 150 mcg (0.15 mg) of iodine, and 150 mcg is the minimum daily requirement for iodine. Depending on the body's needs, iodine status and sensitivity, the amounts for inducing and inhibiting hyperthyroidism vary among different individuals. Note: Graves' patients who are euthyroid or hypothyroid following treatment or spontaneously (and also individuals with Hashimoto's thyroiditis) are susceptible to hypothyroidism upon ingesting between 1.5 to 150 mg/daily or 1,500 mcg to 150,000 mcg of iodine.[7] The average fast food diet is said to provide 1,000 mcg of iodine daily.

Kelp (Laminaria Hyperborea, Laminaria)

Many physicians report that hyperthyroidism and hypothyroidism are similar disorders of thyroid imbalance.[8] Based on this premise, some alternative healers infer that both disorders can be rectified with preparations of kelp or sargassum (seaweed), or other iodine rich herbs such as fucus (bladderwack). However, excess (not adequate) iodine is potentially dangerous for GD patients.

The German Commission E, in its extensive government sponsored study of the safety and efficacy of herbs, lists kelp, sargassum and bladderwack as posing risk in individuals with hyperthyroidism (they have an iodine content >150 mcg).[9] Iodine in excess of 150 mcg, according to the Commission's herbal monographs, can aggravate or induce hyperthyroidism in susceptible individuals. Therefore, any substance capable of delivering 150 mcg of iodine puts individuals with GD at risk and disrupts treatment in patients on ATDs. This does not, however, preclude the prescribed use of therapeutic doses of homeopathic iodine. Nor does it preclude the use of moderate amounts of iodine (<1,000 mcg daily) iodine in GD patients who have become permanently hypothyroid.

Dr. Vogel, writing in *The Nature Doctor*, reports that in some instances the body's natural iodine balance is disrupted by artificial iodine, particularly that found in iodized salt. He reports that iodized salt, with its unnatural composition, may cause palpitations in susceptible individuals although sea salt doesn't have this effect.[10]

Dietary Changes and Supplements

Vitamin and Mineral Supplements

It's important that individuals with GD check supplements for the presence of added iodine or kelp. Patients must also avoid the diet product Triax Metabolic Accelerator or similar preparations containing TRIAC, a potent thyroid hormone produced in one of the intermediary steps of thyroid synthesis. This product can cause heart attacks and strokes and other symptoms of thyrotoxicosis.[11]

Other elements such as manganese, iron, selenium, magnesium, zinc, copper, sulfur and calcium are necessary for proper thyroid function. Excess zinc relative to copper can induce or aggravate symptoms of hyperthyroidism. Zinc supplements must be balanced by supplemental copper in a ratio of 3:1 zinc to copper to correct hyperthyroidism.

Sufficient selenium (at doses of 100 to 200 mcg) is critical for the body's conversion of T4 to T3. Again, more is not better. High concentrations of selenium, like iodine, are reported to cause a decrease in thyroid hormone synthesis although selenium is needed for proper thyroid metabolism. Toxicity occurs at doses greater than 800 mcg.

Some Supplement Recommendations

Kim H, a Graves' patient now in remission after following a natural healing program, reports that her naturopathic practitioner recommended that she take two women's multivitamin capsules with minerals four times daily. Mary B's team of holistic healers advised her to take prenatal vitamins since she was still nursing her daughter. In addition, Mary took vitamin B complex, vitamin C, beta carotene and Ultraclear, a concentrated vitamin and mineral supplement with essential fatty acids and amino acids, as part of her protocol.

Some holistic practitioners recommend testing blood or hair samples for vitamin and mineral levels before they prescribe individual vitamins and minerals. This can help determine individual deficiency states. Most insurance companies cover these tests if the laboratory requisition includes the patient's diagnosis. It's especially important to have levels checked before supplementing with high doses of individual mineral supplements.

Although manganese, magnesium and copper deficiencies are common in GD, there are exceptions. Individual nutritional status is influenced by diet, environment, genetics, and the individual's unique absorption and metabolism of nutrients. Certain enzymes required for mineral metabolism may also be deficient. And some minerals may be stored in tissues rather than blood, for instance copper in Wilson's disease, a genetic disorder of copper metabolism that is aggravated by supplemental copper.

Trace Minerals and Thyroid Autoimmunity

Nutrition experts caution that minerals, unlike vitamins, are to be taken in trace amounts. Consuming 50 mg daily of zinc (the MDR is 15 mg) for several weeks can drive down the body's copper stores. Besides possibly contributing to the development of hyperthyroidism, low copper levels increase the risk of heart and vascular disease.

Nutritionists advise that the safest bet for increasing minerals is to load up on fruits and vegetables, beans and seafood, all of which contain essential trace elements. Although dietary supplements are needed to correct nutrient deficiencies in GD, they shouldn't be counted on to supply all the body's needs.

Immunomodulators

An overactive immune system, as in GD, doesn't mean that it's overly effective. In fact, immune overactivity causes autoimmunity, allergies and inflammation, and sustained periods of hyperimmunity may lead to immune exhaustion and collapse. The goal of therapy in using immuno-modulators is immune system balance, which helps limit autoantibody production and reduces autoimmune symptoms.

Immunomodulators balance or modulate both overactive and sluggish immune systems. In addition, they offer protection from stress-induced immune system depression (for example the immune system depression seen after strenuous exercise). Also, immunomodulators lower the production of pro-inflammatory substances as well as the stress hormone cortisol. The best known immunomodulators are plant sterols and sterolins derived from plant fats such as beta sitosterol. Although fruits and vegetables are natural sources, their sterols are leached out by cooking water or, when frozen, destroyed by enzymes during the thawing process. Besides sterols, several other substances (listed below with dosages) have been found to act as immunomodulators.[12]

PLANT STEROLS/STEROLINS

Dosage: 20 mg capsule of the product which is sold commercial under the name Sterinol may be taken three times daily on an empty stomach. Sterols are also in ingredient of the Polynesian plant *Morinda citrifolia* (Noni, Nonu, Nono). Sterols are contraindicated for individuals who have had tissue or organ transplants. Patients on insulin therapy may experience changes and should have their insulin levels monitored while taking sterols.

REISHI MUSHROOM EXTRACT (GONDERMA LUCIDUM, GANODERMA)

Dosage: Sold as tablets, liquid tonic or as a tea with dosage information accompanying product. Reishi shows significant anti-inflammatory effects, protects the liver and diminishes allergic responses.

GERMAN CHAMOMILE (MATRICARIA RECUTITA)

Dosage: 3 g of dried herb taken as an infusion of tea. May be used four to five times daily between meals. Alternately, six to eight 500 mg capsules may be used. Unlike other forms of chamomile, German chamomile rarely causes allergies. Tea bags made from German chamomile are reported to be effective in reducing swelling when used as compresses over the eyelids. Briefly steep the bags in warm water, cool slightly and place the moist bags over closed eyes for 15 minutes. Note: Only chamomile or black tea should be used.

FLOWER POLLEN EXTRACT (CERNITIN AND PROSTAPHIL PATENT PREPARATIONS)
Dosage: 240 mg of the water soluble extract or 12 mg of the oil soluble extract in capsule or tablet form.

Dietary Influences and Goitrogens

Diet can profoundly alter symptoms of thyrotoxicosis. As a general rule for GD, iodine, saturated fats, caffeine, sugar, wheat and dairy products should be avoided while goitrogens should be increased. Goitrogens, foods that inhibit the uptake of iodine, work much like certain ATDs, inhibiting thyroid hormone synthesis, release or action.

Goitrogens include foods of the Brassica family including broccoli, kale, kohlrabi, rutabaga, Brussels sprouts, turnips, cauliflower, rape and mustard. Non-Brassica Cruciferae with goitrogenic properties include horseradish, cress and radish. Levels of goitrogens are highest in the seeds of these plants. Other goitrogens include peanuts, soy, sweet potatoes, millet, peaches, cabbage, and members of the mint family, including mint, borage, basil, oregano, marjoram, oregano, mustard greens, pears, almonds and spinach, lemon balm, rosemary, lavender and hyssop (also see chapter 3).

Imbalances of Yin and Yang

William Duffy, in his English version of *You Are All Sanpaku* by George Oshawa, includes Graves' disease in the sixth stage or phase of diseases caused by an imbalance of yin and yang. Disorders in the sixth stage are a long time in the making, he writes, but improvement can be seen almost immediately by following a dietary regimen based on macrobiotic principles. For optimal results in severe cases, he recommends a protocol known as Regimen Number 7, which allows only unrefined cereals.

His prescription for healing includes avoiding sugar including fruit and fruit juices, limiting liquids and animal products, including dairy products, especially if you live in a warm climate, avoiding the most yin vegetables, which are tomatoes, potatoes and eggplant, avoiding all processed or imported foods, and avoiding coffee and teas containing dyes and most spices. Fish, shellfish, and wild game are permitted. He recommends that one's daily diet include 60 percent to 70 percent unrefined grains or cereals, and 20 percent to 25 percent baked or cooked vegetables and that every mouthful of food be chewed 50 times.[13]

Mary B's acupuncturist noted that many Graves' symptoms are "hot" or yang conditions. She advised Mary to follow a diet of cold foods including raw fruits, cucumbers, tomatoes, papaya, leafy vegetables, mung beans, bulgar and corn, and steaming or light stir frying rather than boiling or baking. Mary was also encouraged to eat miso, uemoboshi paste, plums, tahini, and the seeds of pumpkin, sunflower, flax and sesame and to use sesame, olive and canola oils.

Another Graves' friend, Carol, noted that her holistic healer recommended using simple raw foods such as pineapple that are easy to digest by virtue of their innate digestive enzymes. This alleviates the stress associated with the digestive process.

Kim's doctor recommended that she eat 1 to 1.5 cups of broccoli or cauliflower and 1.5 cups of soy as soymilk or tofu daily. He also suggested that Kim choose millet as her grain whenever possible and that she use goat milk in place of dairy products.

Natural Iodine

Dr. Vogel recommends growing one's own garden and fertilizing the produce with iodine rich bone meal and other fertilizers containing natural iodine. It's the unnatural composition of iodized salt, he says, that causes problems in individuals with the tendency to develop GD.[14] He recommends that in active GD, only homeopathic *kelpsan* be used.

Avoiding Allergic Foods

In *Spontaneous Healing*, Dr. Andrew Weil recommends using the same guidelines for autoimmune disease and allergy. He suggest a low protein diet providing minimal intake of foods of animal origin including dairy products. He also recommends that organically grown fruits and vegetables should be used and polyunsaturated vegetable oils and hydrogenated fats should be avoided.[15] Foods which trigger allergies should be avoided and foods should be rotated to prevent allergic reactions.

Most general dietary recommendations for GD revolve around a whole foods diet with adequate but not excess protein. Substances to be avoided include sugar, dairy products, caffeine, hot spicy food, and occasionally, wheat. Because of the many nutrient deficiencies associated with GD, high nutrient foods should be selected.

Oral Tolerance

Although oral tolerance is the focus of research at Harvard University and is the basis behind AutoImmune, a company conducting clinical trials for several autoimmune disorders,[16] its origins lie in alternative medicine. In 1911, the response of oral tolerance was first described in a report in which researchers found they could prevent severe allergic reactions in guinea pigs by feeding them proteins before injecting them with these proteins.

The basic concept is that the immune reaction that occurs in the gut causes T cells to either adapt or be destroyed. In the absence of reactive T cells, the body's own proteins are safe. A small amount of protein renders T cells inactive and stimulates regulatory T cells. The regulatory T cells, in turn, release cytokines that dampen killer T cells and curb inflammation. Oral tolerance holds more promise in autoimmune diseases in which T cells (due to their release of cytokines), rather than autoantibodies, cause damage.[17]

Bee Pollen

Bee pollen and its propolis extract are reported to have beneficial effects on GO. Kara, a young computer specialist, reported that several patients reversed proptosis with specially harvested bee pollen. Dr. Vogel confirms the benefits of bee pollen for GO, but he recommends that patients wait to use it until their thyrotoxicosis symptoms are under control since he has observed that bee pollen can raise blood pressure.[18] Note: Patients with pollen allergies should use caution, especially with freshly harvested pollen.

Herbal Medicine

A stellar player in the holistic arena, herbs, by virtue of their antithyroid or sedating effects, are a mainstay in GD treatment. Effects result from their unique plant phytochemical or medicinal properties. Laboratory analysis proves that herbs contain chemicals with structural properties similar to those of synthetic drugs. In fact, many synthetic compounds are designed in an effort to duplicate the healing power of plants. For instance, aspirin or acetylsalicylic acid was formulated to duplicate the salicins in white willow bark, and the heart medicine digoxin is derived from the foxglove plant.

The healing effects of plants have been known for as long as records of civilization exist. Folk medicine records from cultures as diverse as Indian, Chinese, Arabic, Tibetan, Russian, European and Native American describe identical healing effects for thousands of different herbs and plant parts. From a crude system of trial and error passed down through the ages, herbal medicine has evolved into several well documented *materia medicas*. Borrowing from these proven healing formulas, the United States and western European pharmacopoeias are 25 percent plant based.[19] Currently, there are five well defined branches of herbalism, European, Asian-Arabic, Chinese, Indian (Ayurvedic) and Russian.

Adverse Effects and Cautions of Herbal Medicine

Although some people consider herbs little more than weeds, scientists worldwide do not doubt the effects or efficacy of herbs. Most botanical researchers do, however, advise caution, fearing that many consumers do not realize the potency of herbs. A recent report by the Southern Medical Association describes transient episodes of acute hepatitis in two individuals who used large quantities of herbal mixtures for more than six months. In one individual, pure bee pollen was used along with prescription medicines including the barbiturate butalbital, aspirin, caffeine and erythromycin. The other individual used 14 herbal tablets daily along with the beta blocker metoprolol. In both instances, when the herbal medications were discontinued, the symptoms of hepatitis eventually resolved.[20]

Criticism also stems from the lack of regulations currently guiding the herbal industry in the United States. Numerous studies have shown a significant variance in the quantity of active phytomedical substance present in herbal samples manufactured by different laboratories. And many herbs contain more than one active substance.

Standardized Preparations and Safety Issues

In Germany, where about 70 percent of physicians prescribe herbs, herbal preparations are standardized. Capsules listed as standardized (compared by chemical analysis to known or standard concentrations) and said to contain 40 mg of an active substance or extract derived from a given herb can be trusted to contain that amount.

In 1978 the Federal Health Agency in Germany (now known as the Federal Institute for Drugs and Medical Devices) established an expert committee known as Commission E to study the safety and efficacy of herbal preparations. Each herb that is evaluated is subsequently presented as a monograph that includes positive and negative assessments based on chemical analysis, clinical trials, toxicology studies and a number of other stringent guidelines.[21]

In buying herbs it is best to look for standardized extracts unless your practitioner advises that the whole plant or certain plant parts such as the roots are to be used. Different plant parts such as roots and leaves often contain one or more different active ingredients. Their effects may be unrelated or they work synergistically, causing some herbalists to criticize the exclusive use of standardized extracts. The use of herbs for a condition as potentially serious as GD is best managed by an alternative medicine practitioner.

Always check contraindications before trying herbs, especially avoiding known immune system stimulants. Mindy Green, director of education for the Herb Research Foundation in Boulder, Colorado, reports that echinacea, a popular cold remedy, may overly stimulate patients with autoimmune disease and recommends that it not be used by patients with autoimmune disorders.[22]

Note: Dosages listed for the following herbs refer to the dried herbs (drugs), generally listed in grams (g), and not to the amounts in concentrated extracts unless specifically indicated. Some herbs listed below lower both TSH and thyroxine. This may confuse GD patients (whose TSHs are already low). With decreased TSH, less TSH can bind to the TSH receptor. T4 and T3 are consequently decreased. As these levels approach normal, TSH levels rise although it may take several months for this to be reflected in blood levels.

Herbs Used in Graves' Disease Treatment

LACTUCA VIROSA (WILD LETTUCE, PRICKLY LETTUCE, LETTUCE OPIUM, GREEN ENDIVE, ACRID LETTUCE, LACTUCARIUM)

The medicinal parts of *Lactuca* are the dried latex (milky plant contents) and the leaves.

Effects: Analgesic and spasmolytic (reduces spasms or convulsions). Also reported to act as a tranquilizer or narcotic.

Uses: Used to treat whooping cough, bronchial catarrh, asthma and urinary tract diseases. In Graves' disease, lactuca is used for its muscle relaxing effects.

Contraindications: Used only under medical supervision.

Precautions: Drug has a potential for causing allergic reactions.

Dosage: As an alcohol extract only used under medical supervision.

LEONURUS CARDIACA (MOTHERWORT, LION'S TAIL, LION'S EAR, THROW-WORT)

The medicinal parts are the fresh above air parts collected during the flowering season.

Effects: Mildly negatively chronotropic (tempering reproductive hormones), hypotonic (decreasing muscle tension), sedative.

Uses: Cardiac insufficiency, arrhythmia, nervous heart complaints, thyroid hyperfunction, flatulence.

Contraindications: None at recommended therapeutic dosage.

Precautions: None at recommended therapeutic dosage.

Dosage: 4.5 g of herb comminuted for infusions and other oral preparations.

LITHOSPERMUM RUDERALE OR LITHOSPERMUM OFFICINALE

The medicinal parts are the dried roots, flowers, leaves and seeds that contain lithospermic acid and rosmarinic acid. A free dried extract is often used.

Effects: Lithospermum has antithyrotropic (inhibits thyroid hormone and release) and antigonadotrophic (inhibits release of gonadotrophin sex hormones). Reported to also inhibit TSH secretion. *Lithospermum officinale* is also reported to inhibit the peripheral conversion of T4 to T3.

Uses: Mild thyroid hyperfunction.

Contraindications: Lithospermum should not be used in hypothyroidism or in instances of thyroid enlargement not related to thyroid dysfunction.

Precautions: To be used under the guidance of a naturopathic practitioner.

Dosage: Prescribed on an individual basis usually as a tonic also containing *Lycopus virginicus, Mellisa officinalis,* and occasionally *Thymus serpyllum* (no information available on this compound).

LYCOPUS VIRGINICUS (BUGLEWEED, LYCOPI HERBA).

Note: Lycopus europaeus or Gypsywort may also be used.

Lycopus consists of the fresh or dried above-ground parts as well as their preparations. Effects: Lycopus has antigonadotropic and antithyrotropic effects, inhibiting the peripheral conversion of T4 to T3. It also decreases levels of the pituitary hormone prolactin, which induces lactation. It is also reported to inhibit TSH release.

Uses: Mild thyroid hyperfunction with disturbances of the vegetative nervous system; breast pain or tenderness.[23]

Contraindications: Lycopus should not be used in hypothyroidism or in instances of thyroid enlargement not related to thyroid dysfunction. There should not be any simultaneous administration of thyroid hormone preparations.

Precautions: No known hazards or side effects at recommended therapeutic dosage.

Enlargement of the thyroid gland is possible at very high doses of Lycopus. Sudden discontinuation of Lycopus can lead to exacerbation of symptoms.[24]

Dosage: 1 to 2 g of drug for teas or as an ethanol extract equivalent of 20 mg of drug. The German Commission notes that each patient has his own individual optimal level of thyroid hormone. Only rough estimations of dosage are possible for thyroid disorders, in which age and weight must be considered.

MELISSA OFFICINALIS (LEMON BALM, SWEET MARY, DROPSY PLANT, HONEY PLANT, CURE-ALL)

Melissa contains the fresh or dried leaf as well as its preparations.

Effects: sedative, carminative (releases excess gas from the colon).

Uses: Nervous sleeping disorders and agitation, gastrointestinal complaints; memory enhancer; inhibits TSH. In folk medicine, decoctions of the flowering shoots are used for nervous complaints, lower abdominal disorders, gastric complaints, hysteria and melancholia, bronchial catarrh, palpitations, vomiting, migraine and hypertension.[25]

Contraindications: None known.

Precautions: None at recommended therapeutic dosage.

Dosage: 1.5-4.5 g of herb prepared as a tea, up to 8 or 10 g of the drug daily.

PASSIFLORA INCARNATA (PASSION FLOWER, GRANADILLA, MAYPOP, PASSION VINE)

The medicinal parts of passiflora are the dried herb and the fresh aerial parts.

Effects: Sedative.

Uses: Nervousness, insomnia, nervous agitation, nervous gastrointestinal complaints.

In folk medicine, use for depressive states such as hysteria, agitation and insomnia.[26]

Contraindications: None at recommended therapeutic dosages.

Precautions: None at recommended therapeutic dosages.

Dosage: 4 to 8 g of the drug used as infusion taken two to three times daily and half an hour before bedtime.

SCUTTELARIA LATERIFLORA (SCULLCAP, BLUE PIMPERNEL, HELMET FLOWER, HOODWORT, MAD-DOG WEED, MADWEED, QUAKER BONNET)

The medicinal part of Scutellaria is the pulverized herb of the 3 to 4 year old plant, which is harvested in June.

Effects: Sedative, antispasmodic, anti-inflammatory.

Uses: Hysteria, nervous tension, epilepsy, chorea, and other nervous disorders.

Contraindications: None at recommended therapeutic dosages.

Precautions: None at recommended therapeutic dosages.

Dosage: 1 to 2 1 g capsules up to three times daily.[27]

SILYBUM MARIANUM AND SILIBININ (MILK THISTLE, MARIAN THISTLE)

The medicinal parts of milk thistle are ripe seeds or extracts.

Effects: hepatic (liver) aid; alters the structure of hepatocytes (liver cells) in such a way as to prevent penetration of poison into the interior of the cell. Also stimulates liver cell regeneration. *Silymarin* is a collective name for a mixture of flavonoids or flavolignans. Both of these compounds are grouped together with isoflavonoids and phytosterols into a category called phytoestrogens. Flavonoids have physical and chemical properties similar to that of human steroid and thyroid hormones.[28] *Silibinin* strongly inhibits leukotriene production, making it an effective inflammatory agent.

Uses: Used as a tonic for functional disorders of the liver and gallbladder. In traditional Chinese medicine, detoxifying the liver has a healing effect on the eyes. Beneficial for liver symptoms associated with autoimmune disease.

Contraindications: None at recommended dosages.

Precautions: None at designated therapeutic dosages. Reports of nausea when taken on an empty stomach.

Dosage: 12 to 15 g of the drug or an equivalent of 200 to 400 mg of *Silymarin* extract or a combination extract with 150 mg *Silymarin* and 600 mg *Silibinin*.[29]

VALERIANA OFFICINALIS (VALERIAN, AMANTILLA, HELIOTROPE, VANDAL ROOT, ALL-HEAL, CAPON'S TAIL)

The medicinal parts of Valerian are the carefully dried underground parts including roots.

Effects: Sedative, sleep inducer, spasmolytic, muscle relaxant.

Uses: Nervousness, insomnia, restlessness, sleeping disorders due to nervous conditions, mental strain, lack of concentration, excitability, stress, headache, neurasthenia, epilepsy, hysteria, nervous cardiopathy, menstrual related agitation, nervous stomach cramps, angst.

Contraindication: Not to be used for extended periods.

Precautions: None at recommended therapeutic dosage; occasional gastrointestinal and allergic complaints. Long-term use can cause headache, restlessness and cardiac disorders.

Dosage: 15 g of the drug or 1 to 2 mg (1,000 to 2,000 mcg) of .1 percent standardized extract of valerenic acid.

FIXED COMBINATIONS OF PASSIONFLOWER, VALERIAN ROOT AND LEMON BALM

Fixed combinations of passionflower, valerian root, and lemon balm are approved by the German Commission E for conditions of unrest and difficulty in falling asleep.

Dosage: individual compounds should be present at 30 percent to 50 percent of the recommended daily doses for the individual herbs.[30]

Japanese Herbal Medicine, Kampo Preparations

Kampo refers to an ancient Oriental healing approach adhering to the principles of traditional Chinese medicine, which has recently been revived in Japan. The goal of Kampo is to correct imbalances in the body's energy system responsible for disease. By correcting these imbalances, not only are symptoms treated, but the individual's health is restored.

Most formulas are designed to correct excess heat in the liver and gallbladder, which is responsible for energy blockages. Preparations used for GD include the following.

BUPPLEURUM PLUS DRAGON BONE AND OYSTER SHELL DECOCTION
Indications: Used when the primary symptoms are difficulties in concentration and speech as well as irritability, nervousness and rapid pulse.
Precautions: Be sure the traditional ingredient minum (lead oxide) isn't present. Discontinue if existing fever worsens.

EIGHT-INGREDIENT PILL WITH REHMANNIA
Indications: Used for continuous sweating.
Precautions: None listed.

GENTIANA LONGDANCAO DECOCTION TO DRAIN THE LIVER
Indications: Useful when symptoms include irritability, headache and short temper. Useful for women who experience oligomenorrhea (scant menstrual period).
Precautions: Not to be used in women trying to conceive.

HONEY-FRIED LICORICE DECOCTION
Indications: Used for anxiety, irritability and insomnia accompanied by weight loss.
Precautions: None listed.

MINOR BUPLEURUM DECOCTION
Indications: Used as a complementary agent for individuals using prednisone for Graves' ophthalmopathy. Relieves secondary thyroid symptoms, including asthma, chills alternating with hot flashes, and nausea or stomach acid.
Precautions: Fever and skin infection. Not to be used long-term in patent medicine form. Such use may cause headache, dizziness and bleeding gums. These effects are avoided when formula is taken as a tea.

OPHIOPOGONIS DECOCTION
Indications: Increases effectiveness of methylprednisone; occasionally used for proptosis.
Precautions: Use with caution in fever. Discontinue if preexisting fever worsens.[31]

Traditional Chinese Medicine

Traditional Chinese medicine (TCM) is a disciplined science with a formulary of treatments intended for use under the guidance of a doctor of Chinese medicine or an herbalist/acupuncturist. Diagnosis is centered around an intricate process involving an examination of the entire body, especially the tongue. The exam includes visual inspection, listening and smelling, palpation and inquiry. Diseases that are manifested as imbalances in the body's energy system are classified according to their internal or external origin.

Internal causes include emotions and lifestyle, whereas external causes include seasons, and climactic conditions known as the Six Excesses— wind, cold, summer heat, dampness, dryness and fire. These conditions are capable of invading the body with combinations of forces that cause symptoms. Treatment is based on a system of polar opposites with cooling treatment (yin) used to rebalance symptoms of hot disease (yang). Symptoms are an important consideration, but they are always subsidiary to energy healing. A traditional doctor will never contradict the laws of energetic medicine. Instead, he will likely devise a treatment method that works symptomatically through the laws of energy medicine that promote balance of the Five Elements and also yin and yang.

Treatment

Treatment involves a combination of dietary changes, massage, herbal preparations, animal ingredients and acupuncture intended to redistribute opposing forces of qi. If the body's energy is balanced, it's less likely for disease to take hold. Chinese herbs are not intended to work alone but as a protocol including one or more of the other elements listed. The primary goal is restoration of the body's energy known as qi. After TCM treatment is underway, the patient typically develops symptoms of detoxification that would be considered signs of illness under other circumstances. The symptoms, called discharge, occur in three stages and are signs that the body is ridding itself of excesses.

TCM as a Complementary Agent for ATDs

In one recent study, integrationist healers used TCM (replenishing qi and nourishing yin, RQNY) to complement a small dose of Tapazole in an integrative treatment effort directed at treating Graves' disease. The study, conducted at the Institute of Integration of Traditional and Western Medicine in Shanghai, involved two groups of 42 patients, monitored over a period of 18 to 24 months. Results indicate that combination therapy with TCM was much more effective than the use of Tapazole therapy alone.[32]

Chinese Herbal Medicine

In Chinese medicine, herbs may be ground and bound with honey and rolled into pills or pellets. Alternatively, they may be pulverized into a powder that is dissolved in hot water or as a brewed soup consumed like a tea. In general, herbs are taken on an empty stomach once daily upon rising, and no food is consumed for one half hour afterward.

Chinese herbs may be classified as inferior (or medicinal) for use in cases where disease has already taken hold. An example is *coptis* or Chinese goldenseal. Inferior herbs are generally used for infections and inflammation and are taken for short periods. General or preventive herbs such as bupleurum are used to prevent and heal disease that is already present. Superior or promotional herbs are called tonics and may be taken without consulting a herbalist. They can be generally taken over long time periods.

TCM typically uses combinations rather than individual herbs. Although many herbal ingredients in a tonic usually implies that only a minute quantity of each is present, Chinese medicine differs. TCM preparations, using concentrated extracts of each ingredient, are reported to be highly effective. Remedies used to treat Graves' disease are prescribed on an individual basis and may include the following preparations.

CH'AI HU KUEI KAN CHIANG T'ANG

Indications: for yin individuals; treats disorders rooted in the chest including heart palpitations, tightness, hot and cold flashes and insomnia. For heart disease, endocarditis, valvular disease. May be used for one month.[33]

CH'AI HU CH'IA LUNG KU MU LI T'ANG

Indications: for yang individuals, treats tachycardia, seizure disorders, discharges excess energy (chi), hysteria, insomnia, inability to concentrate, benefits the nervous and glandular systems.[34]

LONG DAN XIE GAN WAN

Indications: for yang individuals, treats tachycardia and other symptoms of GD.

TIAN WANG BU XIN WAN[35] (HEART-YIN TONIC)

Indications: for yang individuals, treats tachycardia, benefits the nervous and glandular systems. Individual ingredients include Radix Rehmanniae Glutinosae, Radix Ginseng, Tuber Asparagi, Chochinchinesis, Tuber Ophiopoponis Japanici, Radix Srophulariaee, Ningponensis, Radix Salvaiae Miltiorrhizae, Selerotium Poriac Cocos, Radix Polygalae Tennuifoliae, Radix Schisandrae Chinsensis, Semen Biotae, Orientalis, Semen Zizyphi Sponosae, Radix Platycodi Grandiflori.[36]

JIAOGULAN (XIANCO)

Indications: helps the body adapt to stress, lowers blood pressure, prevents heart disease, acts as an adaptogen strengthening the immune system, nourishes the adrenal glands and raises energy levels. Jiaogulan also helps patients using radiation therapies maintain the immune system cells needed to protect against infection. The dose is reported to be 20 mg taken three times daily.[37]

Homeopathic Preparations

Homeopathy involves treating the patient with highly diluted natural remedies that, if given in larger doses, would cause the particular symptom that is being treated. For instance, a dilute preparation of *nux vomica*, a substance traditionally used to induce vomiting, is used to prevent motion sickness.

Healing Principle

Homeopathy works with and not against nature, using minute dilutions of a substance that is prepared into powders and tablets, granules spun and pressed into sugar, or liquids suspended in a 10 percent or 20 percent ethanol solution taken as drops. Most homeopathic preparations result from 1:100 dilutions and each 1:100 dilution is listed as C. A substance diluted 1:100 six consecutive times would be listed as 6 C. The more dilute the substance the more powerful or potentized the effect is said to be. 1:10 dilutions are listed as X strength, and 1:1000 dilutions are listed as M strength.

Dry or pelleted homeopathic preparations should be rolled gently from their container onto a dry tongue, and in general, food or liquids should not be ingested for 30 minutes before and after the dose. The preparation should be allowed to dissolve on the tongue, not swallowed or chewed. Oil from fingers or food taken simultaneously can interfere with the potency of the preparation as well as its absorption. Liquid preparations are dissolved into water and sipped slowly. In severe disorders, substances may be prescribed to be initially taken every two hours followed by a tapering of dosage.

Diagnostic Applications

A remarkable contribution of homeopathy is its diagnostic approach. Homeopathic practitioners study the patient as a whole, analyzing the trivial complaints and seemingly innocent personality traits that make individuals unique, rather than grasping for a prominent symptom and labeling it as a disease. By categorizing patients by certain prominent characteristics, individuals can be represented as constitutional types. These constitutional types are all related to a particular element deficiency. Remedies, depending on their dosage, are often listed as effective for several seemingly unrelated conditions.

Individualized Treatment

In GD, for example, the uniqueness of each patient is fully appreciated and treatment is prescribed accordingly. The constitutional drug or the one apt to be most beneficial is one that most effectively treats the patient as a total sum of individual strengths and weaknesses, mentally, emotionally and physically.[38]

The most beneficial homeopathic preparations used for hyperthyroidism address the rage at being held down or overlooked, which is considered by some to be the primary cause.[39] *Natrum muriaticum* is the preparation most often recommended. Combined with herbs and acupuncture, full effects should be seen in four weeks. Substances which may be prescribed for Graves' treatment include the following preparations.

Arnica montana for bruising, eyestrain, black eyes, fever (arnica gel or cream applied to eyelids is beneficial for eye swelling and pain. Not to be used on broken skin).

Calcarea phosphoricum for difficulty concentrating, discontentment, bone and teeth pain, weakness and fatigue after illness.

Coffea for insomnia, toothache.

Iodum for symptoms of hyperthyroidism; people needing this have an obsessive desire to keep compulsively busy due to the persistent frightening thoughts they get when forced to remain still.[40]

Kelpasan (1x–6x potency) for Graves' disease.[41]

Lycopodium for nervousness and sleeplessness, alopecia.

Natrum muriaticum for vasomotor disturbances such as the irregular pulse and palpitations of Graves' disease, eczema, acne, and skin blemishes, especially when accompanied by dry mucous membranes.[42]

Pulsatilla for hot flushes disturbing sleep, tendency toward weepiness, fondness for sweets, little thirst.

Sepia (one of the sea remedies) for restlessness related to the menstrual cycle, impatience, menopausal complaints, candidiasis, irritable at home while extroverted with company.

Thyroidinum for symptoms of hyperthyroidism.[43]

Precautions: Preparations of calcarea carbonica used at the 1M strength are reported to boost thyroid function and should be avoided.

Ayurveda

Ayurveda is a 5,000-year-old medical discipline with roots in ancient India, traditionally practiced by 20 percent of the world's population. Recently adopted in the West, it focuses on treating imbalances of the body's doshas, Vata, Pitta, and Kapha.

Imbalances of doshas, seen as constitutional types with characteristic symptoms of the dominant dosha, contribute to disease. The goal of Ayurveda is to balance one's doshas with his environment. For instance, to pacify Pitta, which is characteristically quick and hot, cooling foods such as green salads might be prescribed.

According to Ayurveda, the life energy force known as Prana flows through the body by the force of Vata, which regulates movement. Vata is divided into five parts that regulate different bodily systems. *Prana Vata* regulates the nervous system, for instance, while *Udana Vata* regulates cognition, speech and memory. Imbalances may block energy flow. Drugs in Ayurvedic medicine are not used to tranquilize but to strengthen the nerves. In Ayurvedic medicine, for a remedy to be pure it must be effective, efficacious, and be capable of permanently causing the disorder, not merely the symptoms, to subside from the root or source. Otherwise the remedy is impure. The body is treated as a whole, with no remedy being the same for different individuals with similar conditions.

Treatment Protocols

The interrelationship of the individual to his environment is considered when prescribing treatment. The healing power of food in Ayurvedic medicine is categorized not by carbohydrates or fat content, but by properties of taste such as bitter, salt, sweet, sour, pungent and astringent. Ayurveda also encompasses protocols for detoxification such as fastings and enemas, herbs, drugs, social and mental conditioning, massage, anointing oils and exercise such as yoga, all prescribed on an individual basis.[44]

Ayurvedic preparations are generally contained in a base of brown sugar or honey, which are considered good vehicles for facilitating absorption. Some ingredients commonly used in Ayurvedic medicine are listed below.

Amla: (*Emblica officinalis*): Amla is a fruit with high vitamin C content used as the base of many Ayurvedic preparations. Amla, along with Haritaki (Terminalia chebula) and Bibhitake (*Terminalia belerica*) are blended together in Triphala a compound used to balance, cleanse and nourish the body. Triphala is reported to improve vision and liver function, aid digestion, eliminate toxins and rejuvenate the body.

Gotu kola : (*Hydocotyl asiatica*/Brahmi) Gotu kola, which has recently gained popularity in the United States for its vascular strengthening properties, is used to revitalize nerves and brain cells. Also used as a blood purifier and a memory enhancer.

Shatavari (asparagus root): Shatavari is used as a rejuvenative tonic for women, balancing the reproductive system.

Energy Healing

Energy healing dates back to 500 B.C. when the Pythagoreans recorded observing a halo of light energy surrounding the body. In ancient China, Japan and India, sage healers called this same phenomenon ch'i or qi or prana. In TCM, ch'i is an invisible flowing energy force regulating the body as well as conditions of the environment. Energy, according to TCM, flows or circulates through the body through a system of meridians.

The goal of energy healing is to correct blockages in the flow of ch'i energy along the meridians. In the human body there are 26 or more principal meridians that follow along the front and back of the body. Their midlines correspond to the center of the body. Meridians contain RNA and DNA, which is likely the underlying basis of their action.

Acupuncture

Acupuncture points (acupoints) occur at places where meridians emerge at the surface of the body. Acupuncture restores balance by manipulating acupoints with needles. Although there are 365 different channel points and various systems of charting them, there are approximately 2,000 acupoints.[45] Each acupoint has a mirror image position and a corresponding internal Zang-Fu organ. Zang-Fu organs, while similar to anatomical organs, are more related to clusters of functions working in tandem with other organs to promote whole body healing.

Often, an electro-acupuncture device is used to locate regions of reduced skin resistance or blockage. These regions can be further assessed for states of yin and yang. Acupuncture needles are then guided into specific acupoints and, depending on the manipulation and properties of the needle, are capable of performing more than 150 different actions, including healing, releasing energy blockages and restoring strength.

Treatment

Individual treatment is geared toward correcting imbalance. In addition, by manipulating the flow of ch'i or qi by the insertion of acupuncture needles, the patient can be rendered immune to pain without the use of anesthesia. Acupuncture has been used during surgeries including thyroidectomy, and in China this practice is extensive.

Safety Risks and Precautions

Although acupuncture is generally regarded as safe, the technique has certain risks, which although small, can be serious. One recent study conducted in Münster, Germany, which reviewed data covering more than 30 years, reported 110 serious injuries and four fatalities. Most problems resulted from the piercing of a patient's lung or surrounding tissue.[46] Although most states require acupuncturists to be certified by an exam, experts advise that patients seek a licensed practitioner who is a physician or who has trained at an accredited school. A referral can be obtained from the American Association of Oriental Medicine at (888) 500-7999, http://www.aaom.com.

Acupressure

Acupressure is a form of energy healing that utilizes the same acupoints as in acupuncture, which it refers to as tsubos. Energy flow is manipulated by applying finger pressure to these points. Acupressure isn't as intensive as acupuncture, but is a valuable aid in treating colds, headaches and backaches and boosting energy. Pressure is generally applied for five seconds and then released for five seconds. Sore spots are indicators of ch'i blockage and can be used to diagnose blockage in organs corresponding to the acupoint.

Moxibustion

Another form of energy healing that manipulates energy flow through acupoints, moxibustion, differs in that it also uses heat. The practitioner uses heat from burning substances, usually herbs, and applies them to the acupoints before the acupuncture needles are inserted. Although other herbs may be used, mugwort (artemisia vulgaris) is generally used and is thought to potentiate the effects of acupuncture.

Stress Reduction

Stress depresses immune function by decreasing immune system components that normally stop the autoreactive process before autoantibodies are produced. Stress also causes an increase in white blood cells. Consequently, in stress the immune system remains overactive while its suppressor mechanism is inhibited. Methods for reducing stress such as meditation or breathing exercises also reduce these autoimmune enhancers.

Dr. Walt Stoll describes stored hypothalamic stress as a key player in the development of Graves' disease.[47] Until this stored stress is addressed, he reports, symptoms of autoimmunity will persist.

Role of Stress in Disease

As long ago as 500 B.C., physicians understood that the "passions," which Hippocrates so often refers to, play an important role in disease development. In the last two decades, studies in psychoneuroimmunology

(PNI) have defined a system of communication that exists between the nervous and immune system. PNI effectively established the missing link. Recent animal studies show that impairing this communication either by genetic engineering or with drugs is associated with increased susceptibility of inflammatory diseases, thyroid problems and arthritis.[48]

The waxing and waning of symptoms in GD has been shown to have a psychosomatic component, with exacerbations seen after periods of stress. Recently, scientists have confirmed the early self-healing experiments first described by Dr. Norman Cousins that healed his autoimmune arthritis. Using stress reduction tapes and biofeedback, researchers have employed these same methods to improve symptoms in other arthritic patients.[49]

Julia A in Spain and Mary B have both experienced improvement of their Graves' symptoms by using stress reduction methods such as meditation and yoga. Mary reported noticing a diminishment in her throat's sense of fullness immediately after a yoga session. When she mentioned this to her yoga instructor, he said, "Why, of course." Julia and Mike both recommend Tai Chi Chuan (described in chapter 12) for stress reduction. Although it's long been known that stress depresses the immune system, researchers have only recently learned that positive emotional states can cure the body of serious disease.[50]

The Nature of Stress

Stress does not always cause adverse effects. Nor is it necessarily a result of ominous circumstances. Any condition evoking change, even winning the lottery, causes stress. Stress functions to release two stress hormones, corticotrophin releasing hormone (CRH) via the hypothalamus, and adrenaline by the adrenal glands. CRH causes the pituitary to release adrenocorticotrophic hormone (ACTH). ACTH causes the adrenal gland to release cortisol. All of these hormones cause other organs to pitch in and aid the body in dealing with the stressor agent.

Normally, in response to stress, blood platelets aggregate to prevent massive blood loss in trauma, (although this clotting enhancement is thought to be a cause of some heart attacks), immune cells activate, blood sugar rushes to muscles, the heart rate increases and blood pressure rises. Cortisol, after sustaining the stress response, eventually slows it down so the body can resume its normal functioning.

But sometimes this system goes awry. Over time, the body must deal with an allostatic load (the cumulative effects of long term stress). For our bodies to accommodate these demands, systems are forced to drop out or take short cuts. The stress response in some individuals becomes resistant to the shutdown effect of cortisol. When cortisol can no longer respond, it sends out inflammatory cytokines (signals) in its place. As cytokine levels rise, the immune system is affected. Research studies show that some cytokines, particularly interleukin-2 and interferon-gamma, may be present at higher levels in Graves' disease than in thyroid disease not related to autoimmunity.[51]

Besides traditional stress reduction methods such as biofeedback, meditation and yoga, effectively dealing with stress involves being prepared for certain anticipated life events (having a plan of action like carrying an umbrella when a thunderstorm is expected). It also involves proper attention to diet, avoiding foods such as refined sugar that put us on edge, and taking adequate vitamin and mineral supplements.

Meditation

Evidence left behind on cave walls indicates that man's yearning for spiritual expression began about 17,000 years ago. Early cultures didn't distinguish spiritual from everyday life and regarded spirituality as respect for the mystery of existence. Meditation in contrast to religion fills man's need to illuminate his place in the world without reference to an external entity. In contrast to prayer, Christian meditation focuses on a sacred word used like a mantra. This differs from contemplation, a solitary reflection on spiritual matters. Like prayer, meditation involves stillness, surrender and the longing for wholeness.

Meditation can follow the rules and rituals of various formal disciplines or it can be an uncontrived spontaneous solitary effort to connect with the universe. Formal disciplines include *Vipsayana* or insight meditation, an ancient Buddhist tradition, *Dhyana* or absorption, a Hindu meditation practice where the individual transcends his individuality or meets with the divine, and *Zen*, a Japanese contribution that blends the mysticism of India, the Taoist love of nature and spontaneity and the pragmatism of Confucianism.

Guided imagery and hypnotherapy in particular have been reported to be effective ways to reverse autoimmune disease into remission.[52] Zen meditation accomplishes this goal as the individual attains a state of sustained awareness. Furthermore, any creative effort in which we absorb ourselves to the point of losing track of time has a meditative effect. In several studies, journal writing was shown to have therapeutic benefits.

Yoga

This ancient Hindu word yoga means "to yoke" or to "to join." This refers to the joining of the individual soul to Brahman, which is the ultimate reality and the unifying concept of Hinduism. Brahman is the soul or inner essence of all things. There are several distinctive schools or paths in yoga. Each involves physical training and mental disciplines depending on the spiritual level. Dr. Andrew Weil recommends a yoga posture or asana, called the shoulder stand, to improve thyroid function.[53]

Neural Therapy

Neural or craniosacral therapy is a method that focuses on the movement of energy up and down the spine and assesses how this energy corresponds to the rhythmic pulsations of cerebrospinal fluid. Disruption to the spine's energy flow can be caused by trauma, even circumstances related to birth.

Craniosacral therapy was pioneered by Florida's Dr. John Upledger. While assisting in surgery, Dr. Upledger observed a rhythmic movement of a patient's dura mater. This led him to research what we now know to be the craniosacral system that includes the dura mater, which is attached to facial and skull bones, and the sacrum. Dr. Upledger discovered that he could influence the flow of cerebrospinal fluid by applying pressure to areas of the craniosacral zone and thereby correct energy blockages.[54]

Integrative Medicine

Integrative medical specialists are physicians who integrate alternative medicine into their conventional healing protocols. Responding to patient demand, many doctors are integrating natural healing methods into their conventional protocols.

In cities where integrative centers or physicians aren't available, several Graves' patients have integrated their own services, receiving treatment from conventional physicians and naturopathic practitioners who coordinate their efforts. One 16-year-old girl reported achieving remission within one year using craniosacral therapy along with anti-thyroid drugs (see integrative resources in chapter 13).

10 *Special Considerations in Pregnancy, Children and Teens*

While working in hospital laboratories, I've met thousands of newborns, including many infants who needed hourly blood tests. Long ago, I noticed that after babies experience their first blood test, they appear to remember it. Breaking hearts on subsequent blood draws, some babies stiffen and cringe the minute a laboratory technician approaches their bassinet. Other neonates curl into balls and try to hide their feet. Those with a flair for melodrama squeeze their eyes shut and let out piercing wails.

Despite my keen interest in nursery socialization, until recently, I never gave much thought to the critical role thyroid hormone plays in the newborns' response, a role this chapter focuses on. Chapter 10 discusses the factors influencing fetal thyroid function, including the placenta, maternal thyroid status and circulating autoantibodies. In addition, it describes the development of GD and postpartum thyroiditis in pregnancy, and it discusses changes in thyroid function and treatment concerns associated with pregnancy in both hyperthyroid and hypothyroid Graves' patients as well as their infants.

In the newborn, transient symptoms of thyroid dysfunction can result from placental transfer of both maternal antibodies and medications. Idiopathic thyroid disorders may also develop spontaneously in children. And as you'll learn in this chapter, childhood thyroid disorders have the potential of causing developmental problems when symptoms are not recognized and treated. This chapter concludes with a description of the special diagnostic and treatment challenges of pediatric GD.

The Thyroid in Fetal Development

The first endocrine gland to develop, the thyroid is capable of producing, releasing and circulating low amounts of thyroid hormone to the fetal brain as early as ten to 11 weeks' gestation. The fetal thyroid depends on the mother for its iodine supply, but otherwise, it works independently by about 11 weeks, sending needed hormone to other cells, especially those of the central nervous system.

The development of the thyroid and gastrointestinal tracts are closely related because both of these cell lines develop from the primitive endoderm, the innermost of the embryonic cellular layers that form the digestive tract. This association is demonstrated by their sharing of several functions. For instance, iodine can be concentrated by the salivary and gastric glands as well as the thyroid. Although neither the salivary gland nor the gastric glands respond to TSH stimulation, the salivary glands can also iodinate tyrosine.

Embryonic Origin

The thyroid is the first endocrine gland to develop in mammals. Human thyroid tissue cells are detected in the embryo one month after conception. A developing embryo has three cell layers, the ectoderm, which gives rise to skin and nerves, the mesoderm, which becomes muscle, blood arteries, veins and the heart, and the endoderm, which develops into the stomach lining, the intestines, pancreas, thyroid gland and gastric parietal cells that line the stomach cavity.

The thyroid primordium (early primitive tissue) originates on about day 16 or 17 as epithelial endoderm cells from two distinct regions of the pharynx floor thicken. These thickened cells form a diverticulum (outpocketing of tissue) known as the median thyroid anlage (the thyroid foundation). These inchoate or primitive thyroid cells derived from the pharynx floor emerge adjacent to the cells that simultaneously emerge to form the heart.

As fetal development proceeds, the middle of the diverticulum is displaced, projecting inward. The primitive stalk of tissue connecting this embryonic thyroid tissue to the pharynx elongates forming the thyroglossal duct. While moving inward, the outpocket shape begins to fill with cells, taking on the shape of two lobes. The resulting tissue fuses with the fourth pharyngeal pouch. Because the thyroid develops so close to the emerging heart, its location is influenced by the heart's position. As the heart

descends into the chest, the thyroid is pulled to its position near the base
of the neck.

Ectopic Thyroid Tissue

As it moves into position, remnants of thyroid tissue can lodge in
other locations. Ectopic (away from its normal location) thyroid tissue
occurs in 7 percent to 10 percent of the population.[1] Ectopic thyroid tissue can result from abnormal thyroid migration secondary to changes in
the heart's development. Therefore, when it is present, ectopic thyroid tissue usually occurs in the sublingual region beneath the tongue or in the
region between the neck and heart. In one recent study, a GD patient who
had been ablated had a recurrence of GD nine years later in which medi-
astinal (chest cavity) ectopic thyroid tissue grew (presumably in response
to stimulating TRAb) much like a goiter, causing substernal chest pain.[2]

Two months after conception, the thyroglossal duct normally dis-
solves and fragments. At the junction of the middle and posterior thirds
of the tongue, only a small dimpled remnant of the duct called the fora-
men caecum remains. Cells of the lower portion of the duct differentiate
into thyroid tissue that forms the pyramidal lobe of the thyroid gland. At
ten weeks' gestation, TBG can be detected in fetal serum.

Thyroid Follicle Development

Three months after conception, early thyroid cells form intricate
cord-like arrangements interspersed with vascular connective tissue. These
soon take on the shape of follicles that eventually fill with colloid. By 11
weeks, the follicular cells are able to concentrate iodide and synthesize
thyroxine. Therefore, radioactive iodine given to the mother at this time
would be concentrated by the fetal thyroid and the early fetal thyroid cells
would also be ablated. At ten to 12 weeks, the pituitary begins secreting
TSH and the hypothalamus begins secreting TRH. From then on, rapid
changes in the thyroid and pituitary take place. By 26 weeks' gestation,
fetal TSH levels are higher than those of the mother, perhaps because of
the fetal pituitary's greater sensitivity to TRH stimulation.

Role of Fetal Thyroid Hormone

As the fetus develops, thyroid hormone plays an instrumental role in
the maturation of the skeletal system, the lungs and the brain. Although
T4 is primarily converted to rT3, small amounts of fresh T3 are slowly
deiodinated in the fetal pituitary, brain and brown adipose or fat tissue.
About a week before birth, there's a gradual prenatal surge where T3 levels rise. Two to four hours after birth, these levels abruptly surge (postnatal surge), presumably to meet the increased life demands.

Placental Influences

Fetal development is highly influenced by the placenta. Acting as a semi-permeable membrane between the fetal and maternal systems, the placenta regulates what nutrients, hormones, drugs and other chemicals can cross over to the fetus. Besides supplying iodide, the placenta supplies T4 to the fetus during the first half of gestation when the fetal mechanism is not yet fully functioning. In the euthyroid fetus, transfer of placental T4 is marginal, whereas in hypothyroidism, sufficient maternal T4 may cross the placental membrane in sufficient quantities to bring levels up to half of the normal value seen at birth.

The protective placental tissue is rich in the particular deiodinase enzyme that converts T4 into the benign reverse T3 (rT3, see chapter 3) rather than the more potent T3. Considering the small energy requirements of the fetus, T3 isn't needed until delivery approaches. Excess T3 before then could harm the fetal heart and nervous system, a fact the placenta apparently recognizes. Several weeks before delivery, the placental enzymes shift and the outer ring deiodinase predominates, preparing for the postnatal surge.

The Fetal Pituitary-Thyroid Axis
and Maternal Influences

The fetal pituitary-thyroid axis, which completes its development during late fetal development, functions independently of the mother. Transplacental passage of TSH from the mother is negligible, although the transfer of T4 is significant. At amounts that vary during different stages of gestation, maternal T4 spills over to the fetal circulation and accounts for approximately 30 percent of the serum T4 present in cord blood at term. This maternal contribution is important for normal fetal maturation.

Thyroid Function in the Newborn

Mean T4 levels in the newborn are 12 mcg/ml, a level that would be considered high in an adult. The increase may be due to the elevated TBG normally seen in the newborn. At term, the newborn's levels of FT4 are slightly less than those in maternal serum. Serum T4, T3 and thyroglobulin also continue to rise during the first few hours after delivery, reaching the hyperthyroid range by 24 hours.

Immediately after birth, TSH levels rise rapidly in the newborn, peaking 30 minutes after birth, then dropping to its initial value within 48 hours. This elevation is considered a response to the temperature cooling that occurs at delivery and accounts for the increased levels of T4, T3 and thyroglobulin. D2 type deiodinase present in adipose tissue contributes to the conversion of T4 to T3 rather than rT3. By the fifth day of life, levels of rT3 return to normal, although levels of T3 remain increased for the first year of life, then gradually diminish until they reach the normal range. The normal rates of thyroid hormone production are higher per unit of body weight in infants and children than in adults.

Thyroid Function in Pregnancy

One of the earliest changes in thyroid function during pregnancy involves an increase in the carrier protein TBG brought about by increased estrogens. Also, the type of TBG produced in pregnancy is slightly different in composition and takes longer to be cleared from the circulation. As a result of the increased TBG, the levels of total T4 and T3 are increased accordingly. Although levels of free T4 and free T3 usually remain unchanged, both levels may reflect a slight increase. TSH levels are slightly decreased.

These changes resolve at about five months with levels returning to normal, where they remain throughout the duration of pregnancy. Occasionally, T4 is reduced late in pregnancy, particularly if gestation exceeds 40 weeks, although in iodine rich regions in the United States, the third trimester is associated with T4 levels greater than the upper limit of the normal range.

Human Chorionic Gondatotropin (hCG) Influences

Another hormone released during pregnancy may also contribute to enhanced thyroid function in the first trimester. Levels of human chorionic gonadotropin, commonly referred to as hCG, (the hormone measured in pregnancy tests) rise dramatically during the first trimester. Serum hCG may act as a circulating thyroid stimulator with properties similar to those of TSH. As hCG levels drop in the second trimester, its structure shifts and has less potential to act as a thyroid stimulator.[3]

Gestational Thyrotoxicosis

The thyroid stimulating effects of hCG may contribute to the development of hyperemesis gravidarum, a condition also known as gestational thyrotoxicosis, which is characterized by excessive vomiting and dehydration. In this condition, FT4 is increased and TSH is low, although patients don't exhibit symptoms of thyrotoxicosis, goiter or any of the symptoms typically associated with GD. These biochemical aberrations only last for a few weeks and then resolve, probably as hCG levels decline.[4]

Asian women are at higher risk of gestational thyrotoxicosis than European women.[5]

Increased Renal Clearance

Iodide is normally cleared through the body via both the thyroid and the kidneys. In pregnancy the kidneys speed up their clearance, causing increased urination. Consequently, iodine clearance is also increased and goiter may develop if the diet does not provide adequate stores of iodine. The thyroid is reported to increase in volume by about 10 percent in regions of adequate or excess iodine because of the increase in thyroid stimulating activity.[6]

Maternal iodine diffuses through the placental membrane, supplying the small iodine requirements of the fetus and neonate. In areas of iodine deficiency, both the fetus and neonate (newborn) have reduced iodine stores, which reflect the severity of maternal iodine deficiency. In iodine excess, the developing autoregulatory system is unable to halt thyroid hormone synthesis, and goiter may develop.

Postpartum Thyroid Disorders

Postpartum Graves' disease refers to the development of GD within the first year after delivery. This is a frequent period for GD onset in women, although postpartum GD doesn't occur as frequently as a different disorder known as postpartum thyroiditis. Both disorders are characterized by symptoms of thyrotoxicosis including goiter, although thyroid enlargement is generally greater in GD.[7] GD is associated with an increased RAI-U test, whereas thyroiditis patients have a low RAI-U. Both disorders are associated with high titers of TPO Ab (described in chapter 5). Further confusing the issue, a transient occurrence of postpartum thyroiditis may develop at the same time as relapse from GD.

Postpartum thyroiditis (PPTD) refers to a transient disorder of usually mild hyperthyroidism that occurs in approximately 5 percent to 10 percent of postpartum mothers. It may also occur in the absence of pregnancy. PPTD usually occurs three to 12 months after delivery and lasts two to six weeks. It is often followed by several months of hypothyroidism before there is a return to the euthyroid state. On occasion, a period of hypothyroidism may precede the onset of thyrotoxicosis. Postpartum thyroiditis can coexist with GD, and patients who develop it are likely to experience it again in subsequent pregnancies. More than 33 percent of patients who have positive TPO Ab titers develop PPTD. Some endocrinologists suggest that TPO Ab be included in the routine prenatal workup since this disorder is fairly prevalent.[8]

Postpartum thyroiditis is an immunologic disorder influenced by immune system fluctuations resulting from the resolution of pregnancy involving both delivery and spontaneous or assisted abortion. Considered an inflammatory condition, it is usually treated with anti-inflammatory medications or antibiotics. In general, symptoms resolve within three to nine months after delivery. One study of postpartum depression and mental disturbances found an association between mental disorders and thyroid autoantibodies.[9]

Development of Graves' Disease During Pregnancy

When symptoms of thyrotoxicosis occur during pregnancy, the cause is usually GD. Since symptoms of amenorrhea, increased circulation, thyroid enlargement and increased thyroid hormone levels may occur in both conditions, diagnosis is difficult. Since the RAI-U test is contraindicated in pregnancy, GD is usually confirmed by laboratory tests, including thyroid antibody tests. A suppressed TSH alone may be misleading since increased levels of the hormone human chorionic gonadotropin seen during the eighth and 14th weeks of pregnancy cause thyroid stimulation and decreased levels of TSH.

Immune System Changes During and After Pregnancy

Since the immune system in GD may be stimulated during the first trimester, women with GD who are in remission often have relapses shortly after becoming pregnant. This is thought to be a reflection of the increased thyroid stimulation and iodine uptake caused by hormones (hCG) rather than from the antibody changes.

Pregnant patients are known to have fewer helper T cells and more suppressor T cells in the late stages of pregnancy. This causes a period of immune system suppression (and less antibody production) reflected in the increased susceptibility to infection, enhancement of tumor growth and the prolongation of organ graft rejection seen in pregnancy. Most autoimmune disorders, including GD and HT, tend to wane during gestation. Consequently, patients with GD who are on ATDs often require dosage reductions. On occasion, ATDs are discontinued in late pregnancy.[10]

After delivery, autoimmune diseases tend to relapse. Antibody titers tend to rise, peaking from three to seven months after delivery. Although antibody levels eventually start dropping, one year after delivery they're still higher than before pregnancy. T helper cell levels also rise. Greater rises in antibody titers and T helpers cells are seen in patients who go on to develop postpartum thyroiditis.[11]

Fertility and Pregnancy in Patients
with Active Graves' Disease

Patients with severe active GD have greater difficulty conceiving, and the incidence of spontaneous abortion is increased.[12] The autoimmune process in GD is thought to activate natural killer (NK) cells of the CD 56+ variety and the CD 19+5+ variety. The CD 56+ NK cells produce the cytokine tumor necrosis factor (TNF). TNF causes further inflammation and damage to other organs including the embryo, the womb lining and the placental cells that attach the fetus to the uterus. The CD 19+5+ variety produce antibodies to several hormones, including estradiol, FSH, LH, progesterone and hCG, and to neurotransmitters including endorphins, enkaphlins and serotonin.[13] Women with neurotransmitter autoantibodies are reported to have premature menopause, poor uterine lining responses and poor blood flow responses to the endometrium as the uterus prepares for successful implantation or pregnancy.

Treatment of GD doesn't necessarily bring fertility improvement. Treated women, especially those who become hypothyroid, are said to still suffer poor stimulation cycles, infertility, implantation failures, donor egg failures and miscarriages. Proper diagnosis of these immune disturbances is necessary, followed by preconception treatment that may take up to three months. Tissue slides from previous pregnancy loss can also aid in diagnosis. Depending on the immune system effects, treatment may consist of lymphocyte immune therapy, or intravenous immunoglobulin therapy to suppress NK cell activity.[14]

Treatment of Graves' Disease in Pregnancy

Radioiodine, both ablative and diagnostic, is contraindicated in pregnancy because of its potential to affect the fetus. Surgery during the first and last trimesters is rarely performed since it may induce labor. ATDs are most often used in pregnancy, but they are not without risk. Both methimazole and PTU cross the placental barrier and affect the fetal thyroid. Since PTU crosses the barrier poorly, it causes milder fetal effects and is usually the drug of choice in pregnancy. Another reason for PTU preference is the greater association between methimazole and aplasia cutis in the fetus, although this condition may also rarely occur in mothers using PTU and hyperthyroid mothers not on ATDs.[15] Aplasia cutis causes skin lesions that usually affect the scalp.

ATD DOSAGE EFFECTS

The recommended daily dose of PTU in pregnancy is 200 mg or less. In patients requiring doses greater than 400 mg, subtotal thyroidectomy, particularly in the second trimester, is recommended.[16] Often, however, the ATD dose can be reduced in the second trimester as symptoms spontaneously diminish. Doses as low as 100 mg of PTU are capable of reducing the serum T4 in the fetus and increasing TSH. However, PTU doses below 150 mg/d are rarely associated with fetal hypothyroidism.

With excess ATD in the fetal circulation, Goitrous hypothyroidism can occur. Maternal transfer of T4 is seldom sufficient to compensate. Because of this risk, pregnant patients are kept at the lowest possible ATD dose that keeps FT4 levels at the high end of the normal range. Some physicians advise that hormone levels are not as important as the patient's clinical status.[17] Furthermore, a modest increase in heart rate is reported to be common in pregnancy and not a reason to increase ATD dosage.

In one recent study, fetal goiter was observed in a Graves' patient on PTU. Since maternal thyroid function tests were normal, the patient's PTU was discontinued. Fetal goiter was studied (by ultrasonography) for the following ten weeks at which time fetal thyroid volume diminished and the fetal neck was returned to a normal flexed position. This patient went on to deliver a normal infant. This is the first report to demonstrate that treatment of fetal goiter caused by maternal ATDs may be managed without intervention.[18]

All pregnant patients with GD require careful observation and close monitoring of intrauterine thyroid function, using ultrasound for assessment of fetal growth and fetal heart rate monitoring. Fetal hyperthyroidism can be treated by the use of maternal methimazole, taking advantage of its enhanced ability to cross the placental membrane.

TREATMENT PRECAUTIONS AND CONTRAINDICATIONS

Strong iodine solution should not be used in pregnancy because of its ability to cross over to the placenta. High concentrations of iodine can cause fetal goiter, and an enlarged goiter may interfere with breathing. The use of beta blockers is controversial in pregnancy with some studies showing significant side effects. *The Physician's Desk Reference* (PDR) reports that there are no adequate, well-controlled studies in pregnant women. Under side effects for propranolol, it's noted that newborns whose mothers were using propranolol at the time of delivery have exhibited bradycardia (abnormal heartrhythm), hypoglycemia and respiratory depression.[19] Also, "Intrauterine growth retardation has been reported in neonates whose mothers received propranolol during pregnancy."[20]

Role of Thyroid Antibodies in Pregnancy

TSH receptor antibodies may cross the placental membrane and affect the fetus. Patients with severe thyrotoxicosis, severe GO or infiltrative dermopathy, and patients who have previously had RAI for treatment of

GD, are often monitored for stimulating TRAb. Although only 1 percent of babies born to GD mothers develop fetal thyrotoxicosis, patients with high antibody titers in their first trimester are usually rechecked in their third trimester. Fetal monitoring, however, is more predictive of thyrotoxicosis than antibody titers.

When GD has been treated by ablation, the mother may not have enough remaining thyroid tissue to exhibit symptoms despite having high titers of stimulating TRAb in her blood. Clues to the presence of fetal hyperthyroidism are fetal heart rate consistently above the normal limit of 160 beats per minute and high antibody titers. All women with GD or a history of it should be tested for these antibodies late in pregnancy.[21]

Pregnancy in the Hypothyroid and Euthyroid Graves' Patient

Dosage Adjustments

During pregnancy, hypothyroid patients on thyroid hormone replacement generally require a 50 percent to 100 percent increase in their maintenance doses.[22] Thyroid requirements are increased because of increased TBG, increased body mass and increases in deiodination to rT3 rather than T3. Many physicians increase the patient's maintenance dose by 50 percent as soon as pregnancy is confirmed because the increased requirement begins shortly after implantation and lasts until a few weeks following delivery.[23]

Euthyroid patients in spontaneous remission from GD may have a relapse during pregnancy. This relapse may be due to hormonal changes or it may be triggered by the increased FT4 seen in early pregnancy and the stimulatory effects of hCG. Relapse may be transient with symptoms resolving before delivery, or it may be recurrent.

Drug Treatment During Lactation

Although there have been no side effects reported in nursing infants whose mothers used ATDs, mothers on ATDs have traditionally been advised not to nurse their babies since antithyroid drugs appear in breast milk. However, numerous studies have found ATDs to be safe and there have been no reports of increased neonatal TSH levels occurring with either drug.[24]

Although ATDs haven't been reported to cause abnormally high TSH levels in infants, babies of nursing moms on ATDs are rarely tested for thyroid function. Until recently, the quantity of blood needed to routinely test babies was prohibitive. Before Mary B (on PTU at the time) began nursing her daughter, she checked to make sure her doctor intended to order frequent blood tests on her baby since the effects of hypothyroidism in newborns could be profound before symptoms emerge.

Methimazole crosses into breast milk more readily than PTU, making PTU a better choice for moms who nurse. Several nursing moms, including a few who developed GD or whose symptoms worsened during pregnancy, report that their symptoms significantly improved when they weaned their babies.

Thyroid Dysfunction in the Fetus and Neonate

Hyperthyroidism in the fetus is best diagnosed by ultrasonography to determine if goiter is present and by monitoring fetal heartbeat. In mothers who are on ATDs, the mother is generally switched to methimazole if fetal hyperthyroidism is detected. In children born to mothers with active GD, the onset of neonatal hyperthyroidism usually begins before birth, although symptoms may not appear obvious until a few days after birth. The onset of neonatal GD may also be delayed several weeks or longer.

Symptoms of Neonatal Hyperthyroidism

Hyperthyroid infants are often premature and appear to have stunted intrauterine growth. Goiter is usually present, and the infant appears extremely restless, irritable, hyperactive, unusually alert and anxious. Microcephaly (condition characterized by a small head, which is usually associated with mental defects), ventricular enlargement, tachycardia and an elevated temperature may be present, and the eyes may appear exophthalmic.[25]

In severely affected infants, symptoms may include weight loss despite an increased appetite, hepatosplenomegaly (liver and spleen enlargement), thyrombocytopenia, diarrhea, vomiting, advanced bone age, cranial synostosis (see Symptoms of Childhood GD later in this chapter), jaundice, hypertension, cardiac decompensation and intrauterine death. Serum T4 is markedly elevated and TSH is suppressed. Without prompt treatment of the neonate, intellectual development may be limited and death may occur.[26]

Transient Graves' Disease in the Newborn

When significant concentrations of TSH receptor antibodies pass from the mother's circulation on through the placental membrane and over to the fetal circulation, the newborn may exhibit temporary symptoms of thyrotoxicosis or hypothyroidism depending on the type of antibody. If predominantly stimulating antibodies reach the fetal circulation, symptoms of thyrotoxicosis appear. If blocking receptor antibodies cross the placental membrane, symptoms of fetal hypothyroidism occur. If the neonate is exposed to antithyroid drugs in utero or if blocking TRAb accompany high concentrations of stimulating TRAb, symptoms of hyperthyroidism may be delayed for three to four days.[27]

These effects persist for only as long as the antibodies remain viable, usually six to 12 weeks. However, the disorder may persist longer with high levels of stimulating TRAb. Maternally transferred antibodies do not cause the baby to develop antibodies of his own. Nor do they cause him to develop Graves' disease.

Treatment of Neonatal Hyperthyroidism

Treatment consists of oral administration of propranolol (2 mg/kg/24 hr orally in three divided doses) and PTU (5 to 10 mg/kg/24 hr. given every eight hr.); Lugol's solution (1 drop every eight hr.) may be added. If neonatal hyperthyroidism is severe, intravenous fluid therapy and corticosteroids may also be indicated. In instances of heart failure, digoxin may also be indicated. Once the infant has stabilized and euthyroidism is achieved, only PTU is necessary. Most cases remit within three to four months.[28]

In patients with an impressive family history of GD, neonatal hyperthyroidism may persist into childhood, although TSH stimulating antibodies are absent. If treatment is delayed, significant problems, including mental retardation, may occur. When the cause of hyperthyroidism is not GD but a defect in the TSH receptor gene, surgery is indicated.[29]

Hypothyroidism in the Fetus and Neonate

CAUSES OF FETAL AND NEONATAL HYPOTHYROIDISM

ATDs: Antithyroid drugs used to treat the mother may cross the placental barrier, causing hypothyroidism in the newborn or fetus. PTU does not cross to the placenta as readily as methimazole does. Therefore, PTU is the drug of choice in pregnancy.

TSH Receptor Antibodies: Blocking TSH receptor antibodies may rarely cross into the fetal circulation and bind to the TSH receptor, interfering with TSH. Since the thyroid-hypothalamic-pituitary axis isn't defined until late in pregnancy, the effects and resulting hypothyroidism occur near the end of the gestational period.

Iodine Deficiency and Environmental Causes: Iodine deficiency occurs as a consequence of maternal iodine deficiency or from a maternal diet high in goitrogens or soy. Transient hypothyroidism may also occur in babies who are exposed to substances high in iodine content, such as X-ray dyes and certain skin cleansers, around the time of their birth. In these instances, hypothyroidism may persist for several days to several months.

Untreated Maternal Hypothyroidism: Maternal hypothyroidism is associated with fertility problems and an increased risk of miscarriage, especially in the first trimester.[30] Poor outcome is associated with the severity of the hypothyroidism. Maternal hypothyroidism may have an adverse effect on fetal development. Maternal thyroxine is transferred to the fetal circulation more readily during the first half of pregnancy. Fetal requirements are critical since T4 contributes to the development of the central nervous system. In maternal hypothyroidism, inadequate maternal T4 exacerbates the effects of fetal hypothyroidism, contributing to irreversible nervous system disorders.

PREMATURE BIRTHS AND HYPOTHALAMIC HYPOTHYROIDISM

Infants born prematurely may have hypothalamic hypothyroidism representing developmental immaturity as a consequence of incomplete maturation of the hypothalamic-pituitary-thyroid system. This is demonstrated by low T4 and FT4 levels although the TSH is normal. The severity is inversely related to the developmental age. Infants under 30 gestational weeks have a 50 percent prevalence of low thyroxine (<6 ug/dl) and infants born after 34 to 36 weeks have a 10 percent prevalence.[31]

Treatment of Fetal Hypothyroidism

While the neonate can be treated relatively easily with levothyroxine replacement therapy, there are no commonly available treatment options for fetal hypothyroidism. Administering excess thyroid hormone to the mother produces little change in fetal thyroid levels during the second half of gestation when developmental changes are occurring. Although treatment instituted promptly after birth is effective in preventing the brain damage associated with congenital hypothyroidism, there is debate whether full mental capacity is restored. If the cause of fetal hypothyroidism is maternal antithyroid drugs, discontinuation of the medication (if possible) may cause resolution of the goiter.

INTRA-AMNIOTIC THYROXINE INJECTION

Injecting thyroxine into the amniotic sac (membranous sac containing amniotic fluid that acts as a barrier shield surrounding the placenta) is used in cases of inadvertent maternal radioiodine treatment of GD between 10 and 20 weeks of gestation and for fetal goiter detected by ultrasound.[32]

Pediatric Graves' Disease

Diagnosis

When thyrotoxicosis occurs in children and adolescents, the culprit is usually Graves' disease. Since GD tends to be more severe in children, early diagnosis and treatment are vital. Diagnostic difficulties occur because children are seldom tested for thyroid disorders, and symptoms in children are more difficult to assess. Rarely, Graves' disease is suspected when children are seen for behavioral problems. Dr. Scott Pacer, a child psychiatrist in Cleveland, Ohio, reports that he considers it prudent to test thyroid function in his patients who have a family history of autoimmune thyroid disease.[33]

Family history is generally the best clue when children develop one or more symptoms suggestive of GD. However, many GD symptoms are typical of childhood and aren't noticed unless they're dramatic. Several parents of children with GD report that it was the changes in appearance, energy or behavior that led them to consult a physician. In several instances, another relative who hadn't seen the child in a while remarked on the changes, which in day to day life easily go unnoticed. Similar to what is reported in adults, other conditions are often first suspected.

Incidence

About 5 percent of all patients with GD are less than 15 years old.[34] The peak incidence is adolescence. In children born to mothers with GD, the onset of hyperthyroidism occurred between 6 weeks and 2 years of age. Outside of transient neonatal hyperthyroidism caused by antibody transfer, which affects both sexes equally, childhood Graves' disease occurs four to five times more often in females than males.[35]

Symptoms

Symptoms, which may be cyclic, include weakness, dyspnea, dysphagia, amenorrhea, emotional instability accompanied by motor hyperactivity, mood disorders, personality disturbances and rarely tremors (finger tremor may be seen if the arm is extended). Writing in *Postgraduate Medicine*, Dr. Michael Felz reports that GD in children "usually presents with restlessness, weight loss, and poor school performance, which are often attributed to nonthyroidal factors."[36]

Goiter, sometimes with evidence of bruit and thrill, is seen in more than 90 percent of cases, and the skin is usually warm and moist and the face flushed. Palpitations, tachycardia and systolic hypertension with increased pulse pressure are often seen. Cardiac enlargement and insufficiency are said to cause discomfort but rarely endanger the patient's life.[37]

Because of emotional lability, children with GD become irritable, excitable and cry easily. Their schoolwork may suffer as a result of short attention span.

In one Italian study, researchers described three girls in whom GD developed before age 3 (presumably between an age of 6 to 12 months), although they weren't diagnosed until a mean age of 3.[38] Two of the children consequently had impaired verbal expression and one child had severe mental retardation that is still evident. The children had been previously brought in to the pediatric clinic for symptoms of hyperthyroidism including poor language development, but they weren't tested for GD. The study's authors emphasize the need for psychological assessment in evaluating GD and greater awareness of the consequences on growth and development in the first two years of life.

In two of the children in this study, there was no maternal history of GD although one mother had isolated exophthalmos, and in one child the mother had been diagnosed with GD during pregnancy. Symptoms in all three children included goiter, exophthalmos, tachycardia and hyperactivity, and they all turned out to have consistently high stimulating TRAb. One child showed severe psychomotor delay and had undergone surgery for craniosynostosis.

Craniosynostosis, a condition in which two or more cranial bones mesh to form a single bone, is a known complication of thyrotoxicosis in children. It is attributed to the higher sensitivity to thyroid hormones of membranous bone (bone attached to membrane) compared to enchondral bone (bone connected to bone).[39]

Graves' Ophthalmopathy in Children

Exophthalmos is noticeable in most all children with GD but it is usually mild. Symptoms of GO seen in children and adolescents include lagging of the upper eyelid on downward gaze, impairment of convergence or alignment, upper eyelid retraction, "staring eyes" and infrequent blinking.[40] Infiltrative ophthalmopathy is very rare in children and adolescents, and symptoms usually disappear when euthyroidism is restored. The administration of steroids is restricted to rare severe cases.

Treatment of Pediatric Graves' Disease

Treatment options listed in chapters 8 and 9 are used in children as well as adults. However, because of the risks involved with radioiodine, treatment in children is generally restricted to antithyroid drug therapy or surgery. Alternative healing options are occasionally used in very mild cases or as adjunctive therapy in children on ATDs.

Most pediatric endocrinologists recommend the use of antithyroid drugs.[41] However, whatever treatment is used, the results are reported to be less satisfactory than in adults. Both problems with compliance and the fact that the thyroid cells divide and grow faster in children make treatment more of a challenge.

Antithyroid Drugs

Significant side effects of ATDs are described in chapter 8. Side effects are reported to occur less often with methimazole. ATDs may also cause temporary minor effects. Transient leukopenia (<4,000 white blood cells/mm^3) is common and does not cause symptoms. Nor does it foreshadow agranulocytosis, a condition of decreased white blood cells along with symptoms of sore throat, mouth ulcers, fever or other indications of bone marrow suppression. Transient leukopenia is usually not a reason the discontinue treatment.[42] Transient rashes are also common. When they occur the medication is usually discontinued and the other available ATD started, or the rash is simultaneously treated.

There is considerable debate regarding whether patients on ATDs should be routinely tested for white blood cell determinations. In general, it's recommended that patients be on the alert for symptoms of agranulocytosis, especially during the first three months when side effects of ATDs are most likely to occur.

Because of the high incidence of post-operative hypothyroidism reported in studies of children using other therapies, many endocrinologists recommend initially using a course of one year to two years of antithyroid drug therapy followed by a second course if relapse occurs.[43] However, children using ATDs are reported to have a lower incidence of remission than adults. This may be a compliance issue since many adults complain that ATDs do not taste good and a metallic taste persists. (One woman reported swallowing a mint candy along with her ATDs and claimed that it helps.) Another vote for ATDs comes from reports that GD in children usually resolves in adolescence.

DOSAGE

The initial dosage of PTU is 5 to 10 mg/kg/24 hours given three times daily; the dosage of methimazole is 0.25 to 1.0 mg/kg/24 hr. given once or twice daily.[44] Smaller initial doses are used in early childhood. Patients on ATDs must be carefully monitored with both blood tests and an assessment of symptoms. (See chapter 11 for symptoms of hypothyroidism.) Patients may show signs of an exacerbation of symptoms due to the natural course of the disease or they may show symptoms of hypothyroidism. Ideally, symptoms will be those seen in normal children, and clinical response becomes apparent in two to three weeks. At this time, the dose may be lowered. Adequate control is evident in one to three months and the patient is kept on the dose required to maintain a euthyroid state. Drug therapy may be necessary for five years or longer.

REMISSION

Patients older than 13, boys, patients with a higher body mass index, and patients with small goiters and modestly elevated T3 levels are reported to have earlier remissions. If relapse occurs after remission, it usually occurs between three to six months of the discontinuation of therapy. At this time, ATDs are resumed or other therapy can be decided on.

Radioiodine and Surgery

Because of the enhanced carcinogenic potential of radiation in the thyroid glands of children and the lack of long term studies, many endocrinologists do not recommend the use of radioiodine ablation for children with Graves' disease.[45] Several studies have demonstrated an increased risk for thyroid carcinoma in children receiving X-ray therapy to the head and neck.[46] Also, children and adolescents are considered to be at the greatest risk for genetic damage, damage which may take 30 years or more to show up. Of the various molecules that radiation may damage within the cell, DNA is said to be the most critical since damage to a single gene may irreparably alter or kill the cell.[47]

Furthermore, the prevalence of hypothyroidism in patients following ablation makes radioiodine undesirable for children in whom the effects of hypothyroidism on growth, development and scholastic performance can be critical.[48] When radioiodine is used in children, pretreatment with ATDs should be discontinued five days before ablation. The incidence of recurrence is low and most patients only require one ablation.

Although surgery is a viable option, thyroidectomy in children is associated with a higher risk of hypothyroidism than is seen in adults. This is probably related to the natural course of the disease compounded by the effect of declining thyroid hormone levels on growth. Also, surgical complications such as recurrent laryngeal nerve damage or hypoparathyroidism will have lifelong consequences.

Graves' Disease in Teens

For Brittany, whom you'll meet in chapter 12, GD came as an unwelcome 12th birthday present. But it never stopped her from continuing with gymnastics or becoming a cheerleader or a good student. In remission and now a high school junior after four years on ATDs, she has few complaints. Although Brittany was the first in her family to develop an autoimmune disorder, her mother was recently diagnosed with Hashimoto's thyroiditis.

Graves' disease is hardly the first thing one thinks of when adolescents begin to have problems with weight, increased appetite, emotional lability, nervousness or moodiness. After all, many of the symptoms typical of GD parallel changes seen in puberty. For those whose symptoms remain moderate, behavioral causes may be suspected but the patient is seldom checked to see if underlying causes may be present. Treatment for teens is similar to that of children. As with children, spontaneous remission is said to occur at a rate of about 25 percent every two years.[49]

Treatment Related Hypothyroidism and Relapse

The symptoms and treatment options in hypothyroidism are discussed in the next chapter. However, younger patients will experience lifelong consequences of GD for a longer duration. Thus, their chances for both relapse and progression to spontaneous hypothyroidism are increased, a consideration in choosing GD treatment. Parents of children with GD need to be aware that their children will require lifelong monitoring or treatment with thyroid supplements, or both. Since thyroid status can change even after many years, grown children and their parents must be on the alert for symptoms of both hyperthyroidism and hypothyroidism.

11 Hypothyroidism Associated with Graves' Disease

Most, but not all, patients with Graves' disease will eventually become hypothyroid, either as a consequence of treatment or because they spontaneously develop an autoimmune hypothyroid disorder. Chapter 11 focuses on the causes and symptoms of hypothyroidism and the effects of thyroid hormone deficiency on various bodily systems including progression to myxedema coma. This chapter also discusses the role of laboratory tests in diagnosing hypothyroidism and describes available treatment options.

Primary and Central Hypothyroidism

Most patients with GD will eventually develop primary hypothyroidism, which causes decreased thyroid function. The most common cause of primary hypothyroidism is thyroiditis, usually chronic autoimmune hypothyroidism. Chronic autoimmune hypothyroidism, which is also known as Hashimoto's thyroiditis (HT) or lymphocytic thyroiditis or lymphoadenitis, can be present in the very young, as early as one to two years of age.[1] HT is associated with cell-mediated and antibody mediated destruction of the thyroid gland. Patients with GD are known to occasionally move from autoimmune thyroiditis to GD and back to autoimmune thyroiditis.

Primary hypothyroidism may also occur as a result of the natural progression of GD, resulting in autoimmune hypothyroidism, also known as idiopathic myxedema. It results from an immune system change that causes a predominance of blocking TRAb, or it may occur as a consequence of treatment that causes loss or atrophy of thyroid tissue (postablative hypothyroidism). Postablative hypothyroidism accounts for 30 percent to 40 percent of all instances of primary hypothyroidism. Often, more than one of these causes contributes to the development of hypothyroidism in GD patients.

Central hypothyroidism refers to hypothyroidism that originates in the pituitary, hypothalamus or the hypothalamic-pituitary portal circulation. Central hypothyroidism accounts for approximately 1 percent of the incidences of hypothyroidism. Central hypothyroidism is distinguished by TRH suppression tests. (see chapter 5).

Pre-Graves' Disease Hypothyroidism

Many GD patients are also reported to have a transient period of subtle hypothyroidism prior to the onset of hyperthyroidism. Some patients may experience several years of moderate hypothyroidism before developing Graves' disease.

Less common are patients like Donna J who was diagnosed with HT, a legacy from her mother, while in her late 20s. Ten years later, while teaching college in the Northeast, she began experiencing heat intolerance and unexplained weight loss. Her physician discounted her symptoms and her laboratory results, insisting that she needed to remain on lifelong thyroid replacement therapy, which he continued to prescribe until she began showing symptoms of thyroid storm. Finally diagnosed with GD and rushed into having radioiodine ablation, she quickly became severely hypothyroid.

Autoimmune Thyroid Disease

Autoimmune thyroid disease (AITD) refers to several different thyroid disorders that have an autoimmune component. The list includes:

- Graves' disease (diffuse toxic goiter)
- Hashimoto's thyroiditis (goitrous and atrophic forms)
- Hashitoxicosis
- Thyroid lymphoma
- Fibrous thyroiditis
- Autoimmune thyroid failure
- Primary myxedema
- Thyroid antigen/antibody nephritis

- Transient postpartum hypothyroidism
- Transient postpartum hyperthyroidism

Does It Matter if It's Autoimmune?

In most instances, hypothyroidism is diagnosed on the basis of laboratory tests, and little effort is made to find the cause or category. Since treatment is generally the same, it usually doesn't matter. However, for some patients, the presence of autoantibodies interferes with laboratory results or with thyroid hormone ever getting to the cells.

Although there may be adequate amounts of circulating thyroid hormone, antibodies may block the receptors, preventing thyroid hormone from acting. When this occurs, patients need to be treated on the basis of symptoms, not laboratory results.

Barnes Basal Temperature Test

As long ago as 1940, Dr. Broda Barnes realized that hypothyroidism can be directly correlated to basal body temperature. Basal temperature is the temperature taken immediately on waking (10 minutes axilla or three minutes orally). Normal readings are between 97.8°F and 98.4°F. Temperatures below this range, when taken for 12 consecutive days, indicate hypothyroidism.

In 40 years of research, Dr. Barnes found that a host of illnesses such as high cholesterol and heart disease in patients with low basal temperature responded well to thyroid hormone therapy despite blood tests indicating normal thyroid function. According to the Broda Barnes Foundation, basal temperature, over the years, has proved to more reliable than blood tests results because it shows how the body is using thyroid hormone, not how much is present in the blood.[3]

Myxedema

Hypothyroidism was described in London in the 1870s and termed myxoedema (current usage — myxedema) for the swollen skin and excess mucin content observed (mucin is a jelly-like mucopolysaccharide with an affinity for water, giving the skin a waterlogged or swollen appearance). Although myxedema and hypothyroidism generally refer to the same disorder, myxedema is the end result of a progressive disease leading to total absence of thyroid hormone production.

Symptoms of Hypothyroidism

Often, hypothyroidism is associated with being overweight or feeling cold. However, weight loss and heat intolerance can also occur in

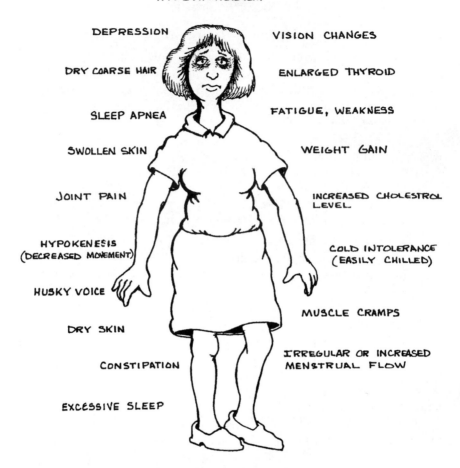

SYMPTOMS OF
HYPOTHYROIDISM

DEPRESSION

VISION CHANGES

DRY COARSE HAIR

ENLARGED THYROID

SLEEP APNEA

FATIGUE, WEAKNESS

SWOLLEN SKIN

WEIGHT GAIN

JOINT PAIN

INCREASED CHOLESTROL LEVEL

HYPOKENESIS (DECREASED MOVEMENT)

COLD INTOLERANCE (EASILY CHILLED)

HUSKY VOICE

DRY SKIN

MUSCLE CRAMPS

CONSTIPATION

IRREGULAR OR INCREASED MENSTRUAL FLOW

EXCESSIVE SLEEP

Postablative Hypothyroidism

hypothyroidism. Symptoms in hypothyroidism run the gamut from cognitive disturbances to sleep apnea. Untreated, hypothyroidism may progress to a potentially fatal condition known as myxedema coma (described later in this chapter), which represents the end state of severe long-standing hypothyroidism. The following list includes the most prominent symptoms associated with hypothyroidism. GD patients who become hypothyroid may also experience symptoms associated with autoimmunity and GD such as vitiligo and emotional lability.

SYMPTOMS OF HYPOTHYROIDISM
- Abdominal pain and distention, colon distention, constipation,

functional bowel disease, malabsorption, constipation, atrophied gastric mucosa, digestive disturbances

- Cardiac manifestations including palpitations, sinus bradycardia, exercise intolerance and increased diastolic blood pressure due to vascular constriction; enlarged heart in severe primary hypothyroidism
- Decreased basal metabolic rate, cold intolerance, decreased drug metabolism, decreased carbohydrate and protein metabolism, elevated serum cholesterol level, decreased conversion of carotenes to Vitamin A, which may cause yellow-orange skin pigmentation (there is no yellowing of the eyes, which distinguishes this condition from jaundice); hyponatremia (decreased serum sodium level), mineral imbalances
- Edema (increased fluid retention caused by glycoprotein [mucin] deposits in the tissues, especially in eyelids, face)
- Hematologic (blood cell) changes, especially anemia
- Hormonal abnormalities including galactorrhea (increased prolactin levels), diminished growth hormone secretion causing stunted growth in children, decreased cortisol secretion, menorrhagia (increased or excessive menstruation), precocious pseudopuberty in children with accelerated genital development, sexual immaturity in infantile hypothyroidism
- Increased skeletal creatine kinase, decreased bone resorption and formation, decreased levels of alkaline phosphatase, arthralgia, joint pain, muscular pains, stiffness of the extremities
- Memory impairment, depression, melancholia, neuropsychiatric disorders, nervousness, anorexia, dyspnea (shortness of breath), headache
- Myopathy, especially of the respiratory muscles and diaphragm; increased muscle mass with diminished muscular activity (Hoffmann syndrome), swollen, heavy calves, leg cramps and restless leg syndrome
- Obstructive sleep apnea, nasal stuffiness, dry throat
- Peripheral neuropathy, carpal tunnel syndrome
- Skin may be dry, coarse, cold, covered with fine scales or a finely wrinkled, parchment-like texture; plugging of hair follicles and sweat glands, pallor of lips and skin, decreased sweating, hair loss, coarseness of hair, brittle, thin, striated nails marked by both horizontal and vertical grooves, slow wound healing, infection, including osteomyelitis
- Slow speech, thick tongue, hoarse voice, voice loss, hearing loss and deafness

- Weakness, lethargy, loss of initiative, slow-wittedness
- Weight gain despite decreased appetite, weight loss, malabsorption.

The Body's Response to Diminished Thyroid Hormone

Hypothyroidism shows little favoritism and affects functions in almost every cell in the body. Many symptoms have a rippling effect. For instance, the accumulation of mucin in tissues causes changes in collagen distribution that lead to slow wound healing. Slow wound healing, in turn, can lead to increased infections, a symptom Dr. Broda Barnes noted seeing in hypothyroid patients. In the following section, I describe the physiological changes caused by thyroid hormone deficiency which are responsible for the symptoms.

The Blood and Nervous System

ANEMIA AND IMPAIRED CLOTTING

Decreased thyroid hormone with its reduced oxygen requirements causes red blood cell production to slow down. This results in mild anemia. Anemia is reported to be present in 30 percent to 40 percent of patents with hypothyroidism.[3] In addition, nutrient deficiencies related to malabsorption may cause iron deficiency anemia. And patients with AITD are more likely to develop pernicious anemia (PA). Overt hypothyroidism is present in 12 percent of patients with PA, and subclinical hypothyroidism is present in 15 percent of PA patients.[4]

The blood's clotting mechanism may also be impaired, resulting in a bleeding tendency, due to decreased levels of factors VIII and IX and increased capillary fragility.[5]

NERVOUS SYSTEM IMPAIRMENT

In hypothyroidism, the nervous system is often characterized by edema with mucinous deposits surrounding the nerve fibers. Consequently, cerebral blood flow is reduced, causing memory impairment and lethargy. In severe hypothyroidism, speech is slow and body movements may be clumsy. Neuropathy, a condition of nerve degeneration, is often seen in hypothyroidism and symptoms are exacerbated by the thickening of connective tissue. Carpal tunnel syndrome and nocturnal paresthesia (hand or foot falling asleep or feeling leaden) with pain in one or both hands are associated symptoms.

The Cardiovascular System

In hypothyroidism, the heart slows down, losing its normal efficiency. Decreased stroke volume, oxygen consumption and heart rate are typically seen. These factors along with an increase in peripheral vascular resistance and a reduction in blood volume cause narrowing of pulse pressure and decreased blood flow to the tissues. Diminished circulation contributes to the cold sensitivity, pallor and cold skin commonly seen.

In severe primary hypothyroidism, the heart is often enlarged, mostly due to mucinous deposits and loss of muscle tone. Accompanied by hypertension, the elevated cholesterol levels of hypothyroidism may contribute to the development of atherosclerosis. Alterations in heart muscle may cause increases in the enzyme creatine kinase (affected by bone and muscle) and changes in its isoenzyme pattern. In hypothyroidism, the pericardial space surrounding the heart is rich in glycoprotein, a component of mucin.

The Respiratory System

Breathing capacity is frequently reduced although lung volumes are typically normal. Obstructive sleep apnea is a common occurrence. Fortunately, especially for the spouses of those of us who have experienced it, it is reversible once adequate treatment is instituted. In severe hypothyroidism there may be retention of carbon dioxide caused by myxedematous involvement of the muscles involved in respiration. This circumstance contributes to the development of myxedema coma.

The Brain and Muscular System

The brain's need for adequate thyroid hormone continues throughout life, affecting neurite growth, synapse development, myelin production, gene expression, and many other processes.[6] Extreme hypothyroidism is associated with myxedematous dementia, a condition characterized by serious deterioration of cerebral function. Common symptoms include extreme somnolence and hypothermia. When other signs of hypothyroidism are absent this condition may be confused with Alzheimer's disease.

In autoimmune hypothyroidism, blocking TRAb may attack the brain tissue instead of the thyroid in a condition known as Hashimoto's encephalopathy, which may also be confused with Alzheimer's disease.

Disorders of muscle function are often the predominant feature of hypothyroidism. In long-standing hypothyroidism, muscular abnormalities known as Hoffman's syndrome may occur. In Hoffman's syndrome, the muscles appear well-developed although the increased muscle volume is accompanied by slow contractions, stiffness and discomfort.

Muscle stiffness and pain are common, and these symptoms are exacerbated by cold temperatures. Muscle contraction and relaxation are both reduced, causing slowness in movement and gait. Muscle strength is usually normal although many treated GD patients may still experience effects of muscle wasting caused by hyperthyroidism.

The electromyogram, which measures muscle activity, frequently shows disordered discharge, hyperirritability and polyphasic action potentials.[7] Many patients with hypothyroidism complain that their calves occasionally feel leaden and swollen despite the large, firm, athletic looking appearance of muscle typically seen in hypothyroidism. In tissue studies, the muscles in hypothyroidism appear pale and swollen. Studies of muscle fibers show swelling and mucinous deposits that may disrupt the normal striation.

Behavioral Aspects

Although the effects of hypothyroidism are more critical in the developing brain, behavioral abnormalities have long been associated with hypothyroidism in adults. Often presenting as the earliest symptoms, subtle behavioral changes may be noted including irritability, agoraphobia, inattentiveness, slowing of thought processes, short term memory impairment, melancholia, cognitive dysfunction and depression.

As hypothyroidism progresses so does the mental decline. Long term memory impairment is common in severe hypothyroidism and visual hallucinations may occur. Sleep requirements increase and responsiveness to others declines. Patients with bipolar disease, especially the rapid cycling malignant variety, have a higher incidence of developing hypothyroidism, although lithium, which is frequently used in therapy for bipolar disease, is a known antithyroid agent and is known to induce or exacerbate hypothyroidism.

The Skin

Reduced secretions of the sweat and sebaceous glands cause dry, coarse skin and hair. In extreme cases the skin may resemble ichthyosis, a skin disorder resembling fish scales. Although the skin may itch, itching is more likely to be seen in hyperthyroidism. Deposits of hyaluronic acid (similar to the GAG seen in pretibial myxedema and GO) accumulate in tissue and bind with water to produce mucin.

Mucin is responsible for the characteristic nonpitting edema that causes the thickened features and puffy, waxy skin known as myxedema. Mucin deposits may also form distinct raised papules on the epidermal surface. Myxedema is most pronounced around the eyes, on the dorsa of the hands and feet, on the tongue, and on the mucous membranes of the pharynx and larynx.

Anemia causes skin pallor, and yellowing is caused by the body's inability to convert carotene to Vitamin A. The reason for the prominent flush often seen in hypothyroidism remains unclear. Changes in nail growth and appearance are related to decreased sebum production and a slowing of the growth rate.

The Skeletal System and Connective Tissue

Skeletal growth is influenced by nutritional, genetic and hormonal factors (thyroid hormone, growth hormone and insulin-like growth factor). Hypothyroidism causes reduced calcium metabolism, which is reflected in diminished bone formation and bone resorption and a decreased serum alkaline phosphatase level. Increased levels of parathyroid hormone in hypothyroidism cause an increase in Vitamin D, which causes increased intestinal calcium absorption. Although serum calcium levels are usually normal in hypothyroidism, there is decreased osteoclast activity.

In early life, hypothyroidism causes delay and abnormalities in the ossification of epiphyseal centers (bone closure). Before puberty, thyroid hormone is critical for bone growth and maturation. In untreated hypothyroidism, the bone pattern is irregular and mottled resulting in a porous texture. This is most pronounced in large cartilage accumulations such as head of the femur. Linear growth is impaired and dwarfism may occur. Decreased bone growth is also evident in dental structures.

Many hypothyroid patients complain of joint and muscle pain as well as stiff extremities. Similar to arthritis, the pain is exacerbated by cold and dampness. Common findings in hypothyroidism include joint effusions (swelling caused by synovial membrane thickening) particularly in the knees and the small joints of the hands and feet. The synovial or joint fluid has increased concentrations of GAG and calcium crystals that cause symptoms of pseudo gout. Compression of nerves by tissue swelling may be responsible for the prevalence of carpal tunnel syndrome in hypothyroidism.

The Digestive System and Metabolism

The digestive process, particularly peristalsis, is decreased, causing constipation and gaseous distention of the abdomen (myxedema ileus), colon and gallbladder. Prolonged constipation may cause fecal impaction (myxedema megacolon). Absorption of nutrients is commonly diminished although the longer digestive process may compensate in part. The pancreas and liver are normal although clearance may be prolonged.

Modest weight gain is a frequent occurrence although frank obesity is rarely attributed to hypothyroidism. Weight gain is attributed to the body's decreased energy consumption and the associated fluid retention. The metabolism of fats, carbohydrates and protein is all reduced. The metabolism of many drugs and hormones is decreased, causing an increase in blood levels in some instances. The half lives of supplemental T4 and T3 are increased as a result of decreased drug clearance.

The production and degradation of lipids, especially LDL (low density lipoproteins) and triglycerides, are decreased causing increased phospholipids, triglycerides and cholesterol although free fatty acid levels are decreased. Insulin metabolism is decreased, causing increased sensitivity to its effects. Protein synthesis is also decreased, causing a reduction in soft tissue and skeletal growth. Alterations in vitamin A metabolism (carotene is not converted to vitamin A) are responsible for the night blindness often seen in hypothyroidism. Increases in Vitamin D and PTH associated with hypothyroidism are responsible for decreased phosphorus concentrations.

The Glandular System

Hypothyroidism influences secretion of all pituitary hormones. Most noticeable in children is the reduction in growth hormone, the effects of which resolve with thyroid supplementation. In females, prolactin, a hormone necessary for lactation, is often increased, causing a condition of galactorrhea with symptoms of oligomenorrhea or amenorrhea (scant or absent menstrual periods), hirsutism (condition of abnormal hair growth, especially of male pattern growth in females) and fertility problems.

In long-standing hypothyroidism, the thyrocytes (pituitary cells that produce TSH), exhibit hyperplasia, which causes pituitary enlargement.

Hormones of the adrenal cortex are also affected by hypothyroidism. Typically, cortisol secretion and metabolism are reduced and adrenocorticotropin (ACTH) increases. However, the mechanism of hormone release in the stress response (see chapter 2) is not affected. Patients with hypothyroidism are more sensitive to the effects of glucocorticoid therapy because of the decrease in cortisol clearance. Glucocorticoid therapy also causes an inhibition of TSH secretion and peripheral conversion of T4 to T3.

Gestational hypertension is often seen in women with postpartum hypothyroidism. Hypothyroidism in boys may interfere with the normal pubertal process but hypothyroidism in adult males appears to have little effect on the reproductive system.

Subclinical Hypothyroidism

Subclinical hypothyroidism refers to a condition of elevated serum TSH and normal levels of FT3 and FT4. Symptoms in subclinical hypothyroidism are usually subtle, although there have been recent reports of an association with increased risks of heart attacks and other cardiac abnormalities, especially in elderly women. In one recent study, older women with subclinical hypothyroidism were more likely to have a history of heart attack or deposits of fatty plaque in the aorta, a condition that may lead to cardiac arrest.[8]

The presence of thyroid antibodies in conjunction with a rising TSH is thought to be predictive of overt hypothyroidism and treatment is generally instituted in this instance of subclinical hypothyroidism. In general, patients with serum TSH values greater than 5 mU/L are treated to prevent overt hypothyroidism from developing.

The Onset of Hypothyroidism

When it occurs spontaneously, the onset of hypothyroidism is generally insidious. In contrast, upon withdrawal of thyroid replacement in hypothyroid patients, and after ablative treatment in GD patients, symptoms of frank hypothyroidism often show up within six weeks. If left untreated, within three months, myxedema is usually full-blown.[9]

Early symptoms of hypothyroidism are frequently nonspecific and differ among the various age groups. In children, there may be impaired growth, and in the elderly, dementia may occur. The most common physical manifestations are tiredness and lethargy. The most common cognitive symptoms are alterations in attention, concentration and speed of thought processing. The most common psychiatric manifestation is depression, although concurrently there may be a melancholic disorder marked by crying and loss of appetite, or a disorganized agitated state. Often, there is a decline in intellectual function that many patients call brain fog. In patients rendered hypothyroid following ablative treatment, cramping of large muscles is often one of the earliest symptoms noticed.

Fibromyalgia

Fibromyalgia is a condition characterized by muscle and joint pain aggravated by stress. Fibromyalgia frequently accompanies hypothyroidism and it is known to be triggered by ablative treatment for an overactive thyroid.[10] Fibromyalgia is often diagnosed within months after a diagnosis of hypothyroidism and nearly 12 percent of all cases are caused by hypothyroidism.[11] Eighty percent of its victims are females between the ages of 20 and 50.

Myxedema Coma

Like thyroid storm in hyperthyroidism, myxedema coma is a rare syndrome representing the end stage of severe hypothyroidism. And like thyroid storm, there are warning signs foreshadowing the event, which usually occurs in the elderly. Certain precipitating factors are similar to those of thyroid storm, including pulmonary infections, cerebrovascualr accidents (strokes) and congestive heart failure. Unlike thyroid storm, even with aggressive treatment, mortality is high with rates reported to be as high as 60 percent.[12]

Certain hypothyroid symptoms may act as precipitating factors or they may occur in conjunction with the development of myxedema coma. These symptom include hypoglycemia or low blood sugar, hyponatremia or low blood sodium, and hypoxemia or low blood oxygen. Precipitating factors include drugs such as narcotics, sedatives, antidepressants and tranquilizers since they act as respiratory depressants. Myxedema coma occurs most frequently in winter, making cold weather a precipitating factor.

The two most prominent symptoms of myxedema coma are hypothermia, frequently without shivering, and unconsciousness. Often, hypothyroidism is undiagnosed and the condition aggravated by infection or systemic illness. Patients in myxedema coma frequently have the typical hypothyroid features of dry, coarse or sparse hair, scaly skin, delayed deeptendon reflexes, orange tinged skin due to their inability to convert carotene into vitamin A, puffy facial features and large tongues.

Years ago, when the high incidence of hypothyroidism following ablative procedures was unknown, it was not unusual for myxedema coma to present in ablated patients with undiagnosed hypothyroidism. Myxedema coma usually runs a course beginning with lethargy and somnolence that progresses to stupor. Typical symptoms of hypothyroidism are generally noted and sometimes exaggerated, and patients often have hypothermia with temperatures as low at 80° F.

Diagnosis of Hypothyroidism

Diagnosis of hypothyroidism is usually based on laboratory tests alone, although TSH levels may be affected by pituitary dysfunction, medications such as glucocorticoids, adrenal insufficiency resulting from longstanding hypothyroidism, the presence of thyroid antibodies or thyroid hormone resistance. Or, following ablation, insufficient time may have passed for TSH to reflect thyroid function. And thyroid antibodies may cause an error rate in thyroid hormone laboratory tests as high as 40 percent.[13]

For these reasons, the International Thyroid Group cautions against relying on laboratory values alone. Furthermore, some endocrinologists recommend measuring TPO and thyroglobulin antibodies when there is a dubious history of hypothyroidism.[14] When a diagnosis of hypothyroidism is questionable, certain other laboratory tests suggestive of hypothyroidism may be relied on. These include elevated cholesterol and triglycerides, creatine kinase, carotene levels, and decreased sodium and alkaline phosphatase.

Laboratory Picture in Hypothyroidism

In uncomplicated hypothyroidism, the TSH level is generally elevated and the level of FT4 or T4 is decreased. In severe hypothyroidism, levels of T3 may also decline.[15] However, after treatment for GD, the TSH level may remain suppressed for many weeks or months after T4 and T3 levels begin to rise. Several patients report that it took 18 months for their TSH levels to adequately reflect their symptoms of hypothyroidism. Occasionally, symptoms of hypothyroidism occur before the level of T4 begins to fall.

Although some endocrinologists recommend waiting to initiate thyroid replacement therapy until TSH levels rise as high as 40 mIU/L to ensure that hypothyroidism isn't transient, most physicians recommend treating hypothyroidism before symptoms become severe since widely fluctuating thyroid hormone levels are associated with GO.

The TSH Myth

In the normal population, TSH is a valuable indicator of thyroid function. For patients with autoimmune thyroid disease, the traditional tests of thyroid function, particularly the TSH, are unreliable as gauges of thyroid function.[16] A low normal TSH does not exclude hypothyroidism. Many people have TSH levels below 1.5 miU/L although their levels of FT3, and sometimes FT4 as well, are below normal. By relying on TSH alone, the vast majority of hypothyroid patients will not be diagnosed and those who are diagnosed, may not receive adequate treatment.

Treatment of Hypothyroidism

In normal individuals, thyroid hormone levels fluctuate according to normal diurnal variation, bodily demands, environmental conditions and dietary influences. Pulsing with fine tuned synchronicity, hormones are released and deiodinated in response to the body's needs and its normal circadian rhythm or diurnal variation. Patients on replacement hormone are not afforded this luxury. The aim in replacement therapy is to provide stable blood hormone levels. Sometimes, replacement hormone is sufficient for the body's needs, while at other times it might not be.

Preparations used therapeutically consist of either glandular animal extracts or synthetic compounds. The goal in therapy is to provide the body with adequate supplies of both free T4 and free T3. Although T4 is thought to act as a prohormone, its need is also critical. T3 utilized by the brain and pituitary must be fresh, that is, made on site by the peripheral conversion of T4 into T3 within these organs.

Synthetic thyroid hormone replacement preparations include levothyroxine (T4), synthetic liothyronine (T3), and combination products that contain both ingredients. Approximately 80 percent of a dose of levothyroxine is absorbed. Of this, approximately 40 percent is converted to T3. T3 with one less iodine atom has a molecular weight of 651 compared to that of T4, which is 777. Consequently, a 1 grain (60 mcg) tablet of glandular extract and a 97 mcg tablet of levothyroxine would both provide 26 mcg of T3, the active thyroid hormone.[17]

Signs of Toxicity

It's important for treated hypothyroid patients to watch for symptoms of both hyperthyroidism and hypothyroidism. Upon the initial use of thyroid hormone or when dosages are increased, there may be temporary side effects while the body adjusts. Signs of toxicity include chest pain, increased pulse rate, palpitations, excessive sweating, heat intolerance and nervousness. Any indication of thyroid hormone toxicity should be reported to your physician immediately. Individual treatment options include the following.

THYROID GLANDULAR EXTRACT

First used in 1892, desiccated thyroid animal extract was for many years the only substance available for the treatment of hypothyroidism. Its major advantage is that it contains all the iodotyronine derivatives, including MIT and DIT, along with calcitonin and other substances normally found in the thyroid gland. However, its use and abuse as a weight loss agent in the 1920s and 1930s when it was the only thyroid preparation available, led to its decline when synthetic thyroxine (considered less apt to induce toxic effects) was introduced. Still, many patients who were switched to synthetic preparations complained that they felt better on glandular extract and requested to be put back on it.[18]

Today, desiccated animal extract is used by approximately 20 percent of thyroid patients.[19] Glandular extract is made from the thyroid glands and thyroglobulin of animals and has a slightly higher ratio of T3 to T4 than that of normal humans. Because of its greater absorption, animal extract may cause immediate increases in T3. Consequently before the drug has equilibrated, symptoms of excess T3 may appear. Some patients report noticing transient palpitations or increased body temperature.

Desiccated thyroid extract provides a medium in which thyroid hormones are available in their natural state attached to a carrier protein. All of the iodothyronines normally found in the blood are present in thyroid extract.

Glandular extracts don't have the stability of synthetic compounds. Their potency declines and they have a shorter shelf-life. For this reason, it's not a good idea to order more than a three month supply at one time. The activity of 1 grain (60 mg) of desiccated thyroid extract can be considered approximately equivalent to 80 mcg of thyroxine with slight variation in individual batches. Because of its T3 content, desiccated thyroid has a greater binding affinity for nuclear receptors than does T4 alone. Overzealous treatment might, therefore, cause cardiac symptoms.

Armour thyroid (Forest pharmaceuticals) consists of porcine derived thyroid powder in a base of anhydrous dextrose) (derived from cornstarch) and cellulose. Armour thyroid tablets are available in amounts ranging from 15 mg (one-fourth grain) up to 300 mg (5 grain). The most common starting dose for hypothyroidism is 90 mg (1.5 grain) taken in divided doses. After one month, blood tests are taken and the dose is adjusted accordingly. Dr. Mercola reports that a small number of large, overweight, thyroid-resistant women may need 6 to 8 grains of Armour thyroid daily.[20]

Nature-Throid

Nature-throid (Jones Medical) tablets are prepared from fresh, desiccated animal thyroid glands. Tablets contain amounts ranging from one half grain to 2 grains.

Levothyroxine

Levothyroxine, the most widely used preparation for the treatment of hypothyroidism, is a synthetic thyroid preparation with a seven day half-life and slow absorption. Because it is made up of entirely T4, it's considered safer, and it's thought that because of it's long half-life, the body's thyroid hormone levels will remain stable even when a dose is missed. The average daily adult replacement dose is 112 mcg. Acting as a prohormone, levothyroxine is deiodinated in peripheral tissues and usually produces sufficient T3 for the body's needs.

According to the U.S. Pharmacopoeia the levothyroxine content of replacement tablets must contain between 90 percent to 110 percent of the stated amount. The typical dose for hypothyroid individuals is 1.4 to 1.6 ug/kg (0.6 to 0.7 ug/lb) ideal body weight. For women, the dose is usually between 75 and 112 mcg daily and for men the usual daily dose is between 125 to 200 mcg.[21]

Because of its long half life, levothyroxine can be taken once daily and when equilibrium is reached, a dose can be missed without undue effects. After six to eight weeks, a constant daily dose provides a steady blood level.

Rarely, allergic reactions have been reported to synthetic T4, likely as a result of a coloring in the tablet. As previously mentioned, some patients may not convert T4 to T3 properly. Most patients experience improvement within two to three weeks.

Levothyroxine is available in Eltroxin (Roberts Pharmaceuticals), Levothroid (Forest Pharmaceuticals), Levoxyl (Daniels Pharmaceuticals) and Synthroid tablets and injection (Knoll Pharmaceuticals). Tablet strengths differ by manufacturers, although most are made in a wide range of products of slightly different increments.

LIOTHYRONINE (TRIIODOTHYRONINE, T3, CYTOMEL)

Liothyronine, a form of synthetic T3, imitates triiodothyronine, boasting a fast half-life that may cause supraphysiological or exaggerated symptoms at two to six hours after ingestion. Because of its propensity for accelerating cardiac activity and because of the body's need for fresh T3, preparations containing T3 alone are rarely used as replacement therapy for GD patients who become hypothyroid. Besides, certain organs, including the brain, require fresh T3 produced from the peripheral conversion of T4. The average daily dose of liothyronine is 25 to 50 mcg. Recent studies show that there are many patients like me who don't convert enough T3 from T4 to cover all the body's needs.

Synthetic preparations are found in Cytomel and Triostat, both manufactured by Smith-Kline Beecham. In euthyroid patients 25 mcg of liothyronine is equivalent to 1 grain of desiccated thyroid or approximately 0.08 to 0.1 mg of levothyroxine.

PREPARATIONS CONTAINING BOTH LIOTHYRONINE AND LEVOTHYROXINE

The Liotrix/Thyrolar combination formula (Forest Pharmaceuticals) contains mixtures of liothyronine (T3) and levothyroxine (T4) in a 1:4 ratio formulated into 1 grain (64 mg) tablets containing 12.5 ug T3 and 50 ug T4. Tablets are available in ranges from one fourth grain up to 3 grains.

LEVOTHYROXINE (T4) AND TRIIODOTHYRONINE (T3) COMPLEMENTARY THERAPY

With levothyroxine was developed, it was assumed that T4 would be converted into sufficient T3 to cover the body's needs. Subsequent studies have shown that in some patients, the dose of T4 needed to convert adequate T3 is higher than expected, indicating that these patients have impaired conversion. In one study where T3 was added to the regimen, most patients felt better, performed better on standard neuropsychological tasks, and their psychological state improved.[22]

This study opened the door to other studies and observations that led to patient demand for T3 supplementation. Given in the body's normal ratio of 4:1 T4:T3, the T3 is usually given in divided doses because of its faster mode of action and short half-life. Many patients who have tried this protocol report an increased sense of well-being although the majority of T3 in the brain is freshly produced by conversion of T4.

Thyroid Hormone Replacement Interferences

In a normal adult, absorption of levothyroxine is 80 percent to 90 percent, and absorption of triiodthyronine is 100 percent. However, the gastrointestinal absorption of thyroid hormone may be impaired in malabsorptive syndromes (which frequently occur in hypothyroidism). For optimal absorption, most endocrinologists recommend that thyroid hormone be taken on an empty stomach two hours before taking other medications. Although it's normally advised that patients abstain from eating for a half hour, certain foods such as fiber and products containing calcium may compete with hormone absorption for up to two hours. Also, thyroid hormone is fat soluble and should be taken with free fatty acids for optimal absorption. In fact, some physicians prescribe free fatty acid supplements for this purpose.

Other substances known to interfere with thyroid hormone absorption include iron sulfate, cholestyramine, aluminum hydroxide (found in antacids and some headache preparations), soybean products, sucralfate, selective serotonin-reuptake inhibitors including sertraline (Zoloft), prenatal vitamins with iron, cholesterol reducing agents and lithium. Goitrogens and soy can interfere with dietary absorption of thyroid hormone and shouldn't be consumed within two hours of thyroid dosage.

Drugs that increase metabolism of T4 causing increased requirements include phenytoin (Dilantin), carbamazepine (Tegretol), rifampin (Rifadin) and phenobarbital. Conversion of T4 to the more potent T3 may be impaired by amiodarone and also by selenium and magnesium deficiency or cirrhosis. In pregnancy, there is usually a 50 percent to 100 percent increase in levothyroxine requirement for patients on thyroid replacement therapy.

Medications Affected by Thyroid
Hormone Replacement Therapy

The initiation of thyroid hormone replacement has an effect on certain medications taken therapeutically. Thyroid hormone may potentiate the effects of sympathomimetic agent such as epinephrine, tricyclic antidepressants (for instance amitriptyline or imipramine), and anticoagulants such as warfarin (Coumadin). Often, the dose of these medications must be decreased.[23] In the case of concomitant oral anticoagulant therapy, the prothrombin time should be measured frequently.

Initiating thyroid hormone replacement therapy may cause increases in insulin or oral hypoglycemic requirements. The daily dosage of antidiabetic medication may need readjustment as thyroid hormone replacement is achieved. If thyroid medication is stopped, antidiabetic medication may require a downward adjustment to prevent hypoglycemia.

Monitoring Thyroid Hormone Replacement

Depending on the progression and severity of their hypothyroidism as well as their age and general health status, newly hypothyroid GD patients will require one or more dosage adjustments at the onset followed by, at the minimum, annual monitoring.

Since all preparations used conventionally contain at least some T4 and it has the longest half-life (seven days), it takes at least six weeks for serum levels of T4 to show a steady state. In a steady state, blood levels remain constant and stable regardless of the time blood is drawn. Improvement of symptoms on patients who are on levothyroxine alone usually occurs within two to three weeks as the peripheral effects of T3 are felt. In preparations containing T3, effects are noticed much sooner, usually within four to six hours, and a maximal response occurs within two days.

To reduce cardiac symptoms, patients are usually started on lower doses than they'll eventually be on, and incremental adjustments are made every six weeks. In younger patients adjustments in up to 50 mcg increments are made, whereas in the elderly adjustments are generally made in 25 mcg increments. In patients with pre-existing cardiac disease, increments of 12.5 mcg are generally made every six to eight weeks.

The first evidence of a response to replacement therapy primarily depends on the dosage prescribed. Older patients are generally started on smaller doses while young, otherwise healthy, patients may start out with a dosage sufficient to correct their symptoms. Small doses are gradually increased in increments of 12.5 to 25 mcg so that any side effects, particularly cardiac manifestations, are minimized. An early clinical sign of response to treatment is significant diuresis (fluid loss) accompanied by an increase in pulse rate and pressure, improvement in appetite and diminishment of constipation.[24]

Side Effects of Thyroid Hormone Replacement

Excessive thyroid hormone replacement may cause osteoporosis in postmenopausal patients. In addition, thyroid hormone excess increases cardiac wall thickness and increases the risk of atrial fibrillation, particularly in elderly patients. Although side effects of therapy in younger individuals are rare, incidences of pseudotumor cerebri (a condition characterized by severe headaches and neuralgia) have been reported in severely hypothyroid children between the ages of 8 and 12 who were treated with initial modest doses of levothyroxine.[25] Thyroid hormone preparations are usually contraindicated in patients with uncorrected adrenal cortical insufficiency, untreated thyrotoxicosis, acute myocardial infarction and hypersensitivity to any of the ingredients, particularly dyes.

Signs of toxicity, including chest pain, increased pulse rate, palpitations, excessive sweating, heat intolerance and nervousness should be immediately reported to the prescribing physician.

Alternative Medical Treatments

Although most ablated GD patients who become hypothyroid require thyroid replacement therapy, untreated patients and patients treated with ATDs may have milder symptoms. For these patients, or as adjunctive therapy in patients with moderate to severe hypothyroidism, a number of alternative medicine options are available. Some of these options both relieve symptoms and help restore thyroid and immune system function.

In *The Ultimate Healing System*, Don Lepore writes that research indicates that many "weak" thyroids are actually strong, but that the pituitary is malfunctioning.[26] The idea that the pituitary-hypothalamic-thyroid regulatory axis becomes inefficient after long periods of thyroid hyperfunction explains the fact that TSH often stays suppressed for many months, long after FT4 and FT3 fall into the normal range. This statement also explains why some alternative medicine practitioners prescribe pituitary extract (pituitropin glandular extract) as a treatment aid in hypothyroidism.

Glandular Extracts

Glandular extracts are commercial preparations containing extracts of animal glands. Thyroid glandular extracts used in alternative medicine do not contain active thyroxine hormone but rather work to stimulate the gland. Lepore recommends corrective nutrients, including thyroid glandular concentrate, the herbs kelp, dulse, vitamin B6 and B complex, the minerals iodine, potassium and sodium and the amino acid tyrosine.

The reasons behind glandular extracts are twofold. Autoantibodies are thought to bind to glandular extracts in a manner much like that described in oral tolerance therapy, preventing the antibodies from attacking the thyroid itself. Secondly, substances normally present in the thyroid or pituitary gland serve as a nutrient source and stimulate thyroid and thyrocyte cell production. (Thyrocytes are the pituitary cells that produce thyrotropin or TSH. In sustained periods of hyperthyroidism, the number of these cells declines).

Dietary Supplements

Many of the symptoms of hypothyroidism are caused by nutrient deficiencies. Nutrient deficiencies in hypothyroidism are related to inadequate absorption and a decreased metabolism. As previously mentioned, many nutrients including manganese, magnesium, free fatty acids, certain B vitamins, and vitamins C and E are essential for proper thyroid function. Vitamin B3 or niacin, in particular, is essential for thyroid function and vitamin B6 is necessary for hormone synthesis. Normal thyroid function is necessary for the body's absorption of vitamin B12. In hypothyroidism, vitamin B12 is deficient.[27]

Copper levels are frequently increased in hypothyroidism while zinc levels are decreased. Imbalances are corrected by properly balanced supplements and eating foods high in zinc such as whole grains and fresh produce. The minimal requirement is 2 mg copper and 16 mg zinc, although to restore balance, higher amounts of zinc may be necessary in the early stages of therapy. Vitamin A supplements of 25,000 IU are required since the hypothyroid body is unable to convert dietary carotenes into vitamin A.

Magnesium levels are frequently low in hypothyroidism. Magnesium controls cell membrane potential, which means that it is regulates the uptake and release of many hormones, nutrients, including iodine and thyroid hormone, and neurotransmitters. Furthermore, insufficient magnesium causes increased potassium and calcium excretion, thereby causing calcium to form deposits in soft tissue and potassium and calcium deficiencies. The minimum requirement for magnesium is 750 mg/day.

Selenium (200 mcg) is necessary for the body's conversion of T4 to T3, and adequate iron and iodine are essential for proper thyroid metabolism. Patients frequently fail to add adequate iodine to their diets when they become hypothyroid. The minimal requirement for iodine is 150 mcg daily and values in excess of 1500 mcg contribute to hypothyroidism, whereas selenium in excess of 400 mcg can contribute to reduced levels of T3. In iodine deficient patients selenium depletes T4 stores by accelerating peripheral conversion of T4 to T3. Proper thyroid function is also dependent on a balance of iodine and manganese. A deficiency of either can cause hypothyroidism.

Dietary Influences

A well balanced diet with adequate protein is necessary for optimal thyroid function. Goitrogenic foods (see chapter 3) in excess can compete with thyroid hormone, and there have been several reports of hypothyroidism being caused by drinking cabbage juice or consuming cabbage soup. A supportive diet includes foods with good stores of natural iodine such as fish, vegetables, especially root vegetables such as potatoes, and foods high in B vitamins, such as raw nuts and seeds, and dark green and yellow vegetables. Foods to avoid include sugar, refined grains, caffeine and processed foods.

Herbal Preparations

Irish Moss used as an infusion steeped for five to 15 minutes; dosage 2 oz. Used two to three times daily.

Dulse and Kelp (150 mcg/tablet) can also be used as sources of iodine.

Dr. J. Christopher's Formula T made by Nature's Way is also effective. See directions on product label.

Homeopathic Preparations

Homeopathy can help regulate thyroid function. Calcareacarbonica (1M calcium carbonate) and homeopathic thyroid extract are reported to stimulate thyroid function. Arsenicum (30C) is also effective used every 12 hours for up to five days while seeking out a licensed homeopath.[28] Other preparations reported to be beneficial include homeopathic Raw Thyroid, Deseret's Thyroplus, and CompliMed's Thyroid.

Digestive Aids and Detoxifiers

Many of the symptoms of hypothyroidism, including nutrient deficiencies, are caused by sluggish digestion. Swedish bitters or extracts of gentian or mugwort are frequently prescribed as digestive aids. Grapeseed extract, using 500 mg three times daily, is used to help detoxify the intestines, and acidophilus capsules are used to help restore friendly bacteria. Products used to eliminate candida overgrowth such as Candistroy by Nature's Secret and the homeopathic remedy Aquaflora are occasionally recommended.

Coexisting Hormonal Deficiencies

Hypothyroidism frequently accompanies deficiencies of other hormones, including estrogen, progesterone and adrenal gland hormones. When thyroid hormone doesn't correct symptoms, other hormonal disorders may be the cause. For this reason, alternative medical practitioners sometimes prescribe nonthyroidal glandular extracts including thymus extract, which contains small amounts of thyroid. Symptoms related to adrenal insufficiency such as multiple allergies and digestive problems are treated with dehydroepiandrosterophe sulphate (DHEA), 10 to 15 mg, and sometimes hydrocortisone. DHEA is considered a master hormone that contributes to the body's production of estrogen and testosterone. Although most practitioners recommend that women use 25 mg daily and men 50 mg, there have been reports of cardiac arrhythmias occurring in patients using 25 to 50 mg daily.[29]

Most instances of hypothyroidism associated with GD have an immune system component. Because food allergies interfere with immune function, some alternative practitioners focus on diagnosing and treating food allergies.

12 *Anecdotes and Testimonies of Graves' Disease Patients*

A wise man should consider that health is the greatest of human bless-ings, and learn how by his own thought to derive a benefit from his illnesses. — Hippocrates

Newly diagnosed Graves' patients often mention feeling bewildered. Frightened by their symptoms, they feel pressured into rushing into treat-ment. Often, their families and friends accuse them of exaggerating their symptoms. It's no wonder that many GD patients mention wishing they could meet someone else with GD. Preferably a sage Gravesian with empa-thy, advice, and most of all, a healing story they're willing to share.

In this chapter, wishes come true. Here, you'll meet patients who went into remission using alternative medicine and patients who had as many as four radioiodine ablations before their symptoms resolved. Having endured, each of these patients has found meaning in their ordeal by open-ing themselves to others. All patient anecdotes in this book are factual, although in some cases the names and background of the individual has been changed to protect their privacy.

Antithyroid Drugs

Jeannette (currently in remission after using ATDs)

New opinions are always suspected, and usually opposed, without any other reason but that they are already common. — John Locke

By the time Jeannette, a marriage and family counselor, was diagnosed with GD, her condition was severe. Her FT3 was 2510 pg/dL with a reference range of 210 to 440 pg/dL. Her T4 was 21.1 ug/dl with a reference range of 4.4 to 12.0 ug/dL. However, within one month of starting Tapazole, her FT3 dropped to 797 pg/dL. Three weeks later it was 569 pg/dL, and within three and one half months, it was down to a normal value of 365 pg/dL.

Jeannette tells us that when she was first diagnosed with GD, she called a doctor who was hosting a local radio show. In response to her inquiry about alternative medicine, he told a story about several GD women who were involved in a study in which none of them could role play returning a defective toaster. Having no doubt heard something about fifth chakra influences, he'd come up with a theory that GD patients were all unassertive. He told Jeannette that when he was younger and more arrogant, he would have tried different things, but now he knew that she needed to have RAI and "get it over with."

Jeannette assertively hung up. Aware that many factors contribute to GD, Jeannette began researching GD on her own and decided she didn't want to destroy her thyroid without first trying ATDs. What this doctor taught Jeannette is to beware of doctors who aim to treat the disease and not the patient. After being on ATDs for two years, Jeannette went into remission and has remained in remission for more than two years.

Kara (hypothyroid for three years prior to developing GD)

Nothing can be done at once hastily and prudently. — Publilius Syrus

Hypothyroid for the previous three years, despite running daily, Kara, a computer programmer in the Midwest, had gained 70 pounds. When her hypothyroidism was finally diagnosed and she was put on replacement thyroid, she was able to lose 25 pounds by dieting. Within a few months, her symptoms changed and she was diagnosed with GD, which knocked off 25 more pounds.

Since her mother and grandmother had both had GD, Kara was familiar with treatment. She writes that her "mother and grandmother both had bulgy eyes, and once their thyroids were removed by thyroidectomy, their eye symptoms disappeared within a month." Realizing that her symptoms weren't as severe as theirs, Kara balked at her doctor's insistence that she have RAI. She has remained euthyroid on ATDs for the past 18 months and has decided that if the medication quits working before she achieves remission, she'll opt for a thyroidectomy.

Randi (on a block and replacement protocol)

Time eases all things. — Sophocles

To ease her symptoms of perimenopause, Randi's gynecologist prescribed hormone replacement therapy. After a few months, Randi was subsequently prescribed an estrogen patch and told to continue using her old pills along with the patch. By the time she realized that the nurse had erred in her dosage instructions, Randi was suffering from classic symptoms of GD and had signs of estrogen toxicity.

Because she also developed GO, Randi opted for ATDs. She was kept on a high dose of ATDs even after experiencing symptoms of hypothyroidism and increased proptosis. When she called to complain of fatigue and weight gain, laboratory tests showed that she was indeed hypothyroid. Rather than lower her dose, her doctor added thyroxin to the regimen, providing the block and replace protocol described in chapter 8. However, when she asked why she would be taking thyroxin, her question went unanswered. Confused, she e-mailed me for an explanation. A bright lady, Randi soon found she had to resort to friends on the bulletin boards if she was to take charge of her healing.

Unfortunately, however, her doctor never took the natural progression of her disease into account and scheduled visits three months apart. Soon, her symptoms of hypothyroidism were back, again confirmed by lab tests that she requested. In a determined effort to keep her from becoming hyperthyroid, Randi's doctor kept her hypothyroid and relied on a TSH alone to monitor her. All the while, her eye involvement worsened. When she requested that he order free T4 and T3 levels, results of both tests were low, despite her normal TSH. Since, Randi's doctor has retired and her new doctor has consented to weaning her off medications so she can see where she's at. Randi feels that her doctor's reliance on a TSH test alone has caused her to have more problems than most people on block and replace therapy would ordinarily have had.

Christine C (on ATDs for 21 years)

The cautious seldom err. — Confucius

Diagnosed with Graves' disease in 1979, Christine tried PTU for one week. Since it upset her stomach, she was switched to Tapazole, which she is still on. For the first 15 years of her therapy, Christine moved several times, and she encountered several new doctors who were reluctant or refused to prescribe Tapazole because she'd been on it so long. Adamant about staying on the low dose that kept her symptoms at bay, Christine made sure she had regular liver function tests and blood counts. In 1995, Christine radically changed her diet to whole, nutritious foods and eliminated foods with iodine, histamine and tyramine. With this change, her palpitations diminished and she lost 90 pounds. Spurred on by these changes, she explored holistic healing suggestions and began a program to reduce stress reduction while continuing on ATDs.

Recently, Christine developed a nodular mass. She refused to have a fine needle aspiration and traveled to another city for a consultation. Her mass was palpated and determined to be merely goitrous. Tests for TRAb showed no evidence of stimulating TRAb although her titer of total TRAb was elevated, suggested that she now had blocking antibodies. She subsequently tried weaning herself off ATDs but her hyperthyroid symptoms returned. She remains euthyroid on ATDs and has no regrets.

Brittany (diagnosed with GD at age 12, achieved remission at age 16)

First say to yourself what you would do; and then do what you have to do. — Epictetus

When Brittany was almost 12 years old, her mother noticed that her appetite was increased and that she was growing thinner. Since she was also growing taller, her mother wasn't concerned. That is, until Brittany's uncle, a physician who hadn't seen her in some time, came to visit. He insisted that she have her thyroid checked. Brittany's pediatrician was skeptical and said it would be highly unusual for someone so young to have a thyroid disorder. But he ran a thyroid profile to appease the family, and to his surprise, Brittany's levels showed that she was indeed hyperthyroid.

Brittany was put on PTU and had no initial problems. However, after four years on the drug, she developed symptoms of drug-induced lupus. She was switched to Tapazole and her symptoms of lupus eventually resolved. After a few months, her Tapazole dose was lowered, and eventually Synthroid was added in an effort to stabilize her levels and prevent symptoms of hypothyroidism.

Brittany has never had any eye involvement and still has perfect vision. The only problems Brittany experienced were muscle weakness during her lupus episode when she was forced to temporarily give up gymnastics. All the while, Brittany's levels of thyroid antibodies have been monitored. When her levels fell into the normal range, Brittany was weaned off her medications and continues to stay in remission.

James (achieved remission four years
after ATDs and Holistic Medicine)

The goal of life is living in agreement with nature. — Zeno

Diagnosed with GD while in his early 30s, James, a business professional from Canada, was considered "grossly" hyperthyroid and told he needed to have RAI immediately. His FT4 level was about seven times normal, and his goiter was three times the size of normal. James asked to try a course of Tapazole first and began treatment with a daily dose of 30 mg. Combining ATDs with dietary changes and what he calls a holistic lifestyle, James soon saw improvement. Eventually, he weaned himself down to 15 mg of Tapazole each week. His labs were monitored every three to six months and he never had any side effects from the drugs, and he never had symptoms of GO. In his fourth year of therapy, he went into remission and has now been in remission for three years.

Alternative Medicine and Holistic Healing

Mary B (allergic to PTU after developing postpartum
GD, she embraced alternative medicine)

In all things of nature there is something of the marvelous. — Aristotle

As previously mentioned, Mary B embraced alternative medicine after experiencing liver problems with PTU. Diagnosed with GD several months after the birth of her daughter, nursing prohibited her from trying a course of Tapazole.

Mary's initial protocol seemed exhausting to me, but not to her since she was the one experiencing the benefits. Under the care of both her physician and a naturopath, Mary's protocol involved taking the beta blocker atenolol, 1 tsp. flaxseeds, and 1,000 mg of Vitamin C on waking. For breakfast, Mary ingested Ultraclear, a detoxifying substance rich in glutathione, cysteine, acetylcysteine, rice protein concentrate, rice syrup solids, high oleic safflower oil, medium chain triglycerides and various vitamins and minerals. An hour later she took a homeopathic preparation. An hour and a half later, she took a herbal blend containing Lenorus, Lycopus, Melissa, and Lactuca. An hour later she took Vitamin B complex and chewed 1 teaspoon of milk thistle seeds.

As her day continued, Mary took beta carotene, three more doses of the herb mixture (up to four times daily is allowed), Vitamin C, Prenatal vitamins, more flaxseeds, Ultraclear, homeopathic remedies and Vitamin B complex.

The mother of two small children, Mary also followed a diet rich in goitrogens and stir fried vegetables. Mary also kept a journal of her symptoms and was able to note when changes in diet exacerbated her condition. Approaching her program with gusto, Mary also had acupuncture treatments and attended weekly yoga classes when she was able.

During one interesting conversation in which Julia described fifth chakra influences (in Tantric tradition, the fifth chakra controls the thyroid and GD is considered a result of stifled verbal expression), Mary confessed that for years she'd kept a secret. And recently, she'd noticed an increase in symptoms just by thinking of her secret. Familiar with Tantric traditions, she sensed it had a harmful effects. She reports that when she learned to let go of her secret and share it with those closest to her, she immediately felt the tension in her thyroid dissolve. She said from that point on she knew she would heal.

Jeremy (followed his wife's advice to try a natural approach)

Keep to moderation, keep the end in view, follow Nature.—Lucan

When Jeremy, an engineer in the Midwest, was diagnosed with Graves' disease, he couldn't decide what conventional option to use. That's when his wife, a dietitian, pointed out that his fast food diet couldn't be helping matters. Finding immediate improvement with nutritional changes, Jeremy ended up consulting a naturopath. Although Jeremy had initially lost 25 pounds, he has been able to regain most of his weight and keep his symptoms in control for more than three years using SSKI, a strong iodine preparation, a course of Clotrimazole, a medication used to treat candida, and dietary changes. Jeremy admits that he has trouble eating as well as he should and for the last year, he has been somewhat lax about taking his SSKI. However, he manages to keep his symptoms at bay and says it would be foolish not to mention that prayer has played a big role in his healing.

Kim H (told she needed RAI, she opted for natural medicine)

If purpose, then, is inherent in art, so is it in Nature also. The best illustration is the case of a man being his own physician, for Nature is like that—agent and patient at once.—Aristotle

When I first met Kim, a biologist, she had recently been diagnosed with GD and had few if any symptoms. Based on her lab tests, her doctor recommended RAI, which she refused. When she asked for alternative medical advice on one conventional on-line bulletin boards, she started a war. Some people warned her she'd go into thyroid storm without aggressive treatment and others told her not to rush into anything.

Living in a large, progressive city, she consulted a different doctor, a medical doctor who specializes in naturopathy. He put her on a natural program that effectively reduced her thyroid hormone levels. After sharing this news, the on-line conflict escalated. Kim wisely realized that the stress generated by the on-line controversy inhibited her healing. Two years later, Kim is no longer as conscientious about following the protocol, avoids thyroid bulletin boards and feels great. She realizes her symptoms can return and feels confident that if that happens she can step up her protocol and again achieve remission.

Kim avoids dairy, adds 1 to 1.5 cups of broccoli and 1.5 cups of soy daily, and uses millet as grain. She also takes herbs in the form of a tonic containing *Lycopus, Lithospermum, Leonurus,* and Siberian ginseng. To regain lost nutrients she initially took a women's multivitamin using two pills four times daily, but has since reduced this dose by half.

Mike P (severely hyperthyroid, he had little success with ATDs before he tried an alternative approach)

Tao invariably takes no action, and yet there is nothing left undone.—
Lao-tzu

Mike was diagnosed with Graves' disease in 1991 while managing a field study for wildlife rabies control. Working 14 to 15 hour days every day, one day he noticed that his normal resting pulse of 65 changed to 120 literally overnight, which led to his diagnosis. After three months on PTU, both Mike and his doctor concluded that it had no effect on him. So he consulted a naturopath physician who designed a therapeutic protocol. Within a few weeks, his heart rate dropped and his other symptoms abated. For five years, Mike took nothing further and made a conscious effort to avoid stress by practicing Taoist tai chi regularly. However, laid off from his job in 1996, his symptoms returned and once again were brought into control by a naturopath.

Mike cautions those considering a natural approach to control their GD symptoms that it's not a free ride or a quick fix and patients must remain under the management of a health practitioner. He finds diet crucial to the program and recommends avoiding table salt and foods with excess iodine and also sugars and caffeine. He also advises that type A individuals have to learn to slow down. He finds tai chi to be particularly beneficial for accomplishing this, and, on his web site (see chapter 13), he says, "Eat well, sleep when you need it, and put yourself first."

Joan R (after a short course of ATDs, she's stayed in remission by adopting a holistic healing approach)

The softest things in the world overcome the hardest things in the world. — Lao-tzu

When Joan, an editor and graduate student, began feeling sick in 1997, she had no idea what was wrong, until she landed in the ER and eventually became diagnosed with Graves' disease. To manage her immediate symptoms, she consented to treatment with atenolol and later added Tapazole. Then she began to search for a cure.

At a complementary clinic, she received several acupuncture treatments and was instructed to eat broccoli and tofu. And she began examining her lifestyle in an attempt to discover what had triggered her GD. She recalled receiving a free bottle of multivitamins when she bought exercise equipment, multivitamins rich in iodine designed to raise her metabolism. She had also been using a natural progesterone cream and taking Siberian ginseng, both of which stimulate the thyroid.

She eliminated all three of these products and began responding to her ATDs only too well. She reported having symptoms of hypothyroidism, which her endocrinologist insisted she was imagining. She, in turn, insisted that he order lab tests, tests that confirmed that she was hypothyroid. Her Tapazole dose was reduced by half, and in a short period, it was reduced again. Within a few months, she had completely tapered off her ATDs. That was five years ago. Joan has remained in remission confirmed by periodic thyroid function tests. She says, "By listening to my body and my own wisdom, and not to the doctors, I was able to get well."

Thyroidectomy Surgery

Julia (she stayed in remission for years after surgery, but eventually had RAI, which she regrets)

Nothing happens to anybody which he is not fitted by nature to bear. — Marcus Aurelius Antoninus

Julia developed Graves' disease in 1980 right after her mother died. She was first prescribed a block and replace ATD protocol, but after two years, Julia's doctors suggested that she have surgery. At the time, RAI wasn't being used in Spain. With no guarantee that surgery would render permanent remission, Julia opted to stay on her medications, and she sought help from a naturalist doctor. The protocol he recommended included a non-toxic diet designed for her specific characteristics, acupuncture, hydrotherapy, a herbal sleeping aid consisting of 40 percent each Hypericum perforatum and Passiflora incarnata, and 10 percent each Valeriana officinalis and Mentha pepperita and a herbal diuretic. She was also advised to take up Yoga and instructed in various exercises, including eye exercises to help with her symptoms of GO. Adding these treatments, she noticed immediate benefits.

One year later, she went into remission although her medical doctor said that she was cured. She continued with follow up visits for six years and then quit seeing doctors since she felt so well. Several illnesses in her family and personal stress caused a recurrence of her GD more than a decade later.

In 1997, Julia visited a naturalistic clinic in Germany where she received various cleansing treatments, lymphatic drainage massages and followed a vegetarian diet. After 16 days at this spa, she felt good. However, after her trip, she experienced a long period of great stress and all her symptoms returned. Her spirits down, she lacked the energy to put any sustained effort into healing herself. She consented to RAI, which is now available in Spain, and she was given a dose of 8 millicuries. This dose, she says, didn't affect her thyroid but it exacerbated her eye disease. In a short time, her eye involvement increased significantly enough to threaten her optic nerve.

Worry and fear led her to make what she describes as two more wrong decisions. She had a subtotal bilateral thyroidectomy and decompression surgery in the early part of 1999. She now suffers from symptoms of hypothyroidism and she continues to have eye problems. Julia is vigilant in her efforts to learn more about natural healing, particularly reflexology, and she regrets having not kept up with yoga and acupuncture and the methods which once brought her to remission. Above all, Julia advises patients to take their time in choosing treatment and learn effective ways of dealing with stress.

Gerry (had surgery 45 years ago and has no regrets)

Healing is a matter of time, but it is sometimes also a matter of opportunity. — Hippocrates

In 1954, at the age of 28, my cousin Gerry was diagnosed with diffuse toxic goiter or Graves' disease ... after being told many times that she was imagining all her symptoms and told that she had an enlarged heart and hypertension, which she "needed to learn how to live with." Her symptoms included increased appetite, severe palpitations lasting as long as 45 minutes, nervousness, insomnia and breathlessness.

Diagnosed by a BMR test, her results were +47 with a normal range of ±10. Her doctor recommended that she see a surgeon and Gerry insisted on a specialist. The specialist she consulted advised her to stay in bed for six weeks because all of the systems in her body were racing. She was also prescribed strong iodine solution, a liquid nerve tonic, and seven phenobarbital tablets daily. She followed this regimen from the end of March until the 21st of June, when she had a thyroidectomy. Her hospital stay was 11 days. For the first three days she had a full-time private nurse. She describes her scar as nice and thin and reports that it can no longer be seen. Although I was a child at the time of her surgery, I never noticed her scar, and I never knew she had GD until I began researching this book.

After her surgery, Gerry had some initial difficulty getting regulated while her doctor switched her from thyroid medication to iodine and back and forth. She admits today's laboratory tests make adjusting dosage much easier. Once she was eventually stabilized, she felt fine for years. She had one brief spell in which her thyroid medication was apparently too strong and she was switched to Synthroid.

Out of curiosity, she quit taking her Synthroid for a year. At her next appointment, her doctor commented that she needed to keep on the same dose since her lab results were so good. When she told him she'd quit taking her medications, he insisted that she needed to stay on them for life. So, she still takes her Synthroid, looks and acts 20 years younger than her age and, like me, complains of occasional leg cramps and severe sugar cravings.

Radioiodine Ablation

Julie U (had RAI at age 24, which she regrets)

He knew the anguish of the marrow. — T.S. Eliot

Only 24 when she was diagnosed with Graves' disease, Julie's symptoms came on suddenly. An avid runner, she was on her usual five mile run when she noticed that her heart was beating too hard. She ignored this and continued on her daily runs until one day when, toward the end of her run, she passed out. She visited a doctor who ran thyroid tests, but all her results, including her TSH, were normal. Pronounced fine, she didn't feel fine. She felt hot all the time and lost her breath easily.

A few months later, Julie married and moved to a new city. Her symptoms continued to worsen. Her eyes began to protrude and her resting heart rate eventually rose to 150 bpm. She consulted another doctor, and by then her TSH level was totally suppressed. She was prescribed propranolol and PTU, but after six months, she was told she'd been on PTU long enough and needed to have RAI. Since she had responded to the PTU and had no side effects, she considered this strange but assumed her doctor knew best.

After RAI, her proptosis increased and her eyelids retracted. She had to see her eye doctor weekly for the first two months and then once a month for the next four months. Within six months, her proptosis receded 6 mm and she was considered out of danger. However, Julie hasn't felt well in the 12 years since she had RAI. Six years after her ablation, her thyroid completely died and she developed swelling, arthritis, sick fatigue, panic attacks, acne, sleep apnea and neuropathies.

Three years after this, Julie became pregnant with the help of a fertility drug. Her doctor never considered that her thyroid status might have contributed to her fertility problems since her TSH level was in the normal range. Consequently, her doctors never ran antibody levels or performed any fetal monitoring. After she delivered, her doctor commented that hers was the smallest placenta he'd ever seen. Although he was never diagnosed with transient GD, for the first six weeks her son slept little and screamed constantly when he was awake. After that, he begin sleeping steadily and calmed down.

Kelly H (severely hyperthyroid, by the time she was finally diagnosed, she ended up having four RAI ablations)

You may drive out Nature with a pitchfork, yet she will hurry back. — Horace

For Kelly Hale, the president and founder of the American Foundation of Thyroid Patients (AFTP), diagnosis did not come easy. When she first complained of nervousness and anxiety, she was given a prescription for tranquilizers. After several months, the tranquilizers quit working. Meanwhile, she dropped from a size 10 to a size 4 and was irritable, crying and shaking most of the time. Constantly ravenous, she had insomnia and felt so stressed out that she quit her job in hospital administration abruptly.

She says she had "heart palpitations, retraction of eyelids, fingernails that peeled like onion skin, limp hair, although it grew furiously. My thighs and upper arms were so weak I had to pull myself up stairs and could not lift a gallon milk jug. My memory was so shot I would go from room to room just trying to recall why I was there or what I had gone to do."

All this before she was finally diagnosed. Even then, her doctor recommended waiting to see how things progressed before starting treatment.

Kelly had to literally beg to be treated. She was put on methimazole (kinder acting on the eyes) for a short period and then requested radioiodine ablation. Afterward, her doctor admitted how close she had been to dying, her symptoms were so severe. It's not surprising that her first ablation of 10 mci did little to resolve her symptoms. Eight months later she was given 7.6 mCi, and eight months after that, she was administered 3.3 mCi. For her fourth ablation, eight months later in July, 1995, she was given 2.0 mCi. Given a short course of prednisone for seven to ten days before her ablations, the GO she had already developed didn't worsen.

After her experience, Kelly has no complaints about her treatment and is very aware of how close she came to dying. She does complain, though, about the length of time it took for her to be diagnosed, time in which her symptoms progressed. In her role as President of the AFTP, Kelly arranges reduced fee thyroid screening fairs and provides a greatly needed educational service to the many GD patients in search of answers.

Donna J (had Hashimoto's thyroiditis before GD; after RAI she could no longer teach)

Even when laws have been written down, they ought not always to remain unaltered. — Aristotle

On thyroid hormone replacement for Hashimoto's thyroiditis, Donna began exhibiting symptoms of hyperthyroidism. Despite laboratory results confirming this, Donna's doctor insisted that once hypothyroid, always hypothyroid. When she began showing symptoms of thyroid storm, her doctor realized she was right. Anxious to remedy the situation, her doctor insisted that Donna have immediate radioiodine ablation. Since, she's been plagued by debilitating symptoms of hypothyroidism.

Elaine (despite mild GD, had RAI without researching treatment options)

Haste in every business brings failures. — Herodotus

Many women worry about the effects their GD has on their children. My children survived growing up during my peak GD years, unscathed. Although I recall exploding if they weren't standing at the curb when I picked them up from school, they don't recall this. And although I remember constantly rushing and driving like a maniac, they recall my always being active and well organized. Both kids say that my obsession with aerobics gave them good habits. They're both overachievers and athletics is a big part of their lives.

My husband, however, clearly recalls how emotional I was in my late 20s and early 30s. He'll never forget the Thanksgiving I had a tantrum, throwing my keys, and flinging myself on the floor and wailing when he tried canceling a trip we'd planned. When people ask whether RAI altered my emotions, I have to say no. I may be less emotionally labile, but I still cry easily. And I still get enraged when I'm confronted with bad drivers or a spouse who forgets my birthday. Only now, I'm too tired to do anything about it.

Becky R (after 6 months on ATDs, she opted for RAI and had it twice)

The greatest griefs are those we cause ourselves. — Sophocles

Only 27 when she was diagnosed with Graves' disease, Becky, a lawyer in the Midwest, had never even heard of the disease before then. Although she had already scheduled radioiodine ablation, Becky postponed it when I suggested that she choose her treatment wisely. She visited some of the on-line thyroid boards and began a course of PTU along with propranolol to help manage her symptoms. Within a month, her level of T4 had dropped considerably and she had gained some weight. And her original RAI-U of 91 percent had dropped to 52 percent. Her doctor expressed surprise at her excellent response but felt that the amount of time on PTU needed to shrink her goiter prohibited its use. She made an appointment with another doctor for a second opinion.

This doctor noticed that she had a pretty loud bruit despite her response to PTU and he also advised RAI. After battling symptoms for four months, Becky opted for ablation. This was her own decision after researching options and trying ATDs. A week after her radioiodine ablation, no longer on ATDs, her symptoms of hyperthyroidism came back worse than before. Since she wasn't warned that this could happen, she was alarmed. To relieve her symptoms, she was put on PTU again and her next blood tests showed considerable improvement. She quit taking the PTU and began only taking propranolol as needed. She continued to have blood tests every three months.

Four months later, she saw another new doctor who suggested that she have another RAI. At this time she was tested for proptosis and her eyes were found to be normal, although she did have spastic eye symptoms. Since her RAI-U was now up to 72 percent, she decided to proceed with a second ablation. Her lab tests, including her FT4, also indicated that she was hyperthyroid. For various reasons, Becky felt it would benefit her to take care of the problem quickly. Although she feels that she was well informed and is already showing symptoms of hypothyroidism a week after her second ablation, she writes that she hadn't realized that RAI could worsen GO, and she didn't realize that the incidence of hypothyroidism after RAI increases each year, with some people not becoming hypothyroid for 10 years.

Glossary

AARDA American Autoimmune and Related Disease Association.

acetylcholine receptor antibodies Autoantibodies to the acetylcholine receptor that block acetylcholine from triggering impulses at cholinergenic synapses, interfering with muscle contraction; usually seen in myasthenia gravis.

Acropachy Dermal manifestation of Graves' disease causing an inflammatory process in soft connective tissue, especially of the fingers and toes.

Addison's disease Autoimmune condition causing adrenal gland insufficiency.

adenohypophysis Anterior region of the pituitary gland or hypophysis.

Adenosine diphosphate (ADP) An ester of adenosine that is reversibly converted to ATP for the storing of energy by the addition of a high-energy phosphate group

Adenosine triphosphate (ATP) Nucleotide of adenosine involved in energy metabolism and required for RNA synthesis; ATP occurs in all of the body's cells and stores energy in the form of high energy phosphate bonds.

Adenyl or adenylate cyclase Enzyme that catalyzes the formation of cyclic AMP from ATP

ADP *see* adenosine diphosphate.

Adrenal glands Endocrine glands located on top of the kidneys that secrete several important hormones including cortisol into the blood.

Adrenergic Substance resembling epinephrine in physiological effect; sympathomimetic.

Agonist A substance capable of binding to a specific cell receptor, causing effects similar to that of the intended substance.

Agranulocytosis Acute blood disorder characterized by a severe reduction in circulating granulocytic white blood cells accompanied by lesions of the throat and other mucous membranes of the GI tract and skin.

AITD Autoimmune thyroid disease.

Albumin Major plasma protein that serves as a transport medium, carrying anions, fatty acids, drugs and hormones to cells throughout the body.

Allele One of a pair of genes that normally occupies a particular locus.

Allopathy Method of treating disease by the use of agents that produce effects antagonistic to or incompatible with those of the disease treated.

Alopecia Autoimmune condition causing baldness or loss of hair, mainly on the head, either in defined patches or completely; the cause is unknown.

Alzheimer's disease A condition in which brain cells degenerate; it is accompanied by memory loss, physical decline and confusion.

Amenorrhea Absence of menstrual periods.

Amiodarone hydrochloride Coronary vasodilator used in the control of ventricular and supraventricular arrhythmias; Cordarone.

amphetamine Racemic drug that stimulates the central nervous system.

ANA *see* antinuclear antibodies.

anaphylaxis Hypersensitive reaction to an allergen with symptoms ranging from respiratory distress to death.

androgen Hormone (such as testosterone) that causes development of male characteristics and sex organs.

anergy A state of unresponsiveness or diminished reactivity, especially to antigen induced in B cells; may cause a delayed response.

angio A combining form referring to blood vessel.

anovulation The absence of ovulation.

antagonists A drug that counteracts the effects of another drug by mimicking the other drug and binding to its receptor, blocking its action.

antibody Immunoglobulin produced by B cells after antigenic stimulation and capable of reacting with the antigen that caused its production.

antibody combining site Cavity formed by the variable segments of an antibody molecule, into which the specific antigenic epitope fits.

anticonvulsant Substance capable of preventing or arresting seizures.

antigen Substance capable of inducing a specific immunologic response and of reacting with the specific antibody produced by that response.

antigen-presenting cells (APCs) Cells capable of presenting antigen to T and B cells.

antigenic determinant Portion of an antigen that determines the specificity of the immune response.

antinuclear antibodies (ANAs) Antibodies directed against nuclear antigens, such as DNA or histones, and associated with a number of autoimmune syndromes.

antiparietal cell antibody Antibodies directed against the parietal cells lining the stomach cavity;

antiphospholipid disease Autoimmune disorder associated with coagulation abnormalities and miscarriage.

antipyretics Substances such as aspirin used for checking or preventing fever.

antithyroid Relating to an agent that inhibits thyroid hormone production.

apathetic hyperthyroidism Form of hyperthyroidism commonly seen in the elderly characterized by depression and an absence of typical hyperthyroid symptoms.

apical Referring to the apex or highest point.

APL *see* antiphospholipid disease.

aplasia cutis Localized failure of development of skin, usually seen on the scalp and less frequently on the trunk and limbs.

apoptosis Normal condition of programmed cell death.

arrhythmia Any disturbance in the rhythm of the heartbeat.

ATD Antithyroid drug.

ATG Antithyroglobulin antibodies.

atherosclerosis Common form of arteriosclerosis in which fatty substances form a plaque deposit on the inner lining of arterial walls.

ATP *see* adenosine triphosphate.

atrial Relating to the atrium (upper heart chambers).

atrial fibrillation An irregular heartbeat in which the upper chambers of the heart (the atria) beat inconsistently and rapidly.

atrophy Reduction in cells leading to general destruction of a tissue or organ.

autoantibody Antibody directed to self antigens.

autoimmune disease Pathological changes resulting from a disordered immune reaction that targets self components.

autoimmune polyglandular syndrome Disorder characterized by a cluster of autoimmune disorders. There are three classes of this syndrome, two of which include autoimmune thyroid disease.

autoimmune thrombocytopenic purpura Autoimmune idiopathic disorder characterized by platelet autoantibodies, resulting in thrombocytopenia, a condition of decreased platelets and disturbances of the normal clotting mechanism

autoimmune thyroid disease (AITD) A number of different autoimmune disorders directed at thyroid cell components, causing abnormal thyroid function.

autoimmunity Condition of immunologic reactivity to self antigens.

autoreactive Intermediate step in autoantibody production; autoreactive cells are either destroyed by the body or they go on to form autoantibodies.

autoregulation Mechanism in which the body regulates levels of certain substances such as iodine in an effort to maintain health.

Ayurveda Ancient Indian medical discipline based on imbalances in doshas.

B cell (B lymphocyte) Immune system white blood cell involved in the humoral response.

Basal metabolic rate (BMR) Measurement of the body's rate of oxygen consumption used as a test of thyroid function.

beta blockers   Beta adrenergic blocking agents are medications such as propranolol used to block the adrenergic response that is associated with cardiac symptoms such as increased heart rate.

bilateral   Affecting both sides of the body or two paired organs.

biliary   Pertaining to bile, the bile ducts or the gallbladder.

binding proteins   Serum proteins that bind substances such as hormones, transporting and carrying these substances through the body.

biosynthesis   Synthesis or production of chemical compounds such as thyroid hormone within the body.

blast cell   Large immature (early stage in development) lymphoid cell with a large nucleus that differentiates into one of the basic cell lines.

blepharoplasty   Plastic surgery of the eyelid.

BMR *see* basal metabolic rate.

calcitonin   Hormone made in the C cells of the thyroid gland that controls calcium levels in the blood by slowing the loss of calcium from bones.

cardiolipin   Phospholipid occurring primarily in mitochondrial inner membranes.

catecholamine   Chemically related neurotransmitters, such as epinephrine and norepineprine, that stimulate the sympathetic nervous system.

cell-mediated immunity (CMI)   Immunity mediated by T cells without a requirement for B cells or antibodies.

cerebral   Relating to the cerebrum, the main portion of the brain.

chemosis   Edema of the bulbar conjunctiva, causing corneal swelling.

chi   The body's vital life or energy source in Eastern medicine.

choroid plexus   Part of the brain that secretes cerebrospinal fluid.

chronobiology   The science of the effect of time, especially rhythms, on life systems.

circumventricular   Pertaining to the area around or in the area of a ventricle, as are the circumventricular organs.

cirrhosis   A chronic disease of the liver in which fibrous tissue invades and replaces normal tissue.

Class I MHC antigens   Histocompatibility antigens encoded by A, B and C MHC loci in humans and by other loci in animals.

Class II MHC antigens   Histocompatibility antigens encoded by HLA-DR, HLA-DP and HLA-DQ antigens in humans and by other loci in animals.

Class III MHC antigens   Histocompatibility markers C2, C4 and complement factor B encoded by genes within the MHC.

clonal   Referring to cell proliferation.

clonal deletion   Removal of clones, primarily as a protective mechanism that is largely responsible for the deletion of self-reactive lymphocytes.

CMV *see* cytomegalovirus.

colloid   Gelatinous substance made up of a system of particles with linear dimensions. Thyroglobulin is the major constituent of thyroid colloid.

complement   Complex series of immune system proteins activated by antigen-antibody complexes and other substances.

computed tomography scanning (CT or CAT scan)   A technique of cross-sectional images in which X-rays are passed through the body at different angles and analyzed by a computer.

Congenital   Existing as a result of birth; hereditary disorders.

Conjunctiva   The clear membrane covering the white of the eye and the inside of the eyelid that produces a fluid that lubricates the cornea and eyelid.

contralateral   Relating to the opposite side, as when pain is felt or paralysis occurs on the side opposite to that of the lesion.

COPD   Chronic obstructive pulmonary disease.

corticosteroids   Natural steroid hormones or synthetic drugs that are used to replace natural hormones; functions to suppress the immune system and help prevent inflammation; includes glucocorticoids and mineralocrticoids.

coupling   The mechanism by which the thyroid hormone precursors MIT and DIT link to form T3 and T4.

cretinism   Condition of stunted growth and mental retardation caused by severe hypothyroidism.

cricoid   Pertaining to a ring-shaped cartilage at the lower part of the larynx.

CT   *see* computed tomography scanning.

CTL   Cytotoxic T lymphocyte.

Cushing's syndrome   Adrenal gland disorder.

cyclic AMP   Cyclic adenosine monophosphate, a chemical acting as a second messenger in the hormonal response.

cytokine   Hormone-like, low molecular weight messenger proteins, which regulate the intensity and duration of immune responses.

cytomegalovirus   Any of several viruses that cause cellular enlargement and formation of eosinophilic inclusion bodies especially in the nucleus and Include some acting as opportunistic infectious agents in immunosuppressed conditions

cytotoxic   Detrimental or destructive to cells.

cytotoxic T cells   T cells with the ability to kill other cells.

D gene region   Diversity segment of the genome that encodes part of the hypervariable region of the immunoglobulin heavy chain.

deiodination   The loss or removal of iodine from a compound as seen in the conversion of T4 to T3; monodeiodination.

deletion   Chromosomal aberration in which a portion of a chromosome is lost. It may also refer to loss of a DNA segment in mutations.

dendritic   Threadlike extensions of the cytoplasm of neurons.

deoxyribonucleic acid   Any of various nucleic acids that are usually the molecular basis of heredity, localized especially in cell nuclei, and are contructed of a double helix held together by hydrogen bonds between purine and pyrimidine bases which project inward from two chains containing alternate links of deoxyribose and phosphate. DNA.

dermatitis herpetiformis Autoimmune disorder characterized by celiac disease and a chronic skin disorder characterized by itchy, occasionally blistering eruptions and hyperpigmention; also known as Duhring's disease.

dermopathy Disorder affecting or involving the skin.

dexamethasone Synthetic glucocorticoid far more potent than cortisol used for treating symptoms of adrenal insuˆciency.

diabetes mellitus (IDDM) Autoimmune disorder of insulin dependent or juvenile diabetes mellitus caused by various antibodies that attack pancreatic cells.

diaphoresis Perspiration, especially when artificially induced or excessive.

Diethylstilbesterol (DES) Synthetic, non-steroidal estrogen compound with estrogenic activity greater than estrone.

diiodotyrosine An intermediate in the biosynthesis of thyroid hormone; DIT.

diphenylhydantoin Phenytoin (Dilantin); an anticonvulsant used in the treatment of seizure disorders, which may interfere with thyroid hormone metabolism.

diplopia Visual disturbance in which an object appears double; double vision.

DIT *see* diiodotyrosine.

DNA *see* deoxyribonucleic acid.

dopamine A chemical neurotransmitter that transmits messages in the brain, which is known to inhibit the secretion of TSH.

Down's syndrome A genetic disorder causing moderate to severe mental handicap.

dysbiosis An imbalanced intestinal ecology that results in a dysfunctional intestinal lining, sometimes referred to as the leaky gut syndrome.

dyshormonogenesis Defect in one or more of the several chemical steps that take place in the manufacture of thyroid hormones.

dysphagia Difficulty swallowing.

dysphoria A mood of general dissatisfaction.

dyspnea Difficulty breathing; shortness of breath.

dystonia Uncontrolled muscle movement due to disordered muscle tonicity.

EBV Epstein Barr virus.

ectopic Located away from its normally occurring position.

edema An abnormal accumulation of fluid in the tissue spaces, cavities or joint capsules of the body, causing swelling of the area.

effector Substances, such as cytokines that are released during the immune response, that act as messengers, inciting other changes.

electrocardiograph A galvanometric device that detects variations in the electric potential that triggers the heartbeat, used to evaluate the heart's rhythms.

endocrine Glands that secrete hormones internally into the blood or lymph.

endocytosis Movement of external substances into a cell, usually by pinocytosis.

endoderm The innermost cell layer of the embryo in its gastrula stage.

enteropathy Any intestinal disorder, for example gluten sensitivity enteropathy (GSE), which is also known as celiac disease.

epinephrine A hormone secreted by the adrenal medulla upon stimulation by the central nervous system in response to stress.

epitope See antigenic determinant.

ER Emergency room.

erythema Abnormal redness of the skin and mucous membranes accompanied by fever and pain.

estradiol An estrogenic hormone produced by the maturing Graaffan follicle that causes proliferation and thickening of the endometrium.

estrogen Relating to any of several major female sex hormones (estriol, estradiol, or estrone) produced primarily by ovarian follicles.

euthyroid Graves' disease Condition in which the characteristic eye disease of GD, Graves' ophthalmopathy, is evident although thyroid function is normal.

euthyroidism A condition in which the thyroid gland is functioning normally as reflected in normal thyroid function tests.

exophthalmos Protrusion of the eyeball from the orbit; proptosis.

extraocular Adjacent but outside the eyeball.

extrathyroidal Outside of or away from the thyroid gland itself.

Fab Antigen-binding fragment or region of an immunoglobulin molecule.

Fas protein Surface protein that acts as a regulator of apoptosis when it's produced at the expense of Fas ligand.

fibroadipose having both fibrous and adipose or fatty characteristics.

fibroblast Immature fibrous connective tissue cell that differentiates into chrondoblasts, collagenoblasts, orbital tissue cells and osteoblasts.

fibromyalgia A condition characterized by muscle and joint pain.

fibrosis Formation of fibrous tissue (such as muscle, tissue containing fibers).

fibrotic Characterized by fibrosis.

folic acid Water-soluble vitamin that is converted to a coenzyme essential to purine and thymine biosynthesis and thyroid function.

follicle Sac or pouch-like depression or cavity; basic structural unit of the thyroid gland.

follicular cells Cells of the thyroid follicles.

free thyroxine (T4) Unbound thyroxine that has been cleaved from its binding protein and is now capable of causing cellular effects.

free triiodothyronine (T3) Unbound triiodothyronine that has been cleaved from its binding protein and is now capable of causing cellular effects.

FT3 *see* free triiodothyronine (T3).

FT4 *see* free thyroxine (T4).

GAG *see* glycosaminoglycan.

galactorrhea An abnormally persistent flow of milk.

GD   Graves' disease.

genome   The total genetic constitution of a cell or organism.

glucagon   A hormone secreted by the pancreas that acts in opposition to insulin in the regulation of blood glucose levels.

glucocorticoid   Any of a class of steroid hormones that are produced by the adrenal cortex under conditions of stress and that inhibit immune reactions.

glycoprotein   Any of a group of complex proteins, as mucin, containing a carbohydrate combined with a simple protein.

Glycosaminoglycan   (GAG)   Any of a class of polysaccharides that form mucins when complexed with proteins. GAG is responsible for the congestive dermal and orbital infiltration in GD.

GO   *see* Graves' ophthalmopathy.

goiter   Enlargement of the thyroid gland.

goitrogen   Substance that induces goiter by decreasing thyroid hormone levels.

gonadal   Referring to the gonads or reproductive organs.

granulomatous   Characterized by aggregates of white blood cells.

Graves' ophthalmopathy (GO)   Characteristic eye disorder associated with Graves' disease that has two components, a spastic disorder and a congestive infiltration.

Guanethidine sulfate   A potent antihypertensive (blood pressure lowering) agent.

halothane   A colorless liquid used as an inhalant for general anesthesia.

haploids   Having a single set of chromosomes.

haplotype   Set of alleles on a single chromosome that are inherited as a closely linked set, generally considered in terms of MHC genes.

hapten   Antigenic determinant of low molecular weight that can act as an immunogen when coupled to an immunogenic carrier molecule.

haptenic determinants   Part of the antigen that determines its antigenic specificity

Hashimoto's thyroiditis (HT)   An autoimmune disorder of the thyroid gland, which may induce thyroid enlargement (goiter) and hypothyroidism.

Hashitoxicosis   A temporary episode of hyperthyroidism in a patient with HT.

hCG   Human chorionic gonadotropin.

Helper T cells (Th)   Subset of T cells, usually bearing CD4, which functions by cooperating with B cells or other T cells.

hematopoietic   Pertaining to the formation of blood cells; of bone marrow origin.

heparin   Synthetic substance with anticoagulant properties used medically to prevent or dissolve blood clots.

hirsutism   Abnormal hairiness usually associated with females having a male pattern of hair growth.

histocompatability   The condition of having similar immune system antigens such that cells or tissues transplanted from a donor to a recipient are not rejected.

HIV   Human immunodeficiency virus (AIDS virus).

HLA (human leukocyte antigens)   Human MHC region and its products located on the short arm of chromosome 6, encompassing the immune system genes.

Hoffman's syndrome   Exaggerated muscle enlargement seen in hypothyroidism characterized by diminished muscle tone and weakness.

homeostasis   The tendency of an organism to maintain health via the coordinated response of its parts to any threatening situation of stimulus.

hormone   Substances secreted by endocrine glands that affect the functions of specifically receptive organs or tissues.

HPP   *see*   hypokalemic periodic paralysis.

HT   *see*   Hashimoto's thyroiditis.

hTG   Thyroglobulin.

humoral   Term applied to soluble substances in body fluids. In immunology, it generally refers to immunoglobulins or complement components (or both).

Hyaluron   Major glycosaminoglycan seen in GD.

hypercalcemia   Condition of excess serum calcium.

hyperdefecation   Condition of increased bowel movements.

hyperglycemia   An abnormally high level of glucose in the blood.

hyperkinesis   An abnormal amount of uncontrolled muscular action; spasm.

hypermetabolism   Increased metabolic state.

hyperplasia   Abnormal multiplication of cells.

hyperthyroidism   A sustained period of thyrotoxicosis.

hypertrophy   Abnormal increase in cell size.

hypoglycemia   An abnormally low level of glucose in the blood.

hypokalemic periodic paralysis   condition of low serum potassium characterized by muscle weakness that may progress to paralysis.

hypomanic   Overexcited state resembling mania but to a lesser intensity.

hyponatremia   Abnormally low blood sodium level.

hypophysis   The pituitary gland.

hypothalamic-pituitary-thyroid axis   Thyroid regulatory system in which there is a negative feedback, which aims to maintain normal thyroid hormone levels.

hypothalamus   The ventral part of the diencephalon in the brain.

hypothyroidism   A sustained period of reduced thyroid hormone.

I   iodine.

I-123   radioiodine isotope 123.

IDDM   Insulin dependent diabetes mellitus (type 1 or juvenile diabetes).

IFN   *see*   interferons.

IFN-α   Interferon, type (alpha).

Ig   *see*   immunoglobulin.

IgA   Immunoglobulin, subclass A.

IL *see* interleukin.

immune complexes Molecular complexes composed of antigen and antibody, with or without complement.

immune system A network of organs, cells and chemicals that protects the body from foreign substances and destroys infected and malignant cells.

immunity The state of being immune from a particular disease.

immunoassays A laboratory method for detecting a substance by using an antibody reactive with it.

immunogen Substance capable of inducing an immune response.

immunoglobulin Protein composed of H and L chains that functions as an antibody.

immunomodulator Substance capable of modulating or balancing the immune system.

immunosuppressive Capable of depressing the immune system.

interferons (IFN) Cytokine with multiple immune regulatory functions.

interfollicular Space between follicles.

interleukin (IL) Cytokine with diverse immunologic and inflammatory activities.

iodine A mineral essential for the production of thyroid hormone.

iodotyrosine Compound formed when an iodine atom combines with tyrosyl residues or the amino acid tyrosine.

islet of Langerhans Any of the clusters of endocrine cells in the pancreas that are specialized to secrete insulin, somatostatin or glucagon.

isoenzyme Subset of an enzyme with certain characteristic functions but with slight difference in chemical structure.

kampo Japanese herbal healing tradition with roots in China.

karyotype The chromosomes of a cell, usually displayed as a systematized arrangement of chromosome pairs in descending order of size.

K cell Killer lymphocyte capable of antibody dependent cytotoxicity.

keratitis Inflammation of the cornea.

ketoacidosis State of imbalance in the body's normal acid-base mechanism characterized by ketones in the blood or urine and an acid Ph.

KI potassium iodide.

lacrimination The secretion of tears, especially in abnormal abundance.

LAF Lymphocyte activating factor.

Leptin Hormone that enhances metabolism while decreasing appetite and caloric intake.

leukocytes White blood cells.

levothyroxine Monosodium salt of the levo isomer of the thyroid hormone thyroxine commonly used in hormone replacement therapy.

LGL Large granulocytic lymphocyte.

ligand Molecule capable of binding to another molecule.

linkage disequilibrium Tendency of certain genes on a chromosome to be inherited as a group and occurring more often than would be seen by chance.

lipolytic Effect of breaking down fat.

Lugol's Solution Liquid solution of strong saturated potassium iodine.

lumen Cavity within a tube or tubular organ.

lupus erythematosus Any of several autoimmune diseases, especially systemic lupus.

lymphocyte Nongranular white blood cell important in antibody production.

lymphokine See cytokine.

lymphoma A tumor arising from any of the cellular elements of lymph nodes.

lysosome A cell organelle containing enzymes that break down proteins and other large molecules into smaller constituents.

lysozyme An enzyme that is destructive of bacteria and functions as an antiseptic, found in tears, leukocytes, mucus, egg albumin and certain plants.

macrophage Large white blood cell that ingests foreign particles and infectious microorganisms by a process called phagocytosis.

magnetic resonance imaging (MRI) A process of producing images of the body regardless of intervening bone by means of a strong magnetic field and low-energy radio waves.

major hisotocompatibility complex (MHC) Cluster of genes on the short arm of chromosome 6 associated with many aspects of immune responsiveness and autoimmunity; in humans, MHC genes are known as HLA antigens.

melanocytes A cell that produces the dark pigment melanin.

menorrhagia Excessive menstrual discharge.

methimazole One of the primary antithyroid agents used in the United States; recently made available in a generic form; brand name Tapazole.

metoprolol Type of cardioselective beta adrenergic blocking agent, Lopressor.

MG *see* myasthenia gravis.

MHC *see* major hisotocompatibility complex.

MIT *see* monoiodotyrosine.

mitochondrion An organelle in the cell cytoplasm that has its own DNA and that produces enzymes essential for energy metabolism.

mitral valve The valve between the heart's left atrium and left ventricle that prevents blood from flowing back into the atrium when the ventricle contracts.

molecular mimicry Cross-reactivity between an antigen and a tissue component; a mechanism for autoimmunity.

monoclonal antibodies Set of identical immunoglobulins produced by one B cell alone.

monoiodotyrosine Thyroid hormone intermediary precursor with one iodine atom; MIT.

MRI Magnetic resonance imaging.

mRNA Messenger RNA.

MS Multiple sclerosis, an autoimmune nervous system disorder.

mucopolysaccharide Former name of glycosaminoglycan.

mucosal immune system Lymphoid tissues associated with the gastrointestinal and respiratory mucosa.

myasthenia gravis A disease of impaired transmission of motor nerve impulses, characterized by episodic weakness and fatiguability of the muscles.

myocardial infarction Heart attack.

myopathy Any abnormality or disease of muscle tissue.

myopia A condition of the eye in which parallel rays are focused in front of the retina, causing nearsightedness.

myxedema A condition of hypothyroidism characterized by thickening of the skin, blunting of the senses and intellect, and labored speech.

naturopathy A method of treating disease that employs no surgery or synthetic drugs to assist the natural healing process.

neurohypophysis Posterior region of the pituitary gland.

neutrophilic Characterized by white blood cells with granular cytoplasm.

nitrofurantoin Synthetic antibacterial agent.

NK (natural killer) cells Cells able to kill certain target cells without previous immunization.

nodule A small node, which can be detected by touch (palpating).

nucleoside Consisting typically of deoxyribose or ribose combined with adenine, guanine, cytosine, uracil or thymine.

nucleoprotein Any of the class of conjugated proteins occurring in cells and consisting of a protein, usually a histone combined with a nucleic acid.

ocreotide Somatostatin analog used in the treatment of GO.

oligomenorrhea Scant menses; infrequent menstrual cycles.

oncogene Gene causing malignant transformation of normal cells.

oncovirus Retrovirus of the subfamily oncovirinae, capable of producing tumors.

onycholysis Separation of the nail from its nail bed; symptom of Graves' disease.

ophthalmopathy Any disease of the eye.

ophthalmoplegia Paralysis of eye muscles, particularly on upward gaze.

optic neuropathy Disorder or compression of the optic nerve.

oral tolerization Autoimmune disease therapy using glandular extracts.

organification Process by which iodide ions are converted to iodine.

orbital decompression Type of surgery used to reduce congestive infiltration of GO

orbital fibroblasts Immature orbital tissue cells.

orbital pseudotumor Non-malignant growth resembling a tumor found in the eye region.

oxyphil   Abnormal white blood cell seen in long-term Graves' disease.

pancytopenia   Suppressed platelet count.

parafollicular   Surrounding the thyroid follicle as in the basement cavity.

paranasal   Situated near the nasal area.

parathyroid   Situated near the thyroid gland.

parenchyma   Functional tissue of an organ, distinct from its stroma.

Parry's disease   Disorder of hyperthyroidism arising in association with toxic multinodular goiter.

PCA   *see* antiparietal cell antibodies.

peau d'orange   Characteristic skin texture with the roughness of an orange.

peptide   A compound containing two or more amino acids in which the carboxyl group of one acid is linked to the amino group of the other.

perchlorate   A salt or ester of perchloric acid, as potassium perchlorate.

peripheral   Away from the normal location or point of origin.

peripheral lymphoid organs or tissues   Lymphoid aggregates or tissues excluding the thymus and bone marrow, the latter considered to be the source of lymphoid stem cells.

pernicious anemia (PA)   A severe anemia associated with inadequate intake or absorption of vitamin B_{12}, caused by an autoimmune mechanism.

peroxidase   Any of a class of enzymes that catalyze the oxidation of a compound by the decomposition of peroxide.

phagocytes   Cells able to ingest particles, including microbes.

phagocytosis   The ingestion by a cell of a microorganism, cell particle or other matter surrounded and engulfed by the cell.

pharmacodynamics   The pharmacological or active mode of drugs.

pharmacopeia or pharmacopoeia   A government or educational publication containing a list of drugs, their formulas, production methods and effects.

pheochromocytoma   Condition caused by a tumor of the adrenal gland(s) that secretes hormones that affect one's blood pressure.

phospholipid   Any of a group of fatty compounds, composed of phosphoric esters, present in living cells.

photophobia   Abnormal sensitivity to or intolerance of light, as in iritis.

phytochemistry   The branch of biochemistry dealing with plants and plant processes.

phytomedical   Chemical or medicinal properties of plants.

pineal gland   An endocrine organ in the posterior forebrain that secretes melatonin; involved in biorhythms and gonadal development.

pinocytosis   Process of cellular ingestion of soluble material.

PIP2   Phospholipase C.

pituitary   Endocrine gland that regulates thyroid function.

plasma cells   Mature B cells capable of intensive antibody production and secretion.

plasmapheresis   Procedure in which blood cells are returned to the bloodstream of the donor and the plasma is removed to reduce antibody levels.

Plummer's disease   Toxic multinodular goiter.

Plummer's nails *see* onycholysis.

PNI   Psychoneuroimmunology.

polyaromatic hydrocarbons (PAH)   Chemicals such as chloroform that are suspected of being hormonal disruptors

polymyositis   A connective tissue disorder with symptoms resembling fibromyalgia.

polypeptide   A chain of amino acids linked together by ten or more peptide bonds and having a molecular weight of up to about 10,000 kD.

postablative hypothyroidism   Hypothyroidism resulting from ablative treatment of hyperthyroidism by surgery or by RAI.

prana   Vital life force in Eastern medicine.

pretibial   Referring to the skin of the lower leg near the shin over the tibia.

pretibial myxedema   A skin condition affecting usually the lower legs and feet.

primary lymphoid tissue   Site of lymphocyte proliferation, generally the bone marrow.

procainamide   A medicine commonly used in the treatment of cardiac arrhythmias.

propranolol   A beta-blocking drug; Inderal.

proptosis   Protrusion of the eyes; exophthalmos.

Propylthiouracil (PTU)   First anti-thyroid compound used in the United States.

prostaglandins   Hormone-like substances released during the inflammatory response.

proteolysis   Cleaving of hormone from its carrier protein.

psychosomatic   Of or pertaining to a physical disorder that is caused or notably influenced by emotional factors.

PTH   Parathyroid hormone.

PTU *see* propylthiouracil.

pyramidal lobe   Remnant of the embryonic thyroglossal duct occasionally seen in the middle region of the thyroid gland.

qi   Chi, the body's vital life force in some Eastern healing traditions.

RA   Rheumatoid arthritis, an autoimmune rheumatic disorder.

radioimmunoassay   One of a group of tests for detecting antigen or antibody where one of the reagents is labeled with a radioactive isotope.

radioiodine   Any of nine radioisotopes of iodine used as radioactive tracers in research and clinical diagnosis and treatment.

radioiodine ablation   Therapeutic destruction of thyroid cells by I-131 used to reduce the amount of functional thyroid cells that produce thyroid hormone.

radioiodine uptake test and scan   Diagnostic measurement of radioiodine and its pattern of distribution quantified after ingestion of a known oral dose of radioiodine.

RAI radioiodine.

RAI-U radioiodine uptake scan.

resorcinol A water-soluble vitamin A derivative used as a skin medication.

retinoid Any of a group of substances related to and functioning like vitamin A.

retrobulbar Behind the orbital cavity.

retrosternal Behind the sternum.

retrovirus RNA virus that uses reverse transcriptase for replication.

reverse transcriptase Enzyme in microorganisms that catalyzes the transcription of DNA from RNA.

rheumatoid factor (RF) Immunoglubulin, usually IgM, directed against IgG, often seen in patients with rheumatoid arthritis or other rheumatic disease.

riboflavin A vitamin B complex factor essential for proper thyroid function.

Riedel's thyroiditis Rare, chronic proliferating inflammatory condition usually involving one thyroid lobe, although it may extend to both lobes and also the trachea.

RNA ribonucleic acid.

rT3 reverse T3.

salicylate A salt or ester of salicylic acid; aspirin.

scintiscan Method of measuring the scanning pattern after RAI-U.

sclerosis An induration, or hardening associated with inflammation.

secondary lymphoid tissue Sites in the body where lymphocytes proliferate in response an immune stimulus.

selenium A mineral essential for the conversion of T4 to T3.

sertaline Zoloft; an antidepressant.

sinus tachycardia Abnormal heart pattern

Sjörgren's Syndrome Autoimmune disorder characterized by oral and ocular dryness.

SLE Systemic lupus erythematosus.

somatostatin A polypeptide hormone, produced in the brain and pancreas.

spironolactone Medication used to lower blood pressure.

SSKI Saturated solution of potassium iodide.

steroidogenic Having properties of a steroid hormone.

sterol Any of a group of solid, mostly unsaturated, polycyclic alcohols, as cholesterol and ergosterol, derived from plants or animals.

stroma Network of supporting tissue or matrix of an organ.

struma ovarri Condition characterized by ectopic thyroid tissue acting as an ovarian tumor.

subacute Somewhat or moderately acute.

subclinical Pertaining to an early stage of a disease; having no noticeable clinical symptoms and only one abnormal lab marker.

sulfonamide   Sulfa drug commonly used as an antibiotic, which has ATD properties.

superantigens   Potent T cell stimulatory molecules that bind to MHC class II molecules.

suppressor T cells   Subset of T cells able to inhibit T cell or B cell reactivity. May be antigen-specific or antigen-nonspecific.

surface receptors   Protein on the cell on the surface membrane that actively reacts with specific hormones or drugs.

sympathomimetic   Mimicking stimulation of the sympathetic nervous system.

T3 *see* triiodothryonine.

T4 *see* thyroxine.

tachycardia   Excessively rapid heartbeat.

TBG   Thyroxine binding globulin.

TBII   Thyrotroin-binding inhibitory.

TBPA   Thyroxine binding prealbumin.

T cell receptor   Antigen-specific complex on a T cell that denotes specificity.

T cells (T lymphocyte)   Lymphocytes subgroup that regulates the immune response.

TCM   Traditional Chinese medicine.

TCR   T cell receptor.

technetium   A synthetic element obtained in the fission of uranium.

TED   Thyroid eye disease.

TgAb   Antithyroglobulin antibodies.

TGI   Thyroid growth stimulating immunoglobulin.

thiamine   A crystalline, water-soluble vitamin B compound; vitamin B_1.

thiocyanate   Medicine used to treat heart problems that has antithyroid properties.

thrombocyte   Blood component that aids coagulation; platelet.

thymoma   Tumor of the thymus.

thymus gland   A ductless gland lying at the base of the neck, formed mostly of lymphatic tissue and aiding in the production of T cells.

thyrocytes   Pituitary cells that produce thyrotropin.

thyroglobulin antibodies   Antibodies mainly directed against the thyroglobulin stored in the thyroid gland.

thyroglossal duct   Embryonic duct connecting the mouth to the thyroid.

thyroid crisis or storm   An acute exacerbation of the symptoms of thyrotoxicosis.

thyroid microsomal antigen   Primary antigenic determinant of the vesicle used to transport thyroglobulin.

thyroid peroxidase (thyroperoxidase)   Enzyme necessary for thyroid hormone production and metabolism.

thyroid stimulating hormone (TSH)   See Thyrotropin.

thyroidectomy   Surgical excision of all or a part of the thyroid gland.

thyroiditis   Inflammation of the thyroid gland.

thyromegaly   Enlarged thyroid

thyrotoxic myopathy   Cardiac muscle involvement associated with thyrotoxicosis.

thyrotoxicosis   Symptoms of excess thyroid hormone.

thyrotropin   Pituitary hormone which regulates thyroid hormone production and release; also known as thyroid stimulating hormone or TSH.

thyrotropin receptor antibodies   Antibodies responsible for symptoms of autoimmune thyroid disease; stimulating antibodies cause the symptoms of Graves' disease.

thyrotropin releasing hormone (TRH)   A hormone of the hypothalamus that controls the release of thyrotropin by the pituitary gland.

thyroxine (tetraiodothyronin)   A hormone of the thyroid gland that regulates the metabolic rate of the body; preparations of it used for treating hypothyroidism; T4.

Thyroxine-binding globulin (TBG)   The most important thyroid hormone carrier protein, carries about 70 percent of thyroxine.

torticollis   A condition in which the neck is twisted and the head inclined to one side, caused by spasmodic contraction of the muscles of the neck.

TPO *see* thyroid peroxidase.

TPO   Ab thyroid peroxidase antibodies.

TRAb *see* thyrotropin receptor antibodies.

transcription   Synthesis of RNA from a DNA template.

translation   Synthesis of a polypeptide protein from an RNA template.

transplacental   Across or passing through the placenta over to the fetal circulation.

transthyretin   Protein which transports thyroid hormone through the blood.

TRBAb   Thyrotropin receptor blocking antibodies.

tremulousness   Characterized by trembling, as from fear, nervousness, or weakness.

TRH *see* thyrotropin releasing hormone.

triiodothyronine   A thyroid hormone, similar to thyroxine but more potent: preparations of it used in treating hypothyroidism; T3.

tRNA   Transfer RNA.

trophic   Hormonal effect produced in a different gland.

TSAb   Thyrotropin receptor stimulating antibodies.

TSBAb   Thyrotropin receptor blocking antibodies.

TSH   Thyroid stimulating hormone (thyrotropin).

TSI   Thyroid stimulating immunoglobulins (stimulating TRAb).

TTR *see* transthyretin.

tumor necrosis factors (TNFs)   Cytokines able to cause tumor cell lysis and other effects, including inflammation.

Turner's syndrome   An abnormal congenital condition resulting from a defect on or absence of the second sex chromosome.

tyrosine   Amino acid that combines with iodine to form thyroid hormone.

tyrosol residues   Tyrosine fragments present in thyroglobulin.

Ultrasonography (ultrasound)   A diagnostic imaging technique utilizing reflected ultrasonic waves to delineate, measure, or examine internal body structures or organs.

unilateral proptosis   Proptosis involving only one eye

uremia   Renal disorder caused by the presence in the blood of excessive urea.

urticaria (hives)   Pruritic skin eruption with edematous wheals.

variable (V) region   Amino-terminus end of an H or L chain where the amino acid sequence differs from one antibody to another.

varicella   Chickenpox virus..

vitiligo   A skin disorder characterized by patches of unpigmented skin.

xenobiotics   non-living substances with biologic properties.

yin and yang   The opposing polarities such as hot and cold which govern man as well as the universe in Eastern medicine.

zoster   Shingles virus.

Notes

Chapter 1

1. Segni, M., et al., "Special Features of Graves' Disease in Early Childhood," Department of Pediatrics, University La Sapienza, Rome, Italy, *Thyroid*, September, 1999; 9(9):871–7.

2. Felz, Michael, M.D., and Peter Stein, M.D. "The Many 'Faces' of Graves' Disease," Part 1 in *Postgraduate Medicine*, Oct. 1, 1999; 106(4):57–64.

3. Burch, Henry, and Colum Gorman, et al., "Graves Ophthalmopathy" in *Werner and Ingbar's The Thyroid, a Fundamental and Clinical Text*, 7th Ed., Edited by Braverman, Lewis E., and Robert D. Utiger, Lippincott-Raven, Philadelphia, 1996, 536.

4. Larsen, P. Reed, Davies, Terry F., and Ian D. Hay, "The Thyroid Gland," in *Williams' Textbook of Endocrinology*, 9th Edition, edited by Wilson, Jean D., W.B. Saunders, Philadelphia, 1998, 438.

5. Op cit., McDougall, 81.

6. Felz, Michael, M.D., and Peter Stein, M.D., "The Many 'Faces' of Graves' Disease, Part 2, "Practical Diagnostic Testing and Mangement Options" in *Postgraduate Medicine*, Vol. 106, No. 5, Oct. 15, '99, 45–52.

7. De Groot, Leslie, M.D., "Graves' Disease and the Manifestations of Thyrotoxicosis," in *Thyroid Disease Manager, The Thyroid and its Diseases*, on-line publication, July 1999,

8. Sato, A., and T. Yamada, "An Elevation of Serum Immunoglobulin E Provides a New Aspec of Hyperthyroid Graves' Disease," *Journal of Clinical Endocrinology & Metabolism*, October 1998; 84(10):3602–3605.

9. Rister, Robert, *Japanese Herbal Medicine, The Healing Art of Kampo*, Garden Park City, NJ, Avery, 1999, 5.

10. Smith, Terry J., "Connective Tissue in Thyrotoxicosis," in Werner and Ingbar's *The Thyroid: a Fundamental and Clinical Text*, 7th Ed., Edited by Braverman, Lewis E., and Robert D. Utiger, Lippincott-Raven, Philadelphia, 1996, 600.

11. Miller, L.J., et al., "Gastric, Pancreatic, and Biliary Responses to Meals in Hyperthyroidism" Medline, National Library of Medicine abstract of article appearing in *Gut*, 1980 Aug.; 21(8):695–700 via the Internet.

12. Boerner, A.R., et al., "Glucose Metabolism of the Thyroid in Graves' Disease Measured by F-18-Fluoro-deoxyglucose Positron Emission Tomography," in *Thyroid*, 1998, Sept.; 8(9):765–72.

13. Loeb, John, "Metabolic Changes in Thyrotoxicosis," in *Werner & Ingbar's The Thyroid: a Fundamental and Clinical Text,* 7th Ed., Edited by Braverman, Lewis E. and Robert D. Utiger, Lippincott-Raven, Philadelphia, 1996, 690.

14. Langer, Stephen E., M.D., with James F. Scheer, *Solved: The Riddle of Illness,* New Canaan, Keats Publishing, Inc., 1984, 30.

15. Op. cit., Larsen, 390–511.

16. Raisz, Lawrence, Kream, Barbara, and Joseph Lorenzo, "Metabolic Bone Disease," in *Williams' Textbook of Endocrinology,* 9th Edition, edited by Jean Wilson, M.D., Philadelphia, W.B. Saunders, 1998, 1229.

17. Op. cit., Langer, 31.

18. Rivlin, Richard S., "Vitamin Metabolism in Thyrotoxicosis" in *The Thyroid: a Fundamental and Clinical Text,* 7th Edition, Edited by Braverman, Lewis E. and Richard D. Utiger, Philadelphia, Lippincott-Raven, 1996, 693–694.

19. Arem, Ridha, M.D., *The Thyroid Solution,* New York, Ballantine/Random House, 1999, 303.

20. Op. cit., Raisz, 1217.

21. Op Cit., Langer, 57.

22. Op. cit., Larsen, 429.

23. Op. cit., Langer, 31.

24. Op. cit., Arem, 67–71.

25. Op. cit., Larsen, 428.

26. Beer, Alan E., M.D., *Thyroid Disorders and Reproductive Problems of Miscarriage, Implantation Failure and In Vitro Fertilization Failure,* Internet World Wide Web Publication of the Reproductive Medicine Program, Chicago, 1999, www.repromed.net/papers/thyroid.html.

27. Longcope, Christopher, "The Male and Female Reproductive Systems in Thyrotoxicosis" in *Werner and Ingbar's The Thyroid: a Fundamental and Clinical Text,* 7th Edition, Edited by Braverman, Lewis E., and Robert D. Utiger, Philadelphia, Lippincott-Raven, 1996, 671–675.

28. DeLong, G. Robert, "The Neuromuscular System and Brain in Thyrotoxicosis" in *Werner and Ingbar's The Thyroid: a Fundamental and Clinical Text,* 7th Ed., Edited by Braverman, Lewis E., and Robert D. Utiger, Philadelphia, Lippincott-Raven, 1996, 645.

29. Klein, Irwin, and Gerald Levey, "The Cardiovascular System in Thyrotoxicosis" in *Werner and Ingbar's The Thyroid: a Fundamental and Clinical Text,* 7th Edition, Edited by Braverman, Lewis E., and Robert D. Utiger, Philadelphia, Lippincott-Raven, 1996, 607–615.

30. Greenspan, Francis, *Basic and Clinical Endocrinology,* 3rd Ed., Norwalk, CT, Appleton & Lange, 1991, 221.

31. Op. cit., Klein, 607–615.

32. Moses, Arnold, and Steven Scheinman, "The Kidneys and Electrolyte Metabolism in Thyrotoxicosis," in *Werner and Ingbar's The Thyroid: a Fundamental and Clinical Text,* 7th Ed., Edited by Braverman, Lewis E., and Robert D. Utiger, Philadelphia, Lippincott-Raven, 1996, 629–630.

33. Ibid., 629.

34. Brunt, I. Michael, "Immunologic Disorders of the Thyroid Gland and Autoimmune Polyendocrinopathies," *Samter's Immunologic Diseaes,* 5th Ed. Vol. 2, edited by Frank, Michael, M.D., New York, Little, Brown, & Company, 1995, 992–993.

35. Suzuki, Hideyo, and Hiroki Shimura, et al., "Exophthalmos, Pretibial Myxedema, Osteoarthropathy Syndrome Associated with Papillary Fibroelastoma in the Left Ventricle," in *Thyroid,* 1999; 9(12):1257–1260.

Chapter 2

1. *Autoimmunity: A Major Women's Health Issue*, publication of the American Autoimmune Related Diseases Association, World Wide Web, the Internet, 1997.

2. Ibid.

3. Selye, Hans, *The Stress of Life*, Revised from 1956 Edition, New York, McGraw-Hill, 1976, 14.

4. Ibid., 480.

5. Ibid, 72–102.

6. Thibodeau, Gary A., *Structure & Function of the Body*, 9th Edition, St. Louis, Mosby Year Book, 1992, 258.

7. Vengelen-Tyler, Virginia, *Technical Manual*, 13th Edition, Bethesda, MD, American Association of Blood Banks, 1999, 241.

8. Smith, Dorinda, and Lori Germolek, "Introduction to Immunology and Autoimmunity" in *Environmental Health Perspectives Supplements*, Oct. '99, 107(5): 661–666.

9. Rose, Noel R., M.D., Ph.D., *Autoimmunity — The Common Thread*, publication of the American Autoimmune Related Diseases Association, Incorporated, Detroit, 1997.

10. Winter, William E., M.D., *Glandular Autoimmune Diseases*, publication of the American Diabetes Association, reprinted by the American Autoimmune Related Diseases Association Incorporated, Detroit, 1993.

11. Locke, Steven, and Douglas Colligan, *The Healer Within: The New Medicine of Mind and Body*, New York, Dutton Publishing Company, 38.

12. Henry, John Bernard, *Clinical Diagnosis & Management by Laboratory Methods*, Philadelphia, W.B. Saunders Co., 1991, 824.

13. Ibid.

14. Op. cit., Greenspan, 221.

15. Borysenko, Joan, *The Power of the Mind to Heal, Renewing Body, Mind and Spirit*, Niles, IL, Nightingale Conant Audio Series, 1993.

16. Colborn, Theo, Dumanoski, Dianne, and John Myers, *Our Stolen Future*, New York, Penguin Publishing, 1996, 63.

17. Claman, Henry, "Environmental Aspects of Autoimmmunity and Other Sensitivity Syndromes", in *Samter's Immunologic Diseases*, Volume II, 5th Edition, edited by Michael Frank, New York, Little, Brown and Co., 1995,1224–1225.

18. Ward, L.S., and G. Fernandes, "Serum Cytokine Levels in Autoimmune and Non-Autoimmune Hyperthyroid States" in *Brazilian Journal of Medical Biology Research*, 2000, Jan.; 33(1):65–69.

19. Thyroid Foundation of America, *Causes of Graves' Disease*, TFA web site via the Internet, www.ckark.net or www.tsh.org June, 1999.

20. Op. cit., Beer.

21. Wenzel, B.E., Chow A., et al., "Natural Killer Cell Activity in Patients with Graves' Disease and Hashimoto's Thyroiditis" in *Thyroid*, Nov. 1998; 8(11) 1019–1022.

22. Ahern, Holly, "The Complement System — Defender Against Microbes," *Advance for Medical Laboratory Professionals*, Vol.10, No. 2, January 19, 1998, 20–26.

23. *Life Extension* staff, "The Immune System," in *Life Extension*, Vol. 5(12), December 1999, 24–25.

24. Hiromatsu, Yuri, et al., "Increased Serum Soluble Fas in Patients with Graves' Disease" in *Thyroid*, 9(4), April 1999, 341–345.

Chapter 3

1. Hoffman, William S., M.D., *The Biochemistry of Clinical Medicine*, 2nd Edition, Chicago, The Year Book Publishers, Inc., 1961, 506.

2. Schwartz, Seymour I., M.D., Editor, *Principles of Surgery*, 7th Edition, Vol. 2, New York, McGraw-Hill, 1999, 1663.

3. Op. cit. Hoffman, 504–505.

4. Op. cit., Brunt, 986.

5. Meissner, William A., *Tumors of the Thyroid Gland*, 4th Fascicle Supplement to the *Atlas of Tumor Pathology*, 2nd Series, Armed Forces Institute of Pathology, Washington D.C., 1984.

6. Carnell N.E., et al., "Thyroid Nodules in Patients with Graves' Disease" in *Thyroid* 8(8), August 1998, 647–652.

7. Ibid.

8. Vogel, H.C.A., M.D., *The Nature Doctor: A Manual of Traditional Complementary Medicine*, English Edition, New York, Instant Improvement, 1991, 158.

9. Ibid., 200–210.

10. Shomon, Mary J., *Living Well With Hypothyroidism, What Your Doctor Doesn't Tell You ... That You Need to Know*, New York, Avon, 2000, 35.

11. Roti, Elio, and Apostolos Vagenakis, "Effects of Excess Iodide: Clinical Aspects" in *Werner and Ingbar's The Thyroid: a Fundamental and Clinical Text*, 7th Ed., Edited by Braverman, Lewis E., and Robert D. Utiger, Philadelphia, Lippincott-Raven, 1996, 324.

12. Woeber, Kenneth, M.D., "Iodine and Thyroid Disease," in *The Medical Clinics of N. America*, Vol. 75(1), *Thyroid Disease*, Edited by Greenspan, Francis, M.D., Jan. 1991, 172.

13. Wood, Lawrence C., M.D., Cooper, David S., M.D., and E. Chester Ridgway, M.D., *Your Thyroid: A Home Reference*, Boston, Houghton Mifflin Company, 1982, 10.

14. Osborne, Sally Eauclaire, "Does Soy Have a Dark Side?" in *Natural Health*, March, 1999; 29(2):110–113.

15. Farwell, Alan P., And Lewis E. Braverman, M.D., "Thyroid and Antithyroid Drugs," In *Goodman & Gilman's The Pharmacological Basis of Therapeutics*, 9th Edition, Edited by Hardman, Joel G., and Lee E. Limbird, New York, McGraw-Hill, 1996, 1390.

16. Chopra, Inder J., "Nature, Source, and Relative Significance of Circulating Thyroid Hormones" in *Werner and Ingbar's The Thyroid: a Fundamental and Clinical Text*, 7th Ed., Edited by Braverman, Lewis E., and Robert D. Utiger, Philadelphia, Lippincott-Raven, 1996, 118.

17. Aziz, Douglas C., M.D., Ph.D., *Use and Interpretation of Tests in Endocrinology*, Santa Monica, CA, Specialty Laboratories, 1997, 141.

18. Arky, Ronald, M.D., Editor, *Physicians' Desk Reference*, 51st Edition, Montvale, NJ, Medical Economics Company, Inc., 1997, 1410–12, 2647–8.

19. Op. cit., De Groot.

20. Harris, S., and K. Goodfellow, *Your Thyroid, What It Does, and What Happens When It Goes Wrong*, International Thyroid Group, 1998 via the Internet.

21. Op. cit., Chopra, 120.

22. Nicoloff, John, and Jonathan LoPresti, "Nonthyroidal Illness" in *Werner and Ingbar's The Thyroid: a Fundamental and Clinical Text*, 7th Ed., Edited by Braverman, Lewis E., and Robert D. Utiger, Philadelphia, Lippincott-Raven, 1996, 286–293.

23. Snyder, Peter, J., "The Pituitary in Thyrotoxicosis" in *Werner and Ingbar's The Thyroid: a Fundamental and Clinical Text*, 7th Ed., Edited by Braverman, Lewis E., and Robert D. Utiger, Philadelphia, Lippincott-Raven, 1996, 653.

24. Op. cit., De Groot

25. Durrant-Peatfield, Barry J., M.D., *The Role of Endocrines in M.E.*, International Thyroid Group web site via the Internet, 1990.

26. Op. cit., Colborn, 85.

27. Vliet, Elizabeth Lee, M.D., *Screaming to Be Heard, Hormonal Connections Women Suspect ... And Doctors Ignore*, New York, M. Evans and Company, 1995, 57–61.

28. Taurog, Alvin, "Hormone Synthesis" in *Werner and Ingbar's The Thyroid: A*

Fundamental and Clinical Text, 7th Edition, edited by Braverman, Lewis E., and Robert D. Utiger, Philadelphia, Lippincott-Raven Publishers, 1996, 49–73.

29. Op. cit., Larsen, 459.

30. Op. cit., De Groot.

31. Singer, Peter A., M.D., "Thyroiditis: Acute, Subacute, and Chronic" in *The Medical Clinics of N. America,* Vol. 75, No. 1, *Thyroid Disease,* edited by Greenspan, Francis, Philadelphia, W.B. Saunders Co., Jan. 1995, 61.

32. Op. cit., Greenspan, 221.

33. Ibid.

34. Op. cit., McDougall, 81.

35. Op. cit., Schwartz, 1674.

36. Op. cit., Larsen, 452–459.

37. Isselbacher, Kurt J., et al., eds., *Harrison's Principles of Internal Medicine,* 13th Edition, McGraw-Hill, New York, 1994, 1942–1943.

38. Op. cit., Arem, 315.

39. Greer, Monte, "Thyrotoxicosis of Extrathyroid Origin" in *Werner and Ingbar's The Thyroid: A Fundamental And Clinical Text,* 7th Edition, Edited by Braverman, Lewis E., And Robert D. Utiger, Philadelphia, Lippincott-Raven, 1996.

40. Op. cit., *Harrison's Principles of Internal Medicine,* 1942.

41. McClatchey, Kenneth D., Editor, *Clinical Laboratory Medicine,* Baltimore, MD, Williams & Wilkins, 1994, 1618–1619.

Chapter 4

1. Op. cit., De Groot.

2. Char, Devron H., M.D., "The Ophthalmopathy of Graves' Disease" in *Medical Clinics of North America,* Vol. 75, No. 1, *The Thyroid,* Edited by Greenspan, Francis, M.D., Philadelphia, W.B. Saunders Co., Jan. 1991, 97–99.

3. Op. cit., Burch, 537.

4. Kennerdell, John, M.D., Pittsburgh, Private correspondence (letter), Sept. 1999.

5. Op. cit., Char, 99

6. Op. cit., Burch, 530–535.

7. Vaidya, Bijayeswar, et al., "Cytotoxic T Lymphocyte Antigen-4 (CTKA-4) Gene Polymorphism Confers Susceptibility to Thyroid Associated Orbitopathy," in *The Lancet,* August 28, 1999, Vol. 354, 743–4.

8. Warwar, R., "New Insights into Pathogenesis and Potential Therapeutic Options for Graves Orbitopathy," in *Current Opinions in Ophthalmology,* 1999 October; 10(5):358–61.

9. Op. cit, Burch, 540–542.

10. Op. cit., Burch, 542.

11. Op. cit., Char, 100.

12. Ibid.

13. Ibid., 101.

14. Ibid., 99.

15. Op. cit, Brunt, 987.

16. Bartalena, L., et al., "Effect of the Treatment Method of Hyperthyroidism on the Course of Graves' Eye Disease" in *New England Journal of Medicine,* 1998 January, 338(2):73–8.

17. Op. cit., Wawar, 359.

18. Mack, W.P., et al., "The Effect of Cigarette Smoke Constituents on the Expression of HLA-DR in Orbital Fibroblasts Derived from Patients with Graves Ophthalmophathy," in *Ophthalmology and Plastic Reconstructive Surgery,* 1999 July; 15(4): 260–271.

19. Fitzgerald, Paul, M.D., 350 Parnassus Ave., San Francisco, CA 94117, (415) 665-1136, "Graves' Disease," via the Internet, *Breaking News.*

20. Mouritis, Maarten, et al., "Radiotherapy for Graves' Orbitopathy: Randomised Placebo-Controlled Study," in *The Lancet*, April 29, 2000, Vol. 355, 1505-1509.

21. Kennerdell, John S., M.D., and Anna Tyutyunikov, M.D., Ph.D., *Graves' Opththalmopathy — What Is It?* Bulletin #36, National Graves' Disease Foundation, Brevard, 1995.

22. Op. cit., Mouritis, 1505.

23. Op cit. Mikkelsen, 8.

24. Soparkar, Charles, M.D., et al., "Thyroid Eye Disease–Surgical Options" in *Thyroid USA*, a publication of the American Foundation of Thyroid Patients, Vol. 6(8), Oct.-Nov.-Dec. 1999, 1.

25. Ibid., 2.

26. Ibid.

27. Ibid.

28. Op. cit., Burch, 546–548.

29. Ibid.

30. Op. cit., Greenspan, 223.

31. Fatourechi, Vahab, "Localized Myxedema and Thyroid Acropachy," in *Werner and Ingbar's The Thyroid: a Fundamental and Clinical Text*, 7th Edition, edited by Braverman, Lewis E., and Robert D. Utiger, Philadelphia, Lippincott-Raven, 1996, 553–556.

32. Ibid.

33. Ibid.

34. Ibid., 557.

35. Op. cit., McDougall, 93.

36. Bystryn, Jean-Claude, M.D., *Questions and Answers about Vitiligo*, by the National Vitiligo Foundation, fact sheet, Jan. 1997, from the National Arthritis and Muculoskeletal and Skin Diseases Information Clearinghouse, through the National Institutes of Health.

37. Ibid.

38. Op cit., Fatourechi, 557.

39. Ibid., 553.

40. Ibid., 557.

Chapter 5

1. Op. cit., Arem, 238.

2. Regalbuto, C., Salamone, C., et al., "Appearance of Anti TSH-Receptor Antibodies and Clinical Graves' Disease after Radioiodine Therapy for Hyperfunctioning Thyroid Adenoma" In *Journal of Endocrinol Invest*, 1999 Feb.; 22(2):147–150.

3. Op. cit., De Groot.

4. Schwid, S.R., et al., "Autoimmune Hyperthyroidism in Patients with Multiple Sclerosis Treated with Interferon beta-1b," *Archives of Neurology*, 1997 Sept.; 54(9): 1169–1190.

5. Giani, Claudio, Bonacci, Rosna and Paola Fierabracci, "Endocrine and Non Endocrine Diseases Associated with Thyroid Disorders," in *Electronic Journal of Surgery*, 1996 1:5–7.

6. Goldman, Arlene, "Thyroid Diseases and Breast Cancer" in *Epidemiologic Reviews*, the Johns Hopkins University School of Hygiene and Public Health, Vol. 12, 1990, 16–28.

7. Op. cit., Locke, 49–50.

8. Rosenthal, M. Sarah, *The Thyroid Sourcebook*, 3rd edition, Los Angeles: Lowell House, 1998, 60.

9. Scriver, Charles, et al., Editors, *The Metabolic and Molecular Bases of Inherited Disease*, 7th Edition, Volume II, New York, McGraw-Hill, 1995, 2887–2890.

10. Op. cit., Greenspan, 225.

11. Op. cit., Larsen, 441.

12. Op. cit., Henry, 316.

13. Leavelle, Dennis, M.D., Editor, *Mayo Medical Laboratories Interpretive Handbook*, Rochester, Mayo Medical Laboratories, 1997, 492.

14. Fisher,Delbert A., M.D., ed., *The Quest Diagnostics Manual: Endocrinology Test Selection and Interpretation*, 2nd ed., 1998, Quest Diagnostics, Inc., Teterbore, NJ, 169.

15. Weiss, Ronald L., M.D., *ARUP Interpretative Guide*, Salt Lake, Associated Regional & University Pathologists, Inc., 1998, 494.

16. Op. cit., Aziz, 145.

17. Op. cit., Leavelle, 490.

18. Op. cit., Aziz, 146.

19. Ibid.

20. Op. cit., Weiss, 484.

21. Op. cit., Fisher, 248.

22. Scanlon, Maurice F., and Anthony D. Toft, "Regulation of Thyrotropin Secretion," in *Werner and Ingbar's The Thyroid: a Fundamental and Clinical Text*, 7th Ed., Edited by Braverman, Lewis E., and Robert D. Utiger, Philadelphia, Lippincott-Raven, 1996, 229.

23. Op. cit., Leavelle, 504–505.

24. Ibid., 253.

25. Op. cit., Aziz, 149.

26. Op. cit., Henry, 319.

27. Op. cit., Aziz, 149.

28. Ibid.

29. McLachlan, Sandra, and Basil Rapoport, "Genetic Factors in Thyroid Disease" in *Werner and Ingbar's The Thyroid*, 7th Edition, Edited by Braverman, Lewis E., and Robert D. Utiger, Lippincott-Raven, Philadelphia, 1996, 483.

30. Op. cit., Fisher, 169.

31. Op. cit. Aziz, 150–151.

32. Ibid., 150.

33. Ibid., 310.

34. Bayer, Monika, M.D, "Effective Laboratory Evaluation of Thyroid Status," in *The Medical Clinics of North America, Thyroid Disease;* 75 (1) Edited by Francis Greenspan, M.D., Philadelphia, W.B. Saunders, 1991, 1–11.

35. Op. cit., Henry, 315–320.

36. Ibid.

37. Ibid.

38. McCowen, K.C., et al., "Elevated Serum Thyrotropin in Thyroxine-Treated Patients with Hypothyroidism Given Sertraline," in *The New England Journal of Medicine*, 1997, Oct. 2; 337(14):1010–1011.

39. Op. cit., De Groot

40. Op. cit., Larsen, 415–430.

41. Fatourechi, Vahab, M.D., "Autoimmune Thyroid Disease," in *Postgraduate Medicine*, Jan. 2000, 7(1) 128–135.

42. Op. cit., Larsen, 415–430.

43. Ibid.

44. Ibid., 410–411.

45. Gofman, John W., M.D., *Radiation & Human Health*, San Francisco, Sierra Club Books, 1991.

46. Maxon, Harry R., and Eugene L. Saenger, "Biologic Effects of Radioiodine on the Human Thyroid Gland" in *Werner and Ingbar's The Thyroid: a Fundamental and Clinical Text*, 7th Edition, Edited by Braverman, Lewis E., and Robert D. Utiger, Philadelphia, Raven-Lippincott, 1996, 342–351.

47. Ibid., 334.

48. Wilson, Michael A., *Textbook of Nuclear Medicine*, Philadelphia, Lippincott-Raven, 1998, 163–166.

49. Jennings, Anthony S., "Non-isotopic Techniques for Imaging the Thyroid" in *Werner and Ingbar's The Thyroid: a Fundamental and Clinical Text*, 7th Edition, Edited by Braverman, Lewis E., and Robert D. Utiger, Philadelphia, Raven-Lippincott, 1996, 433–440.

50. Ibid.

Chapter 6

1. Eisenbarth, George, and Luis Castano, "Diabetes Mellitus" in *Samter's Immunologic Diseases*, 5th Edition, Vol. 2, Edited by Michael Frank, M.D., Little, Brown and Company, New York, 1995, 1007–1032.

2. Ibid., 1015.

3. Maugendre, D., et al., "Antipancreatic Autoimmunity and Graves' Disease: Study of a Cohort of 600 Caucasian Patients" in *European Journal of Endocrinology*, Nov. 1997; 137(5):503–510.

4. Silvergerg, J., and R. Volpe, "Rheumatoid Factors in Graves' Disease," *Annals of Internal Medicine*, 1978; 88:216.

5. Fantry, George, and Stephen James, "Immunology of Hepatobiliary Diseases" in *Samter's Immunologic Diseases*, 5th Edition, Vol. 2, Edited by Michael Frank, M.D., Little, Brown and Company, New York, 1995, 1130–1133.

6. *Primary Biliary Cirrhosis*, publication of the American Autoimmune Related Diseases Association, Inc., East Detroit, MI, 1994.

7. Hoffbuer, Lorenz C., M.D., Spitzweg, Christine, M.D., et al., "Graves' Disease Associated with Autoimmune Thrombocytopenic Purpura," in *Archives of Internal Medicine*, 1997; 157:1033–1036.

8. Vivino, Frederick, M.D., "Diagnosis and Treatment of Sjögren's Syndrome," in *The Female Patient*, Vol. 24, August '99, 65–68.

9. Op. cit., Weiss, 596.

10. Op. cit., De Groot.

11. Op. cit., Larsen, 495.

Chapter 7

1. Weetman, Anthony, "Chronic Autoimmune Thyroiditis," in *Werner and Ingbar's The Thyroid: a Fundamental and Clinical Text*, 7th Ed., Edited by Braverman, Lewis E., and Robert D. Utiger, Lippincott-Raven, Philadelphia, 1996, 739.

2. Op. cit., Larsen, 426–502.

3. Ibid., 431.

4. Op. cit., Isselbacher, 1942.

5. Op. cit., Davies, 525–536.

6. Brix, T.H., and L. Kyvik KO, Hegedus "What Is the Evidence of Genetic Factors in the Etiology of Graves' Disease?" *Thyroid*, August 8, 1998.

7. "Seeking the Genes for Thyroid Disease, More Families Needed for Genetic Studies," reprinted in *Thyroid USA*, publication of the American Foundation of Thyroid Patients, April-May-June, 2000.

8. Davies, Terry F., M.D., "Graves' Disease," in *Werner and Ingbar's The Thyroid: a Fundamental and Clinical Text*, 525–536.

9. Jaspan, Jonathan, et al., "The Interaction of a Type A Retroviral Particle and Class II Human Leukocyte Antigen Susceptibility Genes in the Pathogenesis of Graves' Disease" in *The Journal of Clinical Endocrinology & Metabolism*, 1996, June; 81(6): 2271–2279.

10. "Can Food Bug Cause Arthritis," excerpt from original article in *Nature Medicine* in *In Focus*, publication of the American Autoimmune Related Diseases Association, Inc., Vol. 8(1), March 2000.

11. Op. cit., Davies, 525–536.

12. Ibid.

13. Op. cit., Brunt, 976.

14. Rose, Noel, et al., "Linking Iodine with Autoimmune Thyroiditis" in *Environmental Health Perspectives*, Volume 107, Supplement 5, October 1999.

15. Op. cit., Sato, 1904–1909.

16. Ibid., 977.

17. Op. cit., Davies, 525–536.

18. Op.cit., Colborn, 63.

19. Ibid. 81.

20. Op. cit., Brunt, 977.

Chapter 8

1. Sugino, K., et al., "Postoperative Changes in Thyrotroppin-Binding Inhibitory Immunoglobulin Level in Patients with Graves' Disease: Is Subtotal Thyroidectomy a Suitable Therapeutic Option for Patients of Childbearing Age with Graves' Disease?" in World Journal of Surgery, 1999, July; 23(7):727–731.

2. Op. cit., Larsen, 449.

3. Op. cit., Greenspan, 226.

4. Farwell, Alan, and Lewis E. Braverman, "Thyroid and Antithyroid Drugs," in Goodman and Gilman's *The Pharmacological Basis of Therapeutics*, 9th ed., Health Professions Div. McGraw-Hill, edited by Joel E. Aardman, New York, 1996, 1398.

5. Op. cit., Larsen, 443.

6. Cooper, David, "Treatment of Thyrotoxicosis" in Werner and Ingbar's The Thyroid: a Fundamental and Clinical Text, 7th Ed., Edited by Braverman, Lewis E., and Robert D. Utiger, Lippincott-Raven, Philadelphia, 1996, 717.

7. Op. cit., Larsen, 443.

8. Rakel, Robert E., M.D., Editor, Conn's Current Therapy, W.B. Saunders, Philadelphia, 1999, 657.

9. Op. cit., Cooper, 717.

10. "The 8th Report on Carcinogens 1998 Summary," reported in U.S. Dept. Of Health & Human Services—Public Health Service National Toxicology Program.

11. Arem, Ridha, M.D., "What's New in Thyroid Disease" in Thyroid USA, publication of the American Foundation of Thyroid Patients, Volume 6(6), April-May-June, 1999, 3–4.

12. Yamamoto, M., et al., "Outcome of Patients with Graves' Disease After Long-Term Medical Treatment Guided by Triiodothyronine (T3) Suppression Test," in Clinical Endocrinology (1983) 19, 467–476.

13. Op. cit., Larsen, 444.

14. Op. cit., Langer, 31.

15. Op. cit., Cooper, 718.

16. Op. cit., Farwell, 1400.

17. Op. cit., Larsen, 444.

18. Ibid.

19. Op. cit., Cooper, 720.

20. Op. cit., Schwartz, 1673.

21. Ibid., 1674.

22. Ibid.

23. Op. cit., Larsen, 446.

24. Op. cit., Schwartz, 1673.

25. Op. cit., Larsen, 440–450.

26. Pacer, John, Ph.D., personal communication, April, 2000.

27. Burger, Joanna, "Ionizing Ratiation," in Environmental Medicine, edited by Brooks, Stuart, M.D., Mosby-Year Book, St. Louis, MO, 1995, 527–540.

28. Ibid., 528.

29. Gong, J.K., "A Lifelong, Wide-Range Radiation Biodosimeter: Erythrocytes with Transferrin Receptors," State University of New York at Buffalo, Occupational and Environmental Safety Services, Health Physics, December 1999; 77(6) 713.

30. Op. cit., Cooper, 724–725.

31. Gong, Joseph, Ph.D., Occupational and Environmental Safety Services, State University of New York at Buffalo, NY, private correspondence with author February, March, 2000.

32. Beir, V., Health Effects of Exposure to Low Levels of Ionizing Radiation, National Research Council publication, National Academy Press, Washington, D.C., 1990.

36. Conway, Carolyn, "Radiation Carcinogenic Even Without Hitting Cell Nucleus" in UniSci Science and Research News, via the Internet, 27 April, 1999.

34. Schlichtman, James, M.D., and Mark A. Graber, M.D., "Hematologic, Electrolyte, and Metabolic Disorders: Hyperthyroidism" in University of Iowa Family Practice Handbook, 3rd Edition, Chapter 5 via the Internet, Virtual Hospital.

35. Bajnok, L. et al., "Calculation of the Radioiodine Dose for the Treatment of Graves' Hyperthyroidism: Is More than Seven-Thousand Rad Target Dose Necessary?" in Thyroid, 1999, September; 9(9):865–869.

36. Op. cit., Wilson, 163.

37. Op. cit., Felz, Part 2, 51.

38. Op. cit., Larsen, 448.

39. Ibid., 449.

40. Franklyn, J.A. et al., "Cancer Incidence and Mortality after Radioiodine Treatment for Hyperthyroidism: a Population-Based Cohort Study" in Lancet, 1999 June 19; 353(9170):2111–2115.

41. Franklyn, J.A. et al., "Mortality after the Treatment of Hyperthyroidism with Radioactive Iodine" in The New England Journal of Medicine, March 12, 1998, Vol. 338 (11), 712–718.

42. Op. cit., Ron, 353.

43. Op. cit., Cooper, 724.

44. Chiovatoe, L., et al., "Outcome of Thyroid Function in Graves' Patients Treated with Radioiodine: Role of Thyroid-Stimulating and Thyrotropin-Blocking Antibodies and of Radioiodine-Induced Thyroid Damage" in Journal of Clinical Endocrinology and Metabolism, Vol. 83, No. 1, 1988, 40–46.

45. Op. cit., Larsen, 448.

46. Ibid., 448.

47. Prakash P. et al., "Localization of Radioiodine in the Tissues of Swine: An Autoradiographic Study," in Acta Histochem, 1976; 57(2):282–90, Medline abstract via the Internet.

48. Ibid.

49. Ron, Elaine, et al., "Cancer Mortality Following Treatment for Adult Hyperthyroidism," in JAMA, July 22/29, 1998,Vol. 280(4):347–365.

50. Op. cit., Brunt, 987.

51. Op. cit., Greenspan, 226.

52. Op. cit., Larsen, 446.

53. Op. cit., Brunt, 987.

54. Op. cit., Felz, Part 2.

55. Op. cit., Farwell, 1401.

56. Op. cit., Larsen, 445.

57. Op. cit., Arky, 2837.

58. Yamano, Y., et al., "Differences between Changes in Serum Thyrotropin-Binding Inhibitory Antibodies and Thyroid-Stimulating Antibodies in the Course of Antithyroid Drug Therapy for Graves' Disease" in Thyroid, 1999 August; 9(8):769–773.

59. Paggi, A., et al., "Methimazole Treatment in Graves' Disease: Behaviour of CD5+B Lymphocytes and Regulatory T Cell Subsets" in European Review of Medicine and Pharmacology Science, 1998 January-February; 2(1):11–19.

60. Chung, H.K., et al., "Two Graves' Disease Patients who Spontaneously Developed Hypothyroidism after Antithyroid Drug Treatment: Characteristics of Epitopes for Thyrotropin Receptor Antibodies" in Thyroid 1999 April; 9(4):393–399.

61. Op. cit., Chiovatoe, 45.

62. Nakazato, N., "Antithyroid Drugs Inhibit Radioiodine-Induced Increases in Thyroid Autoantibodies in Hyperthyroid Graves' Disease" in Thyroid, 1999 Aug.; 9(8):775–779.

63. Op. cit., Sugino.

64. Ljunggren, J.G., et al., "Quality of Life Aspects and Costs in Treatment of Graves' Hyperthyroidism with Antithyroid Drugs, Surgery, or Radioiodine: Results from a Prospective Randomized Study" in Thyroid, 1998 Aug.; 8(8):653–659.

65. Pineda, G., et al., "Treatment of Basedow–Graves' Hyperthyroidism: retrospective analysis after 30 years," *Revista Medica de Chile*, Aug. 1998, 126(8): 953–962.

Chapter 9

1. Kroening, Richard J., et al. "Acupuncture: Healing the Whole Person" in *Dimensions in Wholistic Healing, New Frontiers in the Treatment of the Whole Person*, edited by Otto, Herbert A., Ph.D., and James W. Knight, M.D., Nelson-Hall, Inc., Chicago, 1979, 427–439.

2. Op cit., Farwell, 1402.

3. Op cit., Cooper, 721.

4. Op cit., Woeber, 174.

5. Op cit, Farwell, 1402.

6. Op cit, Cooper, 721.

7. Ibid.

8. *An A-to-Z Guide to Common Ailments and Their Best Treatments*, Rodale Press, 1999, 229.

9. Blumenthal, Mark, editor, *The Complete German Commission E Monographs Therapeutic Guides to Herbal Medicine*, The American Botanical Council in cooperation with Intergrative Medicine Communications, Boston, 1998, 683.

10. Op cit., Vogel, 155–65.

11. "What's New in Thyroid Disease" in *Thyroid USA*, newsletter of the American Foundation of Thyroid Patients, Jan.-Feb.-March, 2000, 3.

12. Clovatre, Dallas, Ph.D., "Immunomodulators: The Best Ways to Balance Your Immune System" in *Let's Live*, June, 1999, 49–51.

13. Duffy, William, *You Are All Sanpaku*, English Version of original text by Sakurazawa Nyoiti (George Oshawa), Citadel Press, Secaucus, New Jersey, 1965, 109–111.

14. Ibid., 160–1.

15. Weil, Andrew, M.D., *Spontaneous Healing*, Alfred A. Knopf, New York, 1995, 255.

16. Seachrist, Lisa, "Food for Healing, Oral Tolerance Therapy Aims to Neutralize Autoimmune Diseases," in *Science News*, Sept. 2, 2995, Vol. 148, 158–159.

17. Ibid.

18. Op. cit., Weil, 459.

19. Zevin, Igor Vilevcich, *A Russian Herbal, Traditional Remedies for Health and Healing*, Healing Arts Press, Rochester, 1997, 6.

20 "Acute Hepatitis after Ingestion of Herbs" in *Southern Medical Journal*, 1999, 92(11), article reprint courtesy of Medscape, via the Internet, March, 2000.

21. Ibid., ix, x.

22. Sullivan, Karin Horgan, "Herb Do's and Don'ts" in *Natural Health*, January/February 2000, 97–99.

23. Ibid., 99.

24. *PDR for Herbal Medicine*, Medical Economics Company, Montvale, New Jersey, 1998, 950.

25. Ibid., 969.

26. Op. cit., *PDR for Herbal Medicine*, 1015.

27. Op. cit., Rister, 234.

28. *Life Extension* staff, "Can Silibinin Arrest Cancer Cell Growth," in Life Extension, June, 2000, 27–34.

29. Ibid.

30. Op. cit., Blumenthal, 279.

31. Op. cit., Rister, 234–236.

32. Zha, L.L., "Therapeutic Effect and Its Mechanism Exploration on Mainly Using Traditional Chinese Medicine of Replenishing Qi and Nourishing Yin in Treating Graves' Disease," PubMed abstract of article in *Chung Kuo Chung Hsi I Chieh Ho Tsa Chih*, 1997 June; 17(6):328–330.

33. Op. cit., Hyatt, 75.

34. Ibid.

35. Ibid.

36. Petri, Mary, private correspondence, January 2000.

37. Block, Betsy, "Jiaogulan" in *Natural Health*, November, December, 1999, 41.

38. Blackey, Margery G., *The Patient Not the Cure, the Challenge of Homeopathy*, Woodridge Press Publishing Company, 1978, 7–9.

39. Ballentine, Rudolph, M.D., *Radical Healing*, New York: Harmony Books, 1999, 517.

40. Lockie, Andrew, M.D., and Dr. Nicola Geddes, *The Complete Guide to Homeopathy*, DK Publishing, New York, 1995, 131.

41. Op. cit., Vogel, 424.

42. Ibid, 400.

43. Op. cit., Ballentine, 518.

44. Thakkur, Chandrasekhar G., "Ayurvedic Medicine, Past, Present and Future" in Dimensions in *Wholistic Healing, New Frontiers in the Treatment of the Whole Person*, edited by Otto, Herbert A., Ph.D., and James W. Knight, M.D., Nelson-Hall, Inc., Chicago, 1979, 475–487.

45. Fleischmann, Gary, *Acupuncture: Everything You Ever Wanted to Know*, Barrytown, Ltd., Barrytown, New York, 1998, 61.

46. "Can the Needles Injure You?" in *Health*, April, 2000, 24.

47. Stoll, Walt, M.D., *Saving Yourself from the Disease-Care Crisis*, Sunrise Health Coach, Panama City, FL, 1996.

48. "Emotions and Health, Can Stress Make You Sick" in *Harvard Health Letter*, 23, (6) April, 1998. 1–3.

49. Op. cit., Locke, 113–4.

50. "Supporting the Immune System," in *Healthy Talk*, a publication of the Vitamin Shoppe, December, 1997, 3.

51. Op. cit., Ward, 65–69.

52. Op. cit., Weil, 227–228.

53. O'Brien, Tricia, "Does This Sound Like You?" in *Country Living's Healthy Living*, March/April, 1999, 48–49.

54. Asphar, Judith, et al., ""Healers for the New Millenium," in *Country Living's Healthy Living*, Nov/Dec, 1999, 85.

Chapter 10

1. Basaria, S. and Cooper, D.S., "Graves' Disease and Recurrent Ectopic Thyroid Tissue," *Thyroid*, Dec 99, vol. 12:1261–1264.

2. Ibid.

3. Emerson, Charles, "Thyroid Disease During and After Pregnancy," in *Werner and Ingbar's The Thyroid: a Fundamental and Clinical Text*, 7th Ed., Edited by Braverman, Lewis E., and Robert D. Utiger, Lippincott-Raven, Philadelphia, 1996, 1021.

4. Ibid., 1023.

5. Op. cit., Aziz, 143.

6. Op. cit., Emerson, 1023.

7. Ibid., 1028.

8. Op. cit., Larsen, 457.

9. Op. cit., Emerson, 1029.

10. Ibid., 1028.

11. Ibid.

12. Op. cit., Larsen, 450.

13. Op. cit., Beer.

14. Ibid.

15. Op. cit., Emerson, 1025.

16. Op. cit., Larsen, 450.

17. Ibid., 451.

18. Ochoa-Maya, M.R., et al., "Resolution of Fetal Goiter after Discontinuation of Propylthiouracil in a Pregnant Woman with Graves' Hyperthyroidism," in *Thyroid*, 1999, Nov; 9(11):1111–1114.

19. Op. cit., Arky, 2837.

20. Ibid.

21. Becks, Gregory, M.D., *Thyroid Disorders and Pregnancy*, Thyroid Foundation of America publication, via the Internet, www.tfaweb.org/pub/tfa.

22. Op. cit., Emerson, 1024.

23. Op. cit., Larsen, 473.

24. Op. cit., Emerson, 1027.

25. Ibid.

26. Ibid.

27. Behrman, Richard, M.D., Kliegman, Robert, M.D., and Hal Jenson, M.D., *Nelson Textbook of Pediatrics*, 16th Edition, W.B. Saunders, Philadelphia, PA, 2000, 1709–1712.

28. Ibid.

29. Ibid.

30. Op. cit., Emerson, 1024.

31. Fisher, Delbert, "Thyroid Physiology in the Perinatal Period and During Childhood" in *Werner and Ingbar's The Thyroid: a Fundamental and Clinical Text*, 7th Ed., Edited by Braverman, Lewis E., and Robert D. Utiger, Lippincott-Raven, Philadelphia, 1996, 978.

32. Fisher, D.A., "Fetal Thyroid Function: Diagnosis and Mangement of Fetal Thyroid Disorders," in *Clinical Obstetrics and Gynecology*, 1997 March; 40(1):16–31.

33. Pacer, Scott, M.D., personal correspondence with author, April 2000.
34. Op. cit., Behrman.
35. Hay, William, M.D., et al., *Current Pediatric Diagnosis and Treatment, a Lange Medical Book*, 14th Edition, Appleton & Lange, Stamford, CT, 1994, 824–827.
36. Op. cit., Felz, Part 1, 59.
37. Op. cit., Behrman.
38. Op. cit., Segni, 871–877.
39. Ibid.
40. Op. cit., Behrman.
41. Ibid.
42. Ibid.
43. Ibid.
44. Ibid.
45. Op. cit., Larsen, 451.
46. Favus, M.J., et al., "Thyroid Cancer Occurring as a Late Consequence of Head and Neck Irradiations" in *New England Journal of Medicine*, 1976, 294:1019–1025.
47. Upton, Arthur, "Ionizing Radiation," in *Environmental and Occupational Medicine*, 3rd Ed., Edited by William Rom, Lippincott-Raven, Philadelphia, 1998, 1293.
48. Op. cit., Larsen, 451.
49. Op. cit., Behrman.

Chapter 11

1. Berger, Daniel, M.D., and Inder Chopra, M.D., "Hypothyroidism" in *Conn's Current Therapy*, Edited by Robert E. Rakel, M.D., W.B. Saunders, Philadelphia, 1999, 651.
2. Broda Barnes, M.D., Ph.D., "Profile of a Brilliant Doctor," publication of the International Thyroid Group, Spring, 1996.
3. Ansell, Jack E., "The Blood in Hypothyroidism" in *Werner and Ingbar's The Thyroid: a Fundamental and Clinical Text*, 7th Ed., Edited by Braverman, Lewis E., and Robert D. Utiger, Lippincott-Raven, Philadelphia, 1996, 821.
4. Op. cit., Larsen, 464.
5. Ibid.
6. DeLong, G. Robert, "The Neuromuscular System and Brain in Hypothyroidism" in *Werner and Ingbar's The Thyroid: a Fundamental and Clinical Text*, 7th Ed., Edited by Braverman, Lewis E., and Robert D. Utiger, Lippincott-Raven, Philadelphia, 1996, 826–835.
7. Op. cit., Larsen, 463.
8. Witteman, Jacqueline, M.D., et al., "Thyroid Problems Up Heart Attack Risk in Elderly Women," Reuters Health excerpt of article appearing in *Annals of Internal Medicine*, February 15, 2000.
9. Op. cit., Larsen, 465.
10. Op. cit., Arem, 169–171.
11. Ibid.
12. Wartofshky, Leonard, "Myxedema Coma," in *Werner and Ingbar's The Thyroid: a Fundamental and Clinical Text*, 7th Ed., Edited by Braverman, Lewis E., and Robert D. Utiger, Lippincott-Raven, Philadelphia, 1996, 871.
13. Bodmer, Kerri, and Nan Fuchs, Ph.D., *The Giant Book of Women's Health Secrets*, Soundview Publications, Atlanta, GA, 1998, 119.
14. Op. cit., Berger, 653.
15. Ladenson, Paul, "Diagnosis of Hypothyroidism," in *Werner and Ingbar's The Thyroid: a Fundamental and Clinical Text*, 7th Ed., Edited by Braverman, Lewis E., and Robert D. Utiger, Lippincott-Raven, Philadelphia, 1996, 879.

16. Mercola, Joseph, M.D. "Optimum Diagnosis and Treatment of Hypothyroidism with Free T3 and FT4 Levels," Optimal Wellness Center, www.mercola.com/1999Feb/14/hypothyroidism.treatment.htm.

17. Op. cit., Larsen, 472.

18. Op. cit., Arem, 289.

19. Op. cit., Larsen, 445.

20. Op. cit., Mercola

21. Op. cit., Larsen, 472.

22. Vunevicius, Robertas, "Effects of Thyroxine as Compared with Thyroxine plus Triiodothyronine in patients with Hypothyroidism," in *New England Journal of Medicine*, February 11, 1999; 340(6).

23. Op. cit., Berger, 654.

24. Op. cit., Larsen, 472.

25. Ibid.

26. Lepore, Don, *The Ultimate Healing System*, Woodland Books, Provo, UT, 1988, 244–246.

27. Op. cit., Langer, 29.

28. Monte, Tom, *The Complete Guide to Natural Healing*, Berkley Publishing Company, New York, 1997, 364–367.

29. Ibid.

Resources

Conventional Medicine Resources

Advance for Medical Laboratory Professionals, www.ADVANCEforMLP.com
Bimonthly journal dealing with advances in laboratory testing.

Arem, Ridha, M.D., *The Thyroid Solution, A Mind-Body Program for Beating Depression and Regaining Your Emotional and Physical Health*, New York, Ballantine Books, 1999. Written by an endocrinologist, this book focuses on the emotional aspects of thyroid disease.

Barnes, Broda, M.D. and Lawrence Galton, *Hypothyroidism: The Unsuspected Illness*, New York, Harper & Row, 1976. This book explains how thyroid disorders often escape diagnosis when laboratory tests are used as the sole diagnostic criteria and describes the Barnes Basal Temperature Test as a diagnostic tool.

Baskin, H. Jack, M.D., *How Your Thyroid Works*, 3rd ed., Chicago, Adams Press, 1991. This book provides a good introduction to basic thyroid function.

British Medical Journal, www.bmj.com. Prestigious United Kingdom medical journal; web site offers some full-text articles.

Colborn, Theo, Dumanoski, Dianne, and John Peterson Myers, *Our Stolen Future, Are We Threatening Our Fertility, Intelligence, and Survival? A Scientific Detective Story*, New York, Penguin Publishing, 1997.

CPMC — Thyroid Center, *cpmcnet.columbia.edu/dept/thyroid/.* This site provides information on thyroid cancer, thyroid disease, and parathyroid disease, provided by Columbia Presbyterian Medical Center. Referrals available.

Fagin, Dan, Lavelle, Marianne, and The Center for Public Integrity, *Toxic Deception*, 2nd, Ed. Monroe, Maine, Common Courage Press, 1997.

Hypoparathyroidism Newsletter, Inc., www.hypoparathyroidism.com/default.asp. This quarterly educational newsletter published by a patient has evolved into an international publication for patients with hypoparathyroid disorders. Hypoparathyroidism occasionally occurs in association with GD or as a consequence of its treatment. 2835 Salmon, Idaho Falls, ID 83406, Telephone: (208) 524-3857

INFOCUS, Quarterly newsletter of the American Autoimmune Related Diseases Association, Inc. (AARDA) provides a wealth of information on autoimmune disease that is not easily obtainable elsewhere. Recent issues have included articles on the association of salmonella with autoimmune disease, clinical trials, research registries and opportunities for patients with various autoimmune conditions, and new treatments for Raynaud's syndrome. Although this organization focuses on a large number of autoimmune diseases, I've found articles of value to Graves' patients in every issue I've received.

Journal of the American Medical Association (JAMA), www.ama-assn.org/issues/ current/toc.html

Journal of Clinical Endocrinology and Metabolism. Monthly medical journal revolving around current endocrinology issues. *http://jcem.endojournals.org/*

The Kelly G. Ripken Program at Johns Hopkins, *thyroid-ripken.med.jhu.edu/* The Kelly G. Ripken Program is a patient education program at Johns Hopkins where patients and families with thyroid disorders or concerns can receive information about thyroid disorders and arrange for thyroid screening tests.

Krimsky, Sheldon, *Hormonal Chaos, The Scientific and Social Origins of the Environmental Endocrine Hypothesis*, Baltimore, Md., Johns Hopkins University Press, 2000.

Lancet Highly esteemed British medical journal.

Langer, Stephen, *Solved, The Riddle of Illness*, New Canaan, Conn., Keats Publishing, 1984. This book provides excellent information on nutrient deficiencies that may induce or exacerbate symptoms of both hypothyroidism and hyperthyroidism.

The Mayo Clinic, *www.mayo.org/*. On this site, thyroid related articles and information on Graves' disease can be assessed through their search engine.

National Institutes of Health *Office of Dietary Supplements, www.dietary-supplements.info.nih.gov/*. This site contains fact sheets on vitamins and minerals.

National Women's Health Information Center, *www.4women.gov/*. This is a basic women's health information site. Office of Women's Health, U.S. Department of Health and Human Services, Toll-free: 1-800-994-WOMAN, New England Journal of Medicine (NEJM), *www.nejm.org/content/index. asp*

NGDF News, Quarterly publication of the National Graves' Disease Foundation, offers tips on dealing with eye and hair changes, news about the foundation's educational conventions and basic information geared toward the newly diagnosed Graves' patient. The NGDF also provides a number of excellent informational bulletins on topics related to Graves' hyperthyroidism and GO. Six free bulletins are available to new and renewed memberships, and some lengthier bulletins are also available for a nominal fee.

PubMed, the National Library of Medicine's search service that provides access to over 10 million citations in Medline Plus, Medline, and other related databases, with links to participating on-line journals. Articles can also be located through Medscape's Diabetes and Endocrine subsection, *www.medscape.com.* or through Medline database via the National Library of Medicine, *www.ncbi. nlm.nih.gov/PubMed/*

Rom, William, M.D., M.P.H., Editor, *Environmental & Occupational Medicine*, 3rd ed., Philadelphia, Lippincott-Raven, 1998.

Rosenthal, M. Sarah, *The Thyroid Source Book: Everything You Need to Know,* 3rd ed. Los Angeles, Calif., Lowell House, 1996. This book, written by a thyroid cancer survivor, offers basic information regarding thyroid disorders and their treatment.

Shomon, Mary, *Living Well with Hypothyroidism, What Your Doctor Doesn't Tell You That You Need to Know*, Avon Books, New York, 2000. This book, written by a Hashimoto's thyroiditis patient who is a journalist and thyroid educator, is a must for Graves' patients who have become hypothyroid.

Sticking Out Our Necks, www.thyroid-info.com. Mary Shomon's Free e-mail or paid snail mail newsletter for thyroid patients. This newsletter contains excellent up-to-date information regarding medication interferences, dieting tips, environmental concerns and treatment issues. To subscribe, e-mail news@thyroid-info.com. 1-888-810-9471. Bimonthly subscription version by postal mail, launched in 1999. To receive a free copy by mail, send a stamped (55 cents), self-addressed, #10 size envelope to: Sticking Out Our Necks, Free Issue for Elaine's Readers, P.O. Box 0385, Palm Harbor, FL 34682.

Suite 101 Graves' Disease Site, *www.suite101.com*. This site, which I'm editor of, includes weekly updates regarding current trends in GD research and articles related to the concerns of GD patient.

Thyroid. Medical journal affiliated with the Thyroid Foundation of America; contains conventional thyroid related articles contributed from worldwide sources. Sample issues and subscription information can be found at TFA web site, *www.tsh.org*.

Thyroid Disease Manager *www.thyroidmanager.org*. This site contains a complete thyroid textbook that is frequently updated by its authors, all internationally acclaimed thyroid experts. Although this site is primarily intended for physicians, the chapters relating to Graves' disease contain valuable information relating to both the autoimmune nature of GD and treatment concerns.

Thyroid USA, Quarterly publication of the American Foundation of Thyroid Patients, offers an eclectic blend of current information derived from nutritional and thyroid related article abstracts and interviews. This publication also lists locations where discounted thyroid function laboratory tests are available and presents an overview of pertinent information. Recent topics include ongoing genetic studies that patients with autoimmune thyroid disease can participate in and descriptions of surgical options for patients with Graves' ophthalmopathy.

ThyroWorld, Quarterly publication of the Thyroid Federation International group.

Vliet, Elizabeth Lee, M.D., *Screaming to Be Heard: Hormonal Connections Women Suspect f and Doctors Ignore*, New York, M. Evans & Co., 1995. This book explains how hypothyroidism can occur even when laboratory tests are normal.

Wilson, Jean, Editor, *Williams' Textbook of Endocrinology*, 9th ed., Philadelphia, W.B. Saunders, 1998. Excellent source of GD treatment information.

Woods, Lawrence, M.D., and Chester Ridgway, M.D., *Your Thyroid: A Home Reference*, New York, Ballantine, 1995. This book (available on-line at the Thyroid Foundation of America web site, *www.tsh.org*) offers a general overview of thyroid function in lay terms and provides a good starting point for patients.

Alternative Medicine Resources

Acupuncture.com, *www.acupuncture.com/Referrals/ref2.htm*. This site provides a list of licensed acupuncturists by state.

Alternative Medicine at About.com, *altmedicine.about.com*. This site provides general information about alternative medicine. Within this site, you can search under "thyroid disease" and find links to information on alternative therapy for thyroid disease.

American Botanical Council Online, *www.herbalgram.org/*. This site provides information about the safe and effective use of herbs.

A Woman's Time in Portland, Ore., (503) 222-2322

Ballentine, Rudolph, M.D., *Radical Healing*, New York, Harmony Books, 1999. Author of *Radical Healing*, Dr. Ballentine, an integrative physician, has a background in psychiatry, herbalism, homeopathy and Ayurveda.

Beth Israel Center for Health and Healing in New York City, (212) 420-2496

Blumentahl, Mark, Editor, *The Complete German Commission E Monographs Therapeutic Guides to Herbal Medicine,* Boston, Mass. The American Botanical Council in cooperation with Integrative Medicine Communications, 1998.

Bruce, Eve M.D., Shaman and plastic surgeon. Dr. Bruce conducts workshops on shamanic techniques including dreamwork, psychonavigation and spiritual journeys, and feels there isn't any condition that shamanism can't treat.

Center for Holistic Medicine in New York City, (212)-243-6057

Center for Mind-Body Healing in Washington, D.C., *www.cmbm.org.* (202) 966-7338

The Chopra Center for Well Being in La Jolla, Calif., *www.chopra.com.* (888) 424-6772

Country Living's Healthy Living, www.ccare.hearstmags.com

Dr. Stoll's Health Coach, *www.bcn.net/~stoll.* This site has excellent Graves' disease archives and a very active bulletin board.

Dream Change Coalition in Baltimore, Md., *www.dreamchange.org.* (561) 622-6064

Eleven Eleven Wellness Center in New York City, (212) 255-1800

Gao, Duo, O.M.D., *Chinese Medicine*, New York, Thunder Mouth's Press, 1997.

Gordon, James M.D., Integrative physician and educator. Dr. Gordon is a Harvard trained M.D. and licensed acupuncturist who treats patients suffering from a variety of ailments. Through his center, he presents an ongoing series of 12 week workshops in biofeedback, imagery, meditation and visualization.

Health, www.healthmag.com

Health Central; People's Pharmacy *www.healthcentral.com/peoplespharmacy/ peoplespharmacy.cfm.* This site contains articles, questions and answers, information on the 50 most common herbs, and an archive of newspaper columns.

Herb Med, *www.amfoundation.org/herbmed.htm.* This site contains an electronic database that provides information on herbs.

Hudson, Tori N.D., Naturopathic physician specializing in reproductive health As a leading holistic health practitioner, Ms. Hudson focuses on educating her patients about the variety of natural remedies available to treat common female afflictions. Hudson is author of *Women's Encyclopedia of Natural Medicine*

Institute for Health and Healing in San Francisco, Calif., (415) 202-2562

Kesten, Deborah, Integrative nutritionist. As the former nutrition educator for Dean Ornish, M.D., Ms. Kesten looks beyond food's nutritive content to the way it nourishes the entire body.

Let's Live, www.letsliveonline.com

Life Extension, www.lef.org

Lipman, Frank M.D., L.A.C., Integrative physician specializing in TCM, Dr. Lipman focuses on treating the patient, not the disease, in a holistic practice that provides acupuncture along with nutritional counseling and stress relief.

Lockie, Andrew, M.D., and Dr. Nicola Geddes, *The Complete Guide to Homeopathy*, New York, DK Publishing, 1995.

Merrell, Woodson M.D., L.Ac., Internist and integrative medicine specialist. Dr. Merrell is executive director of the Beth Israel Center for Health and Healing in New York City. This center, which has a clinic and research facility and sponsors outreach and training programs, includes treatments that combine meditation, yoga, acupuncture, herbal remedies and homeopathy with traditional medicine.

Natural Health, www.naturalhealthmag.com

Otto, Herbert A., Ph.D., *Dimensions in Wholistic Healing, New Frontiers in the Treatment of the Whole Person*, Chicago, Ill., Nelson-Hall, Inc., 1979.

Simon, David M.D., Mind/body neurologist. Dr. Simon is the cofounder with Deepak Chopra of the Chopra Center for Well Being and is the clinic's medical director. Simon feels that the traditional role of the physician is not to be all-knowing, but to teach and empower patients so that they can actively participate in the healing process.

Vogel, H.C.A., M.D., *The Nature Doctor: A Manual of Traditional Complementary Medicine*, English Edition, New York, Instant Improvement, 1991.

Yoga Journal, www.yogajournal.com/. 1-800-I-DO-YOGA

National and International Organizations

Accreditation Commission for Acupuncture and Oriental Medicine. This organization can verify which American acupuncture and Oriental Medical schools are accredited. (301)-608-9680.

The American Academy of Medical Acupuncture. This organization provides referrals and requires that its members (all physicians) undergo a minimum of 220 hours of continuing education related to acupuncture.
Telephone: (800) 521-2262

American Association of Clinical Endocrinologists *www.aace.com/indexjava.htm*.
1000 Riverside Ave.; Suite 205
Jacksonville, FL 32204
Telephone: (904) 353-7878; Fax: (904) 353-8185

The American Association of Naturopathic Physicians *www.naturopathic. org/*
2366 Eastlake Avenue East, Suite 322
Seattle, WA 98102
Telephone: 206-323-7610.

The American Association of Oriental Medicine *www.aaom.org/*. This site provides information on locating certified acupuncturists.

American Autoimmune Related Diseases Association (AARDA) *www.aarda. org/*.
This group, founded by a patient, Virginia Ladd, offers a wealth of information on autoimmune disorders. For a nominal fee, this group will send additional informational packets on selected disorders. Annual associate membership dues are $30; membership includes an excellent quarterly newsletter.
National Office
22100 Gratiot Ave., E.
Detroit, MI 48021.
Telephone: (810) 776-3900

The American Foundation for Thyroid Patients *www.thyroidfoundation.org/*.
Founded by Graves' patient Kelly Hale, this group organizes reduced fee blood tests at local hospitals and sponsors a number of support groups throughout

the country. Contact Kelly Hale at thyroid@flash.net for information regarding setting up a support group in your area. Annual memberships dues are $30, which includes a subscription to the group's excellent informational newsletter, *Thyroid USA*.
18634 North Lyford Dr.
Katy, TX 77449
Telephone: 281-855-6608

American Holistic Health Association *www.ahha.org*. This site offers an on-line referral to holistic doctors who are members of this association.
P.O. Box 17400
Anaheim, CA 92817-7400

American Holistic Medical Association *www.ahmaholistic.com*.
6728 Old McLean Village Drive
McLean, VA 22101
E-mail: HolistMed@aol.com

American Thyroid Association, Inc.
Montefiore Medical Center
111 East 210th Street
Bronx, NY 10467
Telephone: (718) 882-6047

Associazone Italiana Basedowiani 3 Tiroidei
C/O Centro Minerva
7 Via Mazzini, 43100
Parma Italy
Telephone/fax 39-521-207771

Australian Thyroid Foundation
P.O. Box 186
Westmead NSW 2145 Australia
Telephone: 61-3-9561-3483; Fax: 61-3-9561-4798
E-mail: snewlands@bigpond.com

British Thyroid Foundation *www.home.ican.net/~thyroid/International/BTF.html*.
PO Box 97
Clifford, Wetherby
West Yorkshire LS23 6XD

Broda Barnes Foundation *www.brodabarnes.org*. The Broda Barnes Foundation is an educational organization dedicated to continuing the efforts of Dr. Broda Barnes in recognizing and treating disorders of hypothyroidism.
Broda Barnes M.D. Research Foundation, Inc.
P. O. Box 98
Trumbell, CT 06611
Telephone: (203) 261-2101

The Endocrine Society *www.endo-society.org/*.
4350 East West Highway, Suite 500
Bethesda, MD 20814-4410
Telephone: (301) 941-0200; Fax: (301) 941-0259

Gland Central *www.glandcentral.com*. Gland Central is a nationwide thyroid education campaign sponsored by the American Medical Women's Association (AMWA). Underwritten by an educational grant from Knoll Pharmaceutical Corporation, this group offers information about the thyroid and its disorders.

The goal of Gland Central is to help individuals identify early signs and symptoms and encourage them to be tested.

Herb Research Foundation *www.herbs.org.* For nominal fees this highly esteemed organization offers a herbal hotline and provides information on herbal support for thyroid function.
1007 Pearl Street, Suite 200,
Boulder, CO 80302
Telephone (800) 748-2617; Herbal Hotline: (303) 449-2265

MAGIC (Major Aspects of Growth in Children) *www.magicfoundation.org*
1327 North Harlem Ave.
Oak Park, IL 60302
Telephone: (708) 383-0808; Toll Free: (800) 3MAGIC3; Fax: (708) 383-0899

The Maharishi Ayurveda Medical Center *www.mapi.com.* This organization serves as an educational resource for Ayurvedic products it manufactures. It offers a newsletter, *Total Health News,* and answers questions regarding therapies.
P.O. Box 49667
Colorado Springs, CO 80949
Telephone: (800) 255-8332

National Association for Rare Disorders (NORD) *www.rarediseases.org/*
P.O. Box 8923
New Fairfield, CT 06812-1783
Telephone: (800) 999-NORD

National Graves Disease Foundation (NGDF) *www.ngdf.org/.* The NGDF was formed in 1990 by Graves' patient Nancy Patterson, with a goal of providing patient information and education at a time when there was little literature available to the lay person. The original intention was to form a constellation of local support groups, and there are indeed 18 groups in the United States. The group has hosted an annual educational conference since 1991. Membership dues are $33, annually which includes a subscription to the group's quarterly newsletter.
P.O. Box 1969
Brevard, NC 28712
Telephone: (828) 877-5251; Fax: (828) 877-5250

Nederlandse Vereniging Van Graves Pati'nten [Dutch Graves' Disease Patients' Organization] *www.ziekenhuis.nl/patntver/graves.htm.*
Secr. N.V.G.P., Dawesweg'
212, 3069 VL Rotterdam/Holland
Telephone: 010-4213390

Schilddreusen Liga Deutschland e.V. *www.thyrolink.com/sd-liga.*
Postfach 800 740, 65907
Frankfurt, Germany
Telephone: 069-31-40-5376; Fax: 069-31-40-5316

Schildklierstichting Nederland
Postbus 138 1620 AC Hoorn
Holland, Netherlands

Thyroid Health and Information Service (THIS) *www.my4tune.u-net.com/.* This site, which is hosted by the organization formerly known as the International Thyroid Group (ITG), contains excellent information on hyperthyroidism, hypothyroidism and adrenal insufficiency. Of particular interest are the articles on environmental concerns and hormonal disrupters.

Society of Nuclear Medicine *www.snm.org/*
  1850 Samuel Morse Dr.
  Reston, VA 20190-5316
  Telephone: (703) 708-9000; Fax: (703) 708-9015
Thyreoidia Landsforeningen *www.netdoktor.dk/patientforeninger/fakta/ thyreoidea/ thyreoidea.html.*
  C/o Lis Larsen, Abakkevej 55, st. tv, 2720
  Vanlose, Denmark
Thyroid Eye Disease (TED) Head Office *home.ican.net/~thyroid/International/ TED.html.*
  34 Fore Street
  CHUDLEIGH — Devon
  TQ13 0HX, United Kingdom.
  Telephone/Fax: 44-1626-852980
  E-mail: tedassn@eclipse.co.uk
The Thyroid Foundation of America *www.clark.net/pub/tfa/; www.tsh. org.* Primarily an organization for physicians, the TFA offers an on-line version of *Your Thyroid, a Home Reference,* and article abstracts from the journal *Thyroid*
  40 Parkman Street
  Boston, MA 02114-2698
  Telephone: (800) 832-8321
Thyroid Foundation of Canada *home.ican.net/~thyroid/Canada.html.*
  96 Mack Street
  Kingston, Ontario
  Canada K7L 1N9
  Telephone: 1-800-267-8822 or (613) 544-8364; Fax: (613) 544-9731
  E-mail: thyroid@kos.net
Thyroid Foundation International *www.thyroid-fed.org/*
  96 Mack Street
  Kingston, Ontario
  Canada K7L 1N9
  Telephone: 613-544-8364; Fax: 613-544-9731
  E-mail: tfi@kos.net
Thyroid Society for Education and Research *www.the-thyroid-society.org.* The Thyroid Society offers a variety of articles on a number of thyroid related topics, which can be obtained through the mail or via their web site.
  7515 South Main Street, Suite 545
  Houston, TX 77030
  Telephone: (800) THYROID; Fax: (713) 799-9919
  E-mail: help@the-thyroid-society.org
Vastsvenska Patientforeningen for Skoldlortelsjoka
  Mejerivalen 8
  439 36 Onsala, Sweden
  Phone/fax 46-30-06-39-12

Individual Web Sites
and Bulletin Boards

Alternative Medicine for Thyroid Disease, *www.delphi.com/ab-altmedoption*
The American Foundation of Thyroid Patients. www.thyroidfoundation.org/
   This site provides a guestbook that patients sign, including information about their thyroid disorder and any concerns they have. Patients correspond with one another through the guestbook and through private e-mail.
Daisy's Graves' Disease Site *www.daisyelaine_co.tripod.com/gravesdisease/*
   My personal GD web site has pages dedicated to environmental concerns, pregnancy, childhood GD, and many other points of interest.
Dianne Wiley's Home Page *www.webpak.net/~deecee/main.htm*
   This is a very informative site that includes an account of Dianne's struggles with Graves' ophthalmopathy.
General Thyroid Support and Info, *www.delphi.com/ab-thyroid*
Graves_support at yahoo *www.yahoogroups.com/group/graves_support*
   Founded by a Graves' patient, this group, where I regularly post, offers tremendous support to newly diagnosed patients and welcomes discussions of new research trends.Graves-alt-search at yahoo *www.yahoogroups.com/groups/graves-alt-search*. Founded by GD patients, this site explores current research news and alternative healing suggestions for GD.
iThyroid *www.iThyroid.com.*
   Founded by John Johnson, a Graves' patient who treated his symptoms of hyperthyroidism using a natural approach, this group focuses on correcting the nutritional imbalances that contribute to the development of thyroid disorders. Open to both newly diagnosed and long-term thyroid patients, this board has numerous links to educational articles contributed by John and other members of this group.
Mary Shomon's About.com Thyroid Web Site *www.thyroid.about.com. www.thyroid-info.com.*
   This site, managed by thyroid patient Mary Shomon, provides a wealth of thyroid related information and has numerous links to articles and forums. Also,

a free monthly newsletter is available via e-mail. This site provides basic information and an overview of current research studies gleaned from the popular press and medical journal article abstracts, and includes information on alternative drugs and treatments including interviews with medical professionals. Mary's lively, patient empowering boards are geared toward the concerns of both new patients and long-term patients. Threads follow a wide variety of topics, including current research and treatment issues as well as environmental concerns. Ongoing topics range from substances interfering with the absorption of replacement hormone to inadequate treatment. Dozens of threads are followed at any one time and various views are welcome.

Mike's Graves' Disease Page *www.webhome.idirect.com/~wolfnowl/thyroid.htm.* This site discusses Graves' disease in layman's terms from the perspective of a male professional who was taken off guard when Graves' disease struck suddenly. Mike's impressive site includes a wealth of provocative links to many environmental articles and an extensive list of thyroid-related links.

The National Graves' Disease Foundation Bulletin Board *www.bb.ngdf.org/bb/new.asp?TC=O.*
This bulletin board is affiliated with the NGDF and support group.com and serves as a gateway to Graves' disease information on the internet. The BB primarily revolves around questions posted by newly diagnosed patients. Responses provide both anecdotal and factual information on thyroid eye disease and hyperthyroidism. Endorsed by both Health on the Net and Medinex Medallion, which regularly review the site, it's the only BB where the posts are monitored by volunteer patient facilitators.

Radioiodine Information *www.egroups.com/community/AtomicWomen. www.clubs.yahoo.com/clubs/atomicwomen*
The following bulletin boards that focus on radioiodine ablation also contain articles on the therapeutic use of radioiodine I-131 for Graves' disease.

Paula Ehler's Home Page *www7.concentric.net/~psychmom/*
This site contains Paula's personal experiences with Graves' disease and her subsequent development of fibromyalgia. Paula's site has a number of links to unusual GD sites.

Spanish Language Thyroid Questions, *www.delphi.com/ab-tiroide*
Thyroid Related Diet, Weight Loss and Nutrition, *www.delphi.com/ab-thyroiddiet*
Thyroid Top Doctors, *www.delphi.com/ab-thyroiddr*

Index